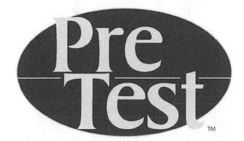

Anatomy, Histology, and Cell Biology

PreTest™ Self-Assessment and Review

D0556641

Notice

Medicine is an ever-changing science. As new research and clinical experience broaden our knowledge, changes in treatment and drug therapy are required. The authors and the publisher of this work have checked with sources believed to be reliable in their efforts to provide information that is complete and generally in accord with the standards accepted at the time of publication. However, in view of the possibility of human error or changes in medical sciences, neither the authors nor the publisher nor any other party who has been involved in the preparation or publication of this work warrants that the information contained herein is in every respect accurate or complete, and they disclaim all responsibility for any errors or omissions or for the results obtained from use of the information contained in this work. Readers are encouraged to confirm the information contained herein with other sources. For example and in particular, readers are advised to check the product information sheet included in the package of each drug they plan to administer to be certain that the information contained in this work is accurate and that changes have not been made in the recommended dose or in the contraindications for administration. This recommendation is of particular importance in connection with new or infrequently used drugs.

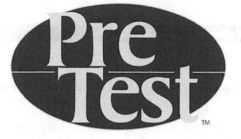

Anatomy, Histology, and Cell Biology

PreTest™ Self-Assessment and Review

Fourth Edition

Robert M. Klein, PhD
Professor of Anatomy and Cell Biology
Associate Dean, Professional Development and Faculty Affairs
University of Kansas, School of Medicine
Kansas City, Kansas

George C. Enders, PhD
Associate Professor and Director of Medical Education
Assistant Dean for Student Affairs
Department of Anatomy and Cell Biology
University of Kansas, School of Medicine
Kansas City, Kansas

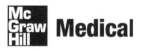 **Medical**

New York   Chicago   San Francisco   Lisbon   London   Madrid   Mexico City
Milan   New Delhi   San Juan   Seoul   Singapore   Sydney   Toronto

The **McGraw·Hill** Companies

Anatomy, Histology, and Cell Biology: PreTest™ Self-Assessment and Review, Fourth Edition

1 2 3 4 5 6 78 9 0   DOC/DOC   14 13 12 11 10

ISBN 978-0-07-162343-8
MHID 0-07-162343-4

This book was set in Berkeley by Glyph International.
The editors were Kirsten Funk and Christine Diedrich.
The production supervisor was Sherri Souffrance.
Project management was provided by Rajni Pisharody, Glyph International.
RR Donnelley was printer and binder.

This book is printed on acid-free paper.

Library of Congress Cataloging-in-Publication Data

Anatomy, histology, and cell biology : PreTest self-assessment and review / [edited by] Robert M. Klein, George C. Enders.—4th ed.
   p. ; cm.
Includes bibliographical references and index.
ISBN-13: 978-0-07-162343-8 (pbk. : alk. paper)
ISBN-10: 0-07-162343-4 (pbk. : alk. paper)
   1. Histology—Examinations, questions, etc.   2. Human anatomy—Examinations, questions, etc.   3. Cytology—Examinations, questions, etc.   I. Klein, Robert M. (Robert Melvin), 1949- II. Enders, George C., 1955-
   [DNLM: 1. Anatomy—Examination Questions.   2. Cytology–Examination Questions.   3. Histology—Examination Questions.   QS 18.2 A53603   2010]
QM554.A52   2010
611'.0076–dc22
                                                            2009044033

McGraw-Hill books are available at special quantity discounts to use as premiums and sales promotions, or for use in corporate training programs. To contact a representative please e-mail us at bulksales@mcgraw-hill.com.

To my wife, Beth, and our children Melanie, Jeffrey, and David, for their support and patience during the writing and revision of this text; and to my parents, Nettie and David, for their emphasis on education and the pursuit of knowledge.

—RMK

To Sally Ling, MD, an incredibly hard working and considerate person whom I am lucky enough to call my wife. She has given us three great children, Carolyn, Tyler, and Robert who keep me on my toes; and to my mother and my father who always encouraged "the boys" to do our best.

—GCE

Student Reviewers

Jodie Bachman
UMDNJ School of Osteopathic Medicine
Class of 2011

Benjamin Chidester
Eastern Virginia Medical School
Class of 2011

Monique Cunningham-Lindsay
UMDNJ School of Osteopathic Medicine
Class of 2011

Jeffrey A. Klein
University of Kansas, School of Medicine
Class of 2010

Andrew Schlachter
University of Kansas, School of Medicine
Class of 2009

J. Eva Selfridge
University of Kansas, School of Medicine
Class of 2012

Gustaf Van Acker III
University of Kansas, School of Medicine
Class of 2012

Contents

Epithelium

Connective Tissue

Specialized Connective Tissues: Bone and Cartilage

Muscle and Cell Motility

Nervous System

Cardiovascular System, Blood, and Bone Marrow

Lymphoid System and Cellular Immunology

Respiratory System

Integumentary System

Gastrointestinal Tract and Glands

Endocrine Glands

Reproductive Systems

Urinary System

Eye and Ear

Head and Neck

Thorax

Abdomen

Pelvis

Extremities and Spine

Preface

In this fourth edition of *Anatomy, Histology, and Cell Biology: PreTest® Self-Assessment and Review*, a significant number of changes and improvements have been made. This PreTest® reviews the anatomical disciplines encompassing early embryology, cell biology, histology of the tissues and organs, as well as regional human anatomy of the head and neck, thorax, abdomen, pelvis, extremities, and spine. Major neuroanatomical tracts are outlined in the High-Yield Facts section, but most pathway questions have been eliminated in favor of more high-yield topics in embryology, histology, and human anatomy. Extensive neuroanatomical tract and pathway-related questions can be found in the new seventh edition of *Neuroscience: PreTest® Self-Assessment & Review*.

This new edition of *Anatomy, Histology, and Cell Biology: PreTest®* represents a comprehensive effort to integrate the anatomical disciplines with clinical scenarios and cases. The development of numerous clinical vignettes, integrating basic science disciplines with clinical medicine, will benefit students enrolled in medical schools with integrated curricula, as well as students in discipline-based programs of study. The sections on cell biology and microscopic anatomy have been updated to include important new knowledge in cell and tissue biology and to focus on cell biological principles relevant to clinical medicine. New and improved light micrographs have been added. Also new for this fourth edition is the addition of more radiographs and MRIs. Those radiological methods have become an important part of medical practice. It is imperative that students be able to recognize structures and relationships as part of their radiological anatomy knowledge base. This fourth edition is designed to help students prepare for USMLE Step 1, Subject Exams in Human Anatomy and Histology, and even USMLE Step 2 in which the NBME plans to integrate more basic science questions.

An updated High-Yield facts section is provided to facilitate rapid review of specific areas of anatomy that are critical to mastering the difficult concepts of each subdiscipline: embryology, cell biology, histology of tissues and organs, regional human (gross) anatomy, pathology, and a brief review of neuroanatomical tracts. Most tables and figures have been moved from individual question feedback to the High-Yield facts section so that all review information is available in one concise location instead of dispersed throughout the book.

Introduction

Anatomy, Histology and Cell Biology: PreTest® Self-Assessment and Review allows medical students to comprehensively and conveniently assess and review their knowledge of anatomy, histology, embryology, and cell biology. The 500 questions provided here in have been written with the goal to parallel the topics, format, and degree of difficulty of the questions found in the United States Medical Licensing Examination (USMLE) Step 1. Although the main emphasis of this PreTest is preparation for Step 1, the book will be very beneficial for medical students during their preclinical courses whether they are enrolled in a medical school with a problem-based, traditional, or integrated curriculum. This *PreTest®* focuses on an interdisciplinary approach incorporating numerous clinical scenarios so it will also be extremely valuable for students preparing for USMLE Step 2 who need to review their anatomical knowledge. Practicing physicians who want to hone their basic science skills and supplement their knowledge base before USMLE Step 3 or recertification will also find this book to be an outstanding resource for their review of the anatomical disciplines.

This book is a comprehensive review of early embryology, cell biology, histology (tissue and organ biology), and human (gross) anatomy with some neuroanatomical topics reviewed in the High-Yield facts section. In keeping with the latest curricular changes in medical schools, as much as possible, questions integrate macroscopic and microscopic anatomy with cell biology, embryology, and neuroscience as well as physiology, biochemistry, and pathology. This *PreTest®* begins with early embryology, including gametogenesis, fertilization, implantation, the formation of the bilaminar and trilaminar embryo, and overviews of the embryonic and fetal periods. This first section is followed by a review of basic cell biology, with separate chapters on membranes, cytoplasm, intracellular trafficking, and the nucleus. There are questions included to review the basics of mitosis and meiosis as well as regulation of cell cycle events. Tissue biology is the third section of the book, and it encompasses the tissues of the body: epithelium, connective tissue, specialized connective tissues (cartilage and bone), muscle, and nerve. Organ biology includes separate chapters on respiratory, integumentary (skin), digestive (tract and associated glands), endocrine, urinary, and male and female reproductive systems, as well as the eye and the ear. The topics in tissue and organ histology and cell biology include light and electron micrographs of appropriate structures that students should be able to identify. The last section of the book contains questions reviewing the basic concepts of regional anatomy of the head and neck, thorax, abdomen, pelvis, and extremities. For each section, appropriate x-rays, including MRIs, are included to assist the student in reviewing pertinent radiological aspects of the anatomy. Where possible, information is integrated with development and histology of the organ system.

Each question in the book is followed by five or more answer options to choose from. In each case, select the one best response to the question. Each answer is accompanied by a specific page reference to a text that provides background to the answer, and a short discussion of issues raised by the question and answer. A bibliography listing all the sources can be found following the last chapter.

Acknowledgments

The authors express their gratitude to their colleagues who have greatly assisted them by providing light and electron micrographs as well as constructive criticism of the text, line drawings, and micrographs. They also acknowledge Eileen Roach and Phillip Shafer for their painstaking care in the preparation of photomicrographs. Thanks to Drs Gregory A. Ator, Amy Klion, Ann Dvorak, Anne W. Walling, Christopher Maxwell, Dale R. Abrahamson, Daniel Friend, David A. Sirois, David F. Albertini, Don W. Fawcett, Linda R. Nelson, Erik Dabelsteen, George Varghese, Giuseppina Raviola, H. Clarke Anderson, J.E. Heuser, John K. Young, Julia Neperud, K. Hama, Kristin M. Leiferman, Kuen-Shan Hung, Louis Wetzel, Michael J. Werle, Nancy E.J. Berman, Per-Lennart Westesson, Robert P. Bolender, Ronal R. MacGregor, Stanley L. Erlandsen, WenFang Wang, Christopher J. Wilbert, Wolfram Sterry, and Xiaoming Zhang for their contribution of micrographs and ideas for question development. Also, thanks to the Jeffrey Modell Foundation and The Primary Immunodeficiency Resource Center for use of the Martin Causubon case. Thanks to Debra Collins for her genetics consult. The authors remain indebted to their students and colleagues at the University of Kansas Medical Center, past and present, who have challenged them to continuously improve their skills as educators.

—RMK

—GCE

High-Yield Facts

Embryology

Embryological development is divided into three periods:

The **first stage** consists of **gamete formation** and maturation, ending in fertilization.

The **embryonic period** begins with fertilization and extends through the **first 8 weeks** of development. It includes implantation, germ layer formation, and organogenesis. This is the critical period for susceptibility to **teratogens.**

The **fetal period** extends from the **third month** through birth.

THE PRENATAL PERIOD

The **development of gametes** begins with the duplication of chromosomal DNA followed by two cycles of nuclear and cell division **(meiosis).**

Genetic variability is assured by **crossing over** of DNA, **random assortment** of chromosomes, and **recombination** during the first meiotic division. Errors can result in duplication or deletion of all or part of a specific chromosome, often with serious developmental consequences.

Spermatogenesis
The process of spermatogenesis is **continuous** after puberty and each cycle lasts about 2 months.

Spermatogonia in the walls of the seminiferous tubules of the testes undergo mitotic divisions to replenish their population and form a group of spermatogonia that will differentiate to form spermatocytes.

Primary spermatocytes are spermatogenic cells that have duplicated their DNA (4N) and enter meiosis.

Secondary spermatocytes result from the first meiotic division (2N).

Spermatids are formed by the second meiotic division (1N).

Spermiogenesis
During this phase, spermatids mature into sperm by losing extraneous cytoplasm and developing a head region consisting of an **acrosome** (specialized secretory granule) surrounding the nuclear material and grow a tail.

1

Oogenesis

Oogenesis begins in the fetal period in females and is a discontinuous process involving mitosis, meiosis, and maturation.

Oogonia undergo mitotic division and duplicate their DNA to form **primary oocytes,** but stop in the prophase of the first meiotic division until puberty.

The second meiotic division is not concluded until fertilization occurs.

Maturational events include retention of protein synthetic machinery in the surviving oocyte, formation of **cortical granules** that participate in events at fertilization, and development of a protective glycoprotein coat, the **zona pellucida.**

Fertilization

Fertilization occurs when sperm and oocyte cell membranes fuse. Following coitus, exposure of sperm to the environment of the female reproductive tract causes **capacitation,** removal of surface glycoproteins and cholesterol from the sperm membrane, enabling fertilization to occur.

Binding of the first sperm initiates the **zona reaction.** Release of **cortical granules** from the oocyte causes biochemical changes in the zona pellucida and oocyte membrane that prevent polyspermy.

EMBRYONIC DEVELOPMENT

The embryo forms one **germ layer** during each of the first 3 weeks. During the first week the **cleavage** divisions form a **morula.** The **blastocyst** forms by **compaction** and precursors of the **inner cell mass (embryoblast)** and **trophoblast** are segregated. The blastocyst must "hatch" or exit the investment of the zona pellucida. Implantation is initiated during the first week of development.

During the second week, the **blastocyst** differentiates into two germ layers, the **epiblast** and the **hypoblast.** This establishes the dorsal (epiblast)–ventral (hypoblast) body axis of the **bilaminar embryonic disc.** Week 2 is the "week of 2s:"

- Two major cell groups exist: embryoblast and trophoblast.

- The embryoblast (inner cell mass) forms the hypoblast layer adjacent to the blastocyst cavity and the epiblast adjacent to the amniotic cavity.

- The trophoblast differentiates into two layers: cytotrophoblast (an inner mononuclear cell layer) and syncytiotrophoblast (an outer multinuclear cell layer).
- Two cavities are established: the amniotic cavity and the primitive yolk sac.
- Uteroplacental circulation develops. Two structures are involved: sinusoid (capillary) = maternal blood vessel in endometrium and lacuna = embryonic blood vessel in syncytiotrophoblast.

During the third week, the process of **gastrulation** occurs, by which epiblast cells migrate toward the **primitive streak** and ingress to form the **endoderm** and **mesoderm** germ layers below the remaining epiblast cells (**ectoderm**). **Somite formation** begins at day 20.

The fourth week of development is characterized by organogenesis as the **primordia of most organ systems** are established. The body tube is formed by **embryonic folding**. **Lateral body folding** at the end of the third week causes the germ layers to form three concentric tubes with the innermost layer being the **endoderm**, the **mesoderm** in the middle, and the **ectoderm** on the surface. **Neurulation** also occurs during the fourth week, leading to the formation of a **neural tube** with overlying surface ectoderm.

GERM LAYER DERIVATIVES

Mesoderm Derivatives

The mesoderm is divided into four regions (from medial to lateral): axial, paraxial, intermediate, and lateral plate.

Chordamesoderm is located in the midline and forms the notochord.

Paraxial mesoderm forms **somites**. Somites are divided into **sclerotomes** (bone and cartilage precursors), **myotomes** (muscle precursors), and **dermatomes** (precursor of dermis).

Intermediate mesoderm gives rise to components of the genitourinary system.

Lateral plate mesoderm forms bones and connective tissue of the limbs and limb girdles (**somatic layer,** also known as **somatopleure**) and the smooth muscle lining viscera and the serosae of body cavities (**splanchnic layer,** also known as **splanchnopleure**).

Intermediate mesoderm is *not found* in the head region, and the lateral plate mesoderm is *not divided* into layers there (Table 1).

TABLE I. GERM LAYER DERIVATIVES

Derivatives	Layers		
Ectodermal	Epithelium of skin (superficial epidermis layer)		
	All nervous tissue (formed from neuroectoderm): Brain and spinal cord (neural tube) Peripheral nerves and other neural crest derivatives		
Endodermal		The gastrointestinal tract	
	Epithelial linings of:	Organs that form as buds from the endodermal tube: Pharyngeal gland derivatives* Respiratory system Digestive organs (liver, pancreas) Terminal part of urogenital systems	
	Hypoblast Endoderm: Gametes migrate to gonads		
Mesodermal	All connective tissue†:	General connective tissue	
		Cartilage and bone	
		Blood cells (red and white)	
	All muscle types:	Cardiac, skeletal, smooth	
	Epithelial linings of:	Body cavities	
		Some organs: Cardiovascular system Reproductive and urinary systems (most parts)	

*Pharyngeal derivatives: palatine tonsils, thymus, thyroid, parathyroids.
†Some connective tissue in the head is derived from neural crest.

Ectoderm Derivatives

Formation of the primitive central nervous system is induced in the ectoderm layer by cells forming the **notochord** in the underlying mesoderm.

The neural plate ectoderm **(neuroectoderm)** forms two lateral folds that meet and fuse in the midline to form the neural tube **(neurulation).**

Cells from the tips of the folds **(neural crest)** migrate throughout the body to form many derivatives, including the peripheral nervous system.

FORMATION OF THE HEAD AND NECK REGION

The branchial (pharyngeal) apparatus consists of arches, pouches, and clefts (Fig. 1)

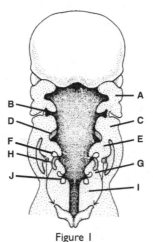

Figure 1
Branchial apparatus.

Branchial Arches:
A = First branchial arch
C = Second branchial arch
E = Third branchial arch
G = Fourth branchial arch
I = Sixth branchial arch

Branchial Pouches:
B = First pouch forming the auditory tube
D = Second pouch forming the palatine tonsil
F = dorsal portion of third pouch (forming the inferior parathyroids)
H = ventral portion of third pouch (forming the thymus)
J = Fourth pouch (dorsal portion forming the superior parathyroids, ventral part joining with a rudimentary fifth pouch to form the ultimobranchial body—C cells of the thyroid)

(Reproduced, with permission, from Sweeney L. Basic Concepts in Embryology: A Student's Survival Guide. New York, NY: McGraw-Hill; 1998.)

The neural crest contributes significantly to the formation of connective tissue elements in the head.

The bony skeleton of the head is comprised of the **viscerocranium** and the **neurocranium.**

The neurocranium (cranial vault) is composed of a base formed by **endochondral ossification** (chondrocranium) and sides and roof bones formed by **intramembranous ossification.**

The chondrocranium is derived from both the **somatic mesoderm** (occipital) and the neural crest.

The viscerocranium (face) is derived from the first two **pharyngeal (branchial) arches** (neural crest in origin).

The cartilages and bones of the face (viscerocranium) develop from the **pharyngeal arches.** Each arch receives its blood supply from a specific aortic arch and its innervation from a specific cranial nerve (special or branchial visceral efferent fibers). The **third aortic arch** provides most of the adult **blood supply to the head and neck.** The **skeletal muscles** of the head and neck primarily arise from the pharyngeal arches and have a unique innervation (special visceral efferent [SVE]).

The face develops from a midline **frontonasal prominence** and bilateral **maxillary and mandibular prominences.** Clefts result from failure of the prominences to fuse.

Teeth originate from both ectodermal (enamel) and neuroectodermal (neural crest: dentin, pulp, cementum, and periodontal ligament) derivatives.

Tables 2 and 3 summarize the adult derivatives of the branchial apparatus that is critical to head and neck development.

TABLE 2. PRINCIPAL BRANCHIAL DERIVATIVES*	
Arch	**Derivative**
I	Mandible, malleus, incus, anterior 2/3 of tongue, muscles of mastication, tensor tympani muscle, tensor veli palatini muscle, mylohyoid muscle, anterior belly of the digastric muscle, mandibular division of the trigeminal nerve
II	Lesser horn of the hyoid, styloid process, stapes bone, muscles of facial expression, stapedius muscle, styloid hyoid muscle, posterior belly of the digastric muscle, facial cranial nerve
III	Greater horn of hyoid, posterior 1/3 of tongue, stylopharyngeus muscle, glossopharyngeal cranial nerve
IV	Thyroid cartilage, cricothyroid muscle, superior laryngeal nerve
VI	Cricoid and arytenoid cartilages, intrinsic muscles of the larynx, recurrent laryngeal nerve

*Each branchial arch contains a nerve, muscle, artery, and cartilage.

TABLE 3. DERIVATIVES OF PHARYNGEAL POUCHES AND CLEFTS		
Pouch/Cleft	**Portion**	**Derivative**
Pouch 1		Epithelial lining of middle ear canals and tympanic membrane; auditory tube
Pouch 2		Epithelial lining of palatine tonsils
Pouch 3	Ventral portion	Epithelial components of thymus gland
	Dorsal portion	Epithelial cells of inferior parathyroid glands
Pouch 4	Ventral portion	Epithelial "C" (parafollicular [interfollicular] cells of the thyroid gland)
	Dorsal portion	Epithelial cells of superior parathyroid glands
Clefts 1		External auditory canal
Clefts 2 → 4		No normal derivatives; abnormal sinuses, fistulae, and clefts

Pituitary

The anterior portion of the pituitary is derived from oral ectoderm arising from the roof of the oral cavity (Rathke pouch) anterior to the buccopharyngeal membrane and migrating through the sphenoid anlagen to unite with a downgrowth of neuroectoderm (posterior pituitary).

Eye and Ear

The eye is derived from three different germ layers:

Neuroectoderm: Vesicular outgrowths of the forebrain differentiate into the retina and the optic nerve.

Surface ectoderm: Contributes to the **lens, cornea,** and epithelial coverings of the lacrimal glands, eyelids, and **conjunctiva.**

Mesoderm: The **sclera** and **choroid** are derived from the **lateral plate mesoderm.**

The **extraocular muscles** are derived from myoblasts of the **cranial somitomeres.**

Structures of the **outer and middle ear** are derived from the **first and second pharyngeal arches** and the **first pharyngeal cleft.**

Structures of the **inner ear** are derived from the **ectodermal otic placode,** *not neuroectoderm.*

Maternal rubella can cause defects in both the eyes (fourth-sixth weeks of gestation) and ears (seventh-eighth weeks) in the developing embryo.

LIMB FORMATION

The limbs form as ventrolateral buds under the mutual induction of the ectoderm (apical ectodermal ridge [AER]) and underlying mesoderm beginning in the fifth week. *The AER influences proximal-distal development.*

Somatic lateral plate mesoderm (somatopleure) forms the bony and connective tissue elements of the limbs and limb girdles while skeletal muscle of the appendages is derived from somites.

Cranio-caudal polarity is determined by specialized mesoderm cells (zone of polarizing activity [ZPA]) that release inducing signals such as retinoic acid.

Homeobox genes are the targets of induction signals. They are named after their homeodomain, called the homeobox, which is a DNA-binding motif. Homeobox genes encode trancription factors that regulate processes such as segmentation and axis formation.

Rotation of the limb buds establishes the position of the joints, the location of muscle groups, and the pattern of sensory innervation (dermatome map).

MATURATION OF THE CENTRAL NERVOUS SYSTEM

Segmentation of the cranial neural tube forms the brain vesicles listed in Table 4:

TABLE 4. BRAIN VESICLES FROM CRANIAL NEURAL TUBE SEGMENTATION		
Primary Brain Vesicle	Secondary Brain Vesicle	Adult Brain Derivative
Prosencephalon (forebrain)	Telencephalon	Cerebral cortex, corpus striatum
	Diencephalon	Hypothalamus, thalamus
Mesencephalon (midbrain)	Mesencephalon	Superior and inferior colliculi
Rhombencephalon (hindbrain)	Metencephalon	Pons and cerebellum
	Myelencephalon	Medulla

Both neurons and glia develop from the original neuroectoderm that forms the neural tube.

Microglia *are the exception.* They develop from the monocyte-macrophage lineage of mesodermal (bone marrow) origin and migrate into the CNS.

Induction of regional differences in the developing CNS is regulated by retinoic acid (vitamin A). Overexposure of the cranial region to **retinoic acid** can result in "caudalization," that is, development similar to the spinal cord. During development, the spinal cord and presumptive brain stem develop three layers: (1) a **germinal layer** or **ventricular zone**, (2) an **intermediate layer** containing **neuroblasts** and comprising gray matter, and (3) a **marginal zone** containing myelinated fibers (white matter).

Other layers are added in the cerebrum and cerebellum by cell migration along glial scaffolds to form cortical regions.

The notochord induces the establishment of **dorsal-ventral polarity** in the neural tube. Ventral portions of the tube will become the **basal plate** and give rise to motor neurons, whereas the dorsal portions become the **alar plates**, derivatives of which subserve sensory functions.

Meninges are formed by mesoderm surrounding the neural tube with contributions to the arachnoid and pia from the neural crest.

Congenital dysmorphologies in the CNS may result from several causes, including high maternal blood glucose levels and vitamin A overexposure, and often involve bony defects (eg, spina bifida and anencephaly). Defects are most common in the regions of neuropore closure. Folic acid, also known as folate, is a B vitamin that can be found in foods such as enriched breads, pastas, rice, and cereals as well as vitamin supplements. Women who take folate before pregnancy have a decreased risk of neural tube defects (NTDs) including spina bifida and anencephaly. The U.S. Public Health Service recommends that all women who could possibly become pregnant take 400 µg (or 0.4 mg) of folic acid every day. It is estimated that such an approach could prevent up to 70% of NTDs.

Fetal alcohol syndrome (FAS) is the most common cause of mental retardation. FAS includes the triad of growth retardation, characteristic facial dysmorphology, and neurodevelopmental abnormalities. Alcohol rapidly crosses the placenta and the fetal blood-brain barrier. Damage is dependent on gestational age, alcohol dosage, and pattern of maternal alcohol abuse. Altered neural crest cell migration, differentiation, and programmed cell death (apoptosis) are hypothesized mechanisms for the congenital dysmorphologies associated with FAS.

FORMATION OF THE PERIPHERAL NERVOUS SYSTEM

Sensory neurons of the spinal ganglia, as well as autonomic postganglionic neurons and their supporting cells, are derived from the **neural crest**.

Focal deficiencies in neural crest cell migration may result in lack of innervation to specific organs or parts of organs. Failure of neural crest cells to migrate to a portion of the colon results in a localized deficiency in parasympathetic intramural ganglia and a loss of peristalsis and bowel obstruction known as Hirschsprung disease or aganglionic megacolon.

FORMATION OF THE CARDIOVASCULAR SYSTEM

All components of the cardiovascular system, including the epithelia, are derived from the **splanchnic lateral plate mesoderm.**

The heart tubes forming on either side of the endodermal tube are brought together by **lateral body folding.**

Looping of the heart tube occurs while the tube is being divided into left and right portions by the interatrial and interventricular septa.

In the interatrial septum, the **septum primum** and **septum secundum** do not close off the **foramen ovale** until birth.

Failure of the **atrioventricular endocardial cushions** to fuse can result in septal and valve defects.

Neural crest cells contribute to septation of the truncus arteriosus and the formation of the aortic and pulmonary outflows, as well as the aortic arches.

The **"Tetralogy of Fallot"** is the most common defect of the conus arteriosus/truncus arteriosus and is due to unequal division of the conus because of anterior displacement of the conotruncal septum. The mnemomic **IHOP** is useful to remember the four cardiovascular alterations that comprise the tetralogy: (1) interventricular septal defect, (2) hypotrophy of the right ventricle, (3) overriding aorta, and (4) pulmonary stenosis. A summary of cardiac congenital dysmorphologies is provided in Table 5.

Vasculature

Vasculogenesis versus Angiogenesis

The endothelial lining of most blood vessels forms by coalescence of vascular endothelial progenitors **(angioblasts)** of mesodermal origin. The endothelial cells proliferate, migrate, differentiate, and organize into tubular structures with subsequent vacuolization to form a lumen. Subsequently, **periendothelial** cells form from local mesoderm and differentiate into muscle and connective tissue elements (ie, **smooth muscle, fibroblasts**, and **pericytes**). This process is known as **vasculogenesis** and occurs

TABLE 5. KEY DEVELOPMENTAL STEPS IN HEART/CIRCULATORY SYSTEM DEVELOPMENT AND RESULTING CONGENITAL DYSMORPHOLOGIES*

Endocardial Cushion Formation	Septation of the Truncus Arteriosus	Atrial Septation	Ventricular Septation	Aortic Arches Formation	Venous System Formation
Persistent atrioventricular canal	Transposition of great vessels	Atrial septal defects	Ventricular septal defects	Coarctation of the aorta	Double inferior vena cava
Ostium primum defect	Persistent truncus arteriosus	Patent foramen ovale	Tetralogy of Fallot	Double aortic arch	Absence of the inferior vena cava
Tricuspid atresia	Pulmonary infundibular stenosis			Right aortic arch	Left superior vena cava
Ebstein anomaly	Tetralogy of Fallot			Patent ductus arteriosus	Double superior vena cava

*Dysmorphologies are listed for key developmental steps of endocardial cushion formation, septation of the truncus arteriosus, atrial septation, ventricular septation, and venous system formation.

11

in both embryonic and adult tissues. Vasculogenesis is the de novo formation of blood vessels and differs from angiogenesis, initiated in a preexisting vessel. Both of those processes are regulated in part by **vascular endothelial growth factor (VEGF)**, which induces chemotactic (migratory) and proliferative responses in endothelial cells. Uterine angiogenesis occurs in adult women during each menstrual cycle. Angiogenesis also is a prominent characteristic of inflammation, pathology such as **diabetic retinopathy**, wound repair, placental development during embryogenesis, and tumor formation. Molecular triggers for angiogenesis include the **cytokines**, small, extracellular signal proteins or peptides that function as local mediators in cell to cell communication. For example, during inflammation or hypoxia, cytokines induce endothelial cell proliferation and differentiation and stimulate **matrix metalloproteinases** that digest type IV collagen in the basement membrane, creating a new branch point in the vessel.

Tumor angiogenesis mimics the process observed during inflammation. Tumor angiogenesis has become a potential target in cancer treatment. Tumors produce **antiangiogenic factors** such as **endostatin** and **angiostatin**, which are derived from type XVIII collagen and plasminogen, respectively. Pharmaceutical agents modeled after these antiangiogenic peptides are being developed to inhibit tumor growth.

Development of the Vasculature
The paired dorsal aortae and the five aortic arches form an early symmetric arterial system. Regression of portions of these vessels later results in the asymmetrical adult arterial system.

The **vitelline arteries** connect the yolk sac to the abdominal dorsal aorta. They will form the arteries of the GI tract: **celiac, superior mesenteric**, and **inferior mesenteric.**

Blood islands are the first sites of **hematopoiesis** and seed other hematopoietic tissues.

The paired **umbilical arteries** develop from the caudal end of the dorsal aorta and invade the mesoderm of the placenta. They carry deoxygenated blood from the fetus to the placenta.

The **caval venous system** is derived mostly from the right anterior and posterior **cardinal veins.**

The **vitelline veins** form the veins of the digestive system, including the **portal vein**, and the terminal part of the inferior vena cava.

No components of the **umbilical veins** remain patent after closure of the ductus venosus.

The pattern of blood supply in the fetus and the changes that occur at birth are shown in Figures 2 and 3.

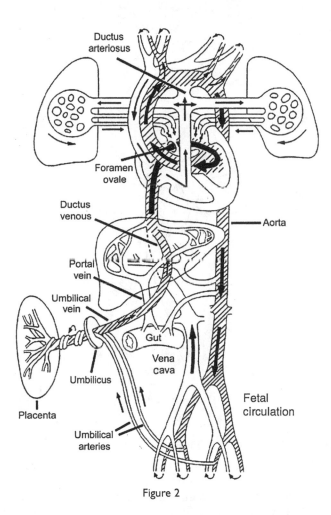

Figure 2

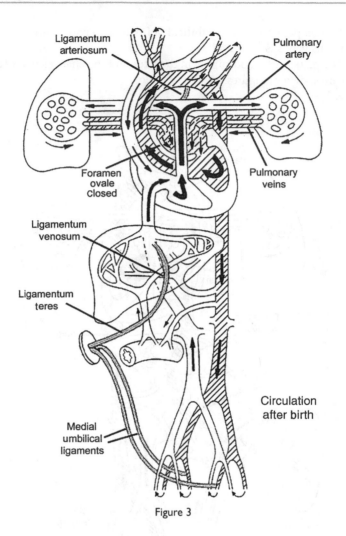

Figure 3

DEVELOPMENT OF THE HEMATOPOIETIC SYSTEM

Onset of **hematopoiesis** is marked by the formation of blood islands in the wall of the **yolk sac** (derived from the hypoblast) during week 3. The islands arise from hemangioblasts, the precursors of hematopoietic stem cells (HSC) that form the blood cells. They also differentiate into angioblasts, the precursors of blood vessel endothelial cells. The HSC seed (colonize) the liver, which is the primary hematopoietic site during the second trimester, and the bone marrow, the definitive blood-forming tissue of the adult, during the third trimester.

All components of hematopoietic organs are derived from the **mesoderm** except for the **epithelium of the thymus**, which is derived from the **endoderm** of the **third pharyngeal pouch.**

DEVELOPMENT OF THE DIGESTIVE SYSTEM

The epithelium of the digestive tract and associated organs is formed by the **endodermal tube,** whereas connective tissue and smooth muscle are derived from **splanchnic lateral plate mesoderm.** The mesoderm induces regional specialization in the endoderm.

The midgut endoderm is the last to fold into a tube and remains connected to the yolk sac via the yolk stalk.

Formation of the mesodermal **urorectal septum** divides the cloaca into the **urogenital sinus** and **primitive rectum.**

Cell proliferation results in closure of the endodermal tube lumen during week 6. The lumen is reopened by **recanalization** in week 8.

Failure to recanalize can result in **stenosis,** preventing the passage of amniotic fluid swallowed by the fetus, causing **polyhydramnios.**

Peristalsis begins in week 10 when neural crest cells invade the muscular layer to form the enteric nervous (autonomic) system. Failure of neural crest cell migration to the distal hindgut results in **aganglionic megacolon (Hirschsprung disease),** which may cause fatal intestinal obstruction.

The adult pattern of GI organ distribution is achieved by **physiologic herniation** and then retraction of the midgut during the second month.

Failure of the midgut loop to return to the abdominal cavity may result in an **omphalocele** or **umbilical hernia.**

Associated digestive organs (liver, gallbladder, and pancreas) originate as outgrowths of the endodermal tube. Connective tissue components of the liver are derived from both splanchnic and somatic **(septum transversum)** lateral plate mesoderm. Lateral plate mesoderm also forms the peritoneum and mesenteries of the abdominal cavity.

FORMATION OF THE RESPIRATORY SYSTEM

The first part of the respiratory system is lined by ectoderm derived from the nasal **ectodermal placodes.**

In the fourth week, a **respiratory diverticulum** arises as an outgrowth of the ventral **endodermal tube.**

Endoderm will form the respiratory epithelium, whereas **splanchnic lateral plate mesoderm** will form connective tissue elements including cartilage, smooth muscle, and blood vessels.

Mesoderm directs the branching pattern of the developing airways.

The **diaphragm** forms from the **septum transversum**, the two **pleuroperitoneal membranes**, the **dorsal mesentery** of the **esophagus** (where the **crura** develop), and the muscular parts of the **dorsal and lateral body wall.**

Although most **alveoli** do not form until after birth, the lungs are capable of sufficient gas exchange after 6.5 months of gestation. **Respiratory distress syndrome (RDS)** develops in premature infants because of immaturity of the type II pneumocytes that produce **surfactant.** Surfactant is essential for expansion of the pulmonary alveoli; it lowers the **air-interface surface tension** and prevents the alveoli from collapsing at the end of expiration. Without surfactant, premature babies suffer from RDS with rapid breathing, chest wall retractions, grunting noise with each breath, and nasal flaring.

Abnormal septation of the trachea and esophagus can result in stenosis, atresia, or tracheoesophageal fistulas (TEFs).

DEVELOPMENT OF THE URINARY SYSTEM

Epithelial structures of the urinary system are derived from two sources: **intermediate mesoderm** and **urogenital sinus endoderm.**

Three pairs of kidneys develop in cranio-caudal sequence in the urogenital ridge of intermediate mesoderm: **pronephros, mesonephros,** and **metanephros.**

The caudal end of the mesonephric duct gives rise to the ureteric bud. The **ureteric bud** induces the surrounding intermediate mesoderm to form the **metanephric cap,** which forms the excretory units of the kidney. The ureteric bud will form the collecting ducts.

During kidney development, **epithelial-mesenchymal interactions** occur reciprocally between the epithelium of the ureteric bud and the mesenchyme of the metanephric cap (blastema) to convert the **mesenchyme** of the metanephric cap into an **epithelium.** Those complex inductions are regulated by a cascade of growth factors that allow a **dialogue between the epithelium and mesenchyme** and the eventual formation of urine-producing (nephron) and collecting portions (ie, collecting ducts, calyces, and pelves) of the developing kidney.

The epithelial lining (transitional epithelium) of the **ureters,** as well as their muscular and connective tissue components, are derived from the **intermediate mesoderm.**

The transitional epithelium of the **bladder** and most of the **urethra** are derived from the hindgut **endoderm of the urogenital sinus.** Connective tissue and muscle are derived from splanchnic lateral plate mesoderm.

DEVELOPMENT OF THE REPRODUCTIVE SYSTEMS

Intermediate mesoderm forms the epithelia, connective tissues, and smooth muscle of the indifferent **sex cords** and their ducts.

The **endoderm of the urogenital sinus** gives rise to the epithelia of distal organs of the reproductive system and the external genitalia. As in the urinary system, connective tissue and smooth muscle of these terminal elements are provided by splanchnic lateral plate mesoderm.

Germ cells migrate from their origins in yolk sac endoderm into the indifferent sex cords of the **urogenital ridge** by week 6. Further differentiation of both the immature sex cords and the germ cells occurs.

The **SRY (sex-determining region Y) gene** on the **Y chromosome** directs the differentiation of the medullary sex cords into **testes.** If this gene *is not* present, the cortical sex cords will develop as ovaries.

Sertoli cells produce **Müllerian inhibiting substance,** which causes the apoptosis of **paramesonephric (Müllerian) duct** structures in the male fetus.

Leydig cells produce **testosterone** and other sex hormones that regulate further male differentiation.

In the absence of testosterone, **follicular cells** and **oogonia** develop.

Two pairs of genital ducts develop in both sexes. **Mesonephric (Wolffian) ducts** develop first as part of the urinary system.

Paramesonephric (Müllerian) ducts develop next and are open to the pelvic cavity at their cranial ends, and connect to each other and then to the urogenital sinus via a sinovaginal bulb at their caudal ends. The mesonephric system will persist in the male and the paramesonephric system in the female. In males, the mesonephric system gives rise to the efferent ductules, epididymis, ductus deferens, seminal vesicles, and ejaculatory ducts. In females the paramesonephric system gives rise to the oviduct, uterus, and upper part of the vagina.

In **males,** the **urogenital sinus endoderm** gives rise to the epithelia of the **urethra** and associated **prostate** and **bulbourethral glands.**

In the **female,** the endoderm of the **urogenital sinus** is the origin of the epithelium of the **lower vagina,** the upper portion being formed by the **paramesonephric ducts.**

Male differentiation of external genitalia requires androgens. Female differentiation is the intrinsic pathway and occurs in **the absence of androgens and/or functioning androgen receptors.**

DEVELOPMENT OF THE PLACENTA AND FETAL MEMBRANES

The fetal portion of the placenta forms from the **trophoblast.**

Syncytiotrophoblast cells are in direct contact with maternal tissue, whereas the embryo proper is separated from the **cytotrophoblast** by **extraembryonic mesoderm** (together, the **chorion**).

Primary villus: Syncytiotrophoblast with a cytotrophoblast core.

Secondary villus: Cytotrophoblast core invaded by extraembryonic mesoderm.

Tertiary villus: Fetal blood vessels invade the mesoderm (week 3).

The presumptive **umbilical blood vessels** form in the wall of the **allantois,** an endodermal outpocketing of the urogenital sinus.

The **amnionic membrane** develops from **epiblast** and is continuous with embryonic ectoderm. The lining of the **yolk sac** develops from **hypoblast** and is continuous with embryonic endoderm.

The yolk sac gives rise to the first **blood islands** that will form the **vitelline vessels.**

Passive immunity is transferred to the fetus by transport of **immunoglobulin G** (IgG) from the maternal to the fetal circulation.

Excess amniotic fluid is swallowed by the fetus, absorbed by the fetal GI tract, transferred to the fetal circulation, and finally crosses the placental membranes to the maternal circulation.

Hormones secreted by the placenta include chorionic gonadotropin (HCG), estrogen, progesterone, and chorionic somatostatin (placental lactogen).

High-Yield Facts

Histology and Cell Biology

CELL (PLASMA) MEMBRANES

Cell membranes consist of a **lipid bilayer** and associated proteins and carbohydrates. In the bilayer, the hydrophilic portions of the lipids are arranged on the external and cytosolic surfaces, and the **hydrophobic tails** are located in the interior. **Transmembrane proteins** are anchored to the core of the bilayer by their hydrophobic regions and can be removed only by detergents that disrupt the bilayer. **Peripheral membrane proteins** are attached to the surface of the membrane by weak electrostatic forces and are easy to remove by altering the pH or ionic strength of their environment. The general structure of the cell membrane is shown in Figure 4.

Receptors on the cell membrane are the target of signal molecules such as hormones and neurotransmitters. Steroid hormones are an exception as signal molecules that cross the plasma membrane and interact with intracellular receptors. There is a large family of cell surface receptors that share

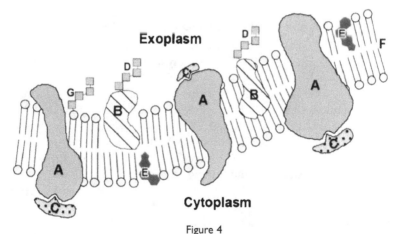

Figure 4
General structure of the cell membrane.

A = Integral membrane protein, B = Glycoprotein, C = Peripheral membrane protein (more abundant on cytosolic surface), D = sugar, E = cholesterol, F = hydrophobic fatty acid chains (hydrophilic polar head groups are not labeled), G = glycolipid

a common multipass transmembrane motif of **seven transmembrane α-helices**. An example is the β-adrenergic receptor, which is activated by epinephrine and norepinephrine and pharmacological agents used in the treatment of hypertension, pulmonary, and cardiovascular disease. Signals are transduced from these **G-protein-coupled receptors (GPCR)** to an intracellular **G (GTP-binding) protein** (Table 6).

SIGNAL TRANSDUCTION (G PROTEINS)

TABLE 6. TRIMERIC G PROTEINS AND THEIR FUNCTIONS	
G Protein	**Function**
G_s	Activates adenylyl cyclase
G_{olf}	Activates adenylyl cyclase (in olfactory neurons)
G_I	Inhibits adenylyl cyclase
G_o	Activates phospholipase C and K^+ channels; inactivates Ca^{2+} channels
G_t (transducin)	Activates cGMP (specific to rod photoreceptors)
G_q	Activates phospholipase C

CYTOPLASM AND ORGANELLES

Cytoplasm is a dynamic fluid environment bounded by the cell membrane. It contains various membrane-bound organelles, nonmembranous structures (such as lipid droplets, glycogen, and pigment granules), and structural or cytoskeletal proteins in either a soluble or insoluble form. The **endoplasmic reticulum (ER)** is a continuous tubular meshwork that may be either **smooth (SER), or rough (RER)** where studded with ribosomes. RER is involved in protein synthesis while the SER is involved in steroid synthesis and detoxification. The discoid stacks of the **Golgi apparatus** are involved in the packaging and routing of proteins for export or delivery to other organelles, including lysosomes and peroxisomes. There is a specific topography to the Golgi apparatus: *cis*-Golgi-network (CGN), *cis*, medial, *trans*, and *trans*-Golgi network (TGN) as one moves from the RER-side to the secretory vesicle-side. The Golgi apparatus is involved in packaging and routing proteins for export or delivery to other organelles, including lysosomes and peroxisomes. **Lysosomes** degrade intracellular and imported debris, and **peroxisomes** oxidize a variety of substrates, through β-oxidation and are the sole source of **plasmalogens**. Targeting sequences include **KDEL**, which targets ER proteins from the Golgi to the ER, and **mannose 6-phosphate**, which targets proteins to the lysosome. **Mannose-6-phosphate receptors** are found in the Golgi and in lysosomes. In the absence of mannose 6-phosphate on lysosomal enzymes **(I-cell disease)** they follow the default pathway and are secreted from the cell. Lysosomal enzymes are specific for substrate; the absence of specific enzymes results in **lysosomal storage diseases** such as **Tay-Sachs disease**. Secretory granules leave the **TGN** to dock with the plasma membrane. In this process, **v-SNARE** (vesicle-soluble NSF attachment protein receptors) on the vesicle docks with **t-SNARE** (target-soluble NSF attachment protein receptors) on the cell membrane and requires **Rab GTPase**-activity, linking to tethering proteins, and eventually binding to a receptor protein in the cell membrane. **Receptor-mediated endocytosis** is the process that permits selective uptake of molecules into the cell using **clathrin-coated pits and vesicles**. Molecules not recycled to the cell membrane enter **early endosomes** and subsequently **late endosomes** by way of **multivesicular bodies (MVBs)**. The late endosome is more acidic than the early endosome and generally leads to degradation of the molecules in lysosomes. There are several major pathways for shuttling of receptors and ligands.

- The internalized ligand-receptor complex dissociates in the early endosome with recycling of receptors (eg, low density lipoprotein [LDL]-LDL-receptor complex).
- Receptor and ligand are recycled (eg, iron-transferrin-transferrin receptor-complex).
- The internalized ligand-receptor complex dissociates in the late endosome and is degraded in the lysosome (eg, growth factors such as epidermal growth factor).
- Internalized ligand-receptor passes through the cell (transcytosis) and is released at another surface (eg, IgA uptake by small intestinal enterocytes).

There are other coating proteins. COP-I (**CO**at **P**rotein-**I**) coats vesicles involved in retrograde transport from Golgi → RER and COP-II (**CO**at **P**rotein-**II**) is the coat protein for vesicles transported in an anterograde direction from the RER → Golgi.

Only the **nucleus**, which is the repository of genetic information stored in deoxyribonucleic acid (DNA), and the **mitochondria**, which are the storage sites of energy for cellular function in the form of adenosine triphosphate **(ATP)**, are enclosed in double membranes. Also included in the cytoplasm are three classes of proteins that form the **cytoskeletal infrastructure: actin bundles** that determine the shape of the cell; **intermediate filaments** that stabilize the cell membrane and cytoplasmic contents; and **microtubules (tubulin)**, which use molecular motors (ie, dynein and kinesin) to move organelles within the cell.

NUCLEUS

The nucleus consists of a **nuclear envelope** that is continuous with the ER membrane, chromatin, matrix, and a **nucleolus**, the site of ribosomal ribonucleic acid (rRNA) synthesis and initial ribosomal assembly.

The nucleolus is a highly organized, heterogeneous structure, with distinct regions visible by EM: (1) fibrillar centers, the nucleolar organizer regions where transcription does **not** occur; (2) dense fibrillar components (*pars fibrosa*) where RNA molecules are transcribed; and (3) a granular component (*pars granulosa*) where ribosomal subunits undergo maturation. The nucleolar organizer contains clusters of rRNA genes (DNA). The size and number of nucleoli differ with the metabolic activity of cells.

The nuclear envelope contains pores for bidirectional transport and is supported by intermediate filament proteins, the **lamins.** Chromatin consists of **euchromatin** (eu = true), which is an open form of DNA that is actively transcribed, and **heterochromatin** that is quiescent. There is a sequential packing of chromatin beginning with the DNA double helix, which is combined with **histones** to form the **nucleosomes,** the smallest unit of chromatin structure. This is the **"beads on a string"** structure with the histones forming the octamer arrangement of paired H2A, H2B, H3, and H4. **H1** is the **linker histone.** The nucleosomes are connected by strands of protein-free DNA, so called **linker DNA.** Nucleases degrade the linker DNA, but nucleosome particles are protected against micrococcal nuclease activity because of the close interaction of DNA with histone proteins. The next orders of packing are the 30 nm chromatin fibril, the chromatin fiber with loops of chromatin fibrils, and chromatin fibers loosely or tightly packed in euchromatin and heterochromatin, respectively.

During **cell division,** DNA is accurately replicated and divided equally between two daughter nuclei. Equal distribution of chromosomes is accomplished by the **microtubules of the mitotic spindle.** The separation of cytoplasm **(cytokinesis)** occurs through the action of an **actin** contractile ring. The cell cycle consists of interphase (G_1, S, and G_2), and the stages of mitosis (M): prophase, prometaphase, metaphase, anaphase, and telophase.

The events that occur during the specific phases of the cell cycle are summarized in Table 7:

TABLE 7. DEFINING EVENTS OF CELL CYCLE PHASES

Phase of Cell Cycle	Defining Event(s)
Interphase (G_1, S, and G_2 phases)	Duplication of centrioles and DNA synthesis (S phase)
Prophase	Nucleolus disappears
Prometaphase	Nuclear envelope breaks down
Metaphase	Alignment of chromosomes in metaphase plate
Anaphase	Separation of sister chromatids; initiation of cytokinesis
Telophase	Nuclear envelope reforms; completion of cytokinesis

(Reproduced, with permission, from McKenzie JC, Klein, RM. *Basic Concepts in Cell Biology and Histology*. New York, NY: McGraw-Hill; 2000.)

The cell cycle is regulated at the G_1/S and G_2/M boundaries (checkpoints) by phosphorylation of complexes of a protein kinase (**cyclin-dependent kinase [Cdk] protein**) and a cyclin (cytoplasmic oscillator). For example, the G_2/M interface is regulated by **M-Cdk complex** (formerly called **mitosis promoting factor, MPF**), which is responsible for the phosphorylation of **spindle proteins, histones, and lamins.** Phosphorylation of **lamins** results in their breakdown as well as the dissolution of the nuclear envelope. There are different cyclins and Cdks for each of the cell cycle checkpoints. Overarching the Cdks are the **Cdk inhibitors** that form an additional regulatory layer at each of the cell cycle checkpoints. Study of the cell cycle is critical to an understanding of the regulation of abnormal proliferation occurs in cancer cells. Two **tumor suppressor genes** that have been well studied are **retinoblastoma gene (***Rb***)** and *p53*. Rb is active (suppressing growth) in the hypophosphorylated state and inactive in the hyperphosphorylated form. In its nonphosphorylated form Rb serves as a brake on the cell cycle at the G_1/S interface by binding to the **transcription factor, E2F.** Stimulation by growth factors results in phosphorylation and release of the brake; E2F is free to turn on transcription of cell cycle genes, allowing cells to traverse the G_1/S interface. **Mutations in Rb occur in** tumors; a mutation has the same effect as inactivating Rb, leading to uncontrolled cell proliferation as E2F transcribes cell cycle genes. *p53* **is a protective gene,** or molecular policeman, which prevents the replication of damaged DNA and stimulates repair. *p53* acts as a transcription factor and also works through the Cdk inhibitors to arrest the cell cycle at the G_1/S interface. *p53* **mutations are found in many human tumors.**

INTRACELLULAR TRAFFICKING

The key event in exocytosis is translocation of newly synthesized protein into the cisternal space of the rough ER (**signal hypothesis**). Proteins and lipids reach the Golgi apparatus by vesicular transport. Using carbohydrate-sorting signals, proteins are sorted from the *trans*-face of the Golgi apparatus to secretory vesicles, the cell membrane, and **lysosomes.** Lysosomal enzymes are sorted by using a **mannose-6-phosphate** signal recognized by a receptor on the lysosomal membrane. Absence of mannose 6-phosphate results in **default to the secretory pathway and release of enzymes by exocytosis.** Nuclear and mitochondrial-sorting signals (positively charged amino acid sequences) are recognized by those organelles.

Endocytosis involves transport from the cell membrane to lysosomes using endosome intermediates. The process originates with a **clathrin-coated pit** that invaginates to form a **coated vesicle** that fuses with an **endosome.** This internalization can be **receptor-mediated** (eg, uptake of cholesterol). Endosomes subsequently fuse with lysosomes. Internalized receptor/ligand complexes may be conserved, degraded, or recycled.

EPITHELIUM

Epithelial cells line the free external and internal surfaces of the body. Epithelia have a paucity of intercellular substance and are interconnected by **junctional complexes.** Components of the junctional complex include the *zonula occludens* (tight junction), which prevents leakage between the adjoining cells and maintains apical/basolateral polarity; *zonula adherens,* which links the actin networks within adjacent cells; and *macula adherens* (desmosome), which links the intermediate filament networks of adjacent cells. Epithelial cells also form a firm attachment to the **basal lamina,** which they secrete. **Gap junctions** permit passage of small molecules directly between cells. Junctional complexes are summarized in Table 8.

The components of the basal lamina/basement membrane that underlies the epithelium are summarized in Table 9.

TABLE 8. JUNCTIONAL COMPLEXES

Classification	Type	Function	Interactions
Occluding	Zonula occludens (tight junction)	Prevents passage of luminal substances; confers epithelial tightness or leakiness; maintains apical vs basolateral polarity	Intramembranous sealing strands occlude the space between cells (number of strands directly proportional to tightness of) epithelium
Anchoring	Zonula adherens	Mechanical stability—cohesive function of cell groups, important during embryonic folding; transmits motile forces across epithelial sheets	Link actin filament network between cells, cadherins are transmembrane linkers
	Focal contacts	Attach cells to the extracellular matrix (ECM)	Link actin filament network of cell to integrins in ECM; actin-binding proteins form link
Anchoring	Desmosome (macula adherens)	Spot welds (rivets) provide high tensile strength and resist shearing forces, numerous in stratified squamous epithelia	Link intermediate filaments to transmembrane proteins (cadherins: desmogleins and desmocollins). Linkage through plaque proteins (desmoplakins)
	Hemidesmosome	Increased stability of epithelia on ECM	Link intermediate filaments in the cell to the ECM through integrins rather than cadherins
Communicating	Gap junction (nexus)	Selective communication in the form of diffusible molecules between 1 and 1.5 kD	Connexons in hexameric arrangement with central pores in adjacent cells align

TABLE 9. COMPONENTS OF THE BASEMENT MEMBRANE

Molecular Component	Component Arrangement	Function
Type IV collagen	3 α-chains	Insoluble structural support
Laminin	3 (α, β, and γ)-chains	Bridge between the cells and type IV collagen
Heparan sulfate	Protein core (polypeptide chain) with glycosaminoglycan side chains	Electrostatic charge (anionic sugar side chains repel one another)
Entactin (nidogen)	Single polypeptide chain	Bridge between two networks: laminin and type IV collagen

Apical specializations are prominent in epithelia and include **microvilli** that increase surface area; **stereocilia,** which are long, non-motile modified microvilli; and **cilia and flagella,** which are motile structures. Cilia and flagella have the classic "9 + 2" microtubular arrangement emanating from **basal bodies.** The basal surface may be modified with infoldings that house numerous mitochondria, as found in proximal and distal tubule cells of the kidney and striated duct cells of the salivary glands. Those cells are involved in extensive ion transport.

Epithelia occur in simple (one layer) and stratified types. Table 10 lists functions and locations of epithelia.

CONNECTIVE TISSUE

Connective tissue consists of cells and a matrix (fibers and ground substance). The cells include **fibroblasts** (the source of collagen and other fibers), **plasma cells** (the source of antibodies), **macrophages** (the cells responsible for phagocytosis), **mast cells** (the source of heparin and histamine), and a variety of transient blood cells: **lymphocytes (B and T), eosinophils, basophils,** and **neutrophils (PMNs).** B cells are involved in **humoral immunity** and T cells in **cell-mediated immunity** as well as humoral immunity (helper T cells). Neutrophils phagocytose bacteria; the dead neutrophils are a major component of pus. Basophils, like mast cells, release histamine, although they originate from a different bone marrow stem cell. Eosinophils are involved in response to parasitic infection. Eosinophilic granules contain a crystalline core of major basic protein, which is toxic for parasites and histaminase, which breaks down histamine

TABLE 10. EPITHELIAL TYPES, LOCATION, AND FUNCTION		
Epithelial Type	Location	Function
Simple		
Simple squamous	Endothelium of blood vessels	Transport, absorption, secretion
Simple cuboidal	Collecting ducts of kidneys	Transport, reabsorption, secretion
Simple columnar	Epithelium of the gut: stomach, intestines	Absorption, protection, lubrication (mucus)
Stratified		
Stratified cuboidal	Sweat ducts	Transport
Stratified columnar	Excretory ducts of salivary glands	Transport
Stratified squamous (keratinized)	Epidermis	Protection, water conservation
Stratified squamous (nonkeratinized)	Esophagus, anus, vagina	Protection, lubrication, secretion
Pseudostratified	Respiratory system (trachea with cilia), male reproductive system (no cilia)	Movement of material across epithelial surface
Transitional	Urinary system: ureter, bladder	Stretch, protection

and limits the allergic response. The function and origin of the connective tissue cells are summarized in Table 11.

Leukocytes **extravasate** from the blood to the lymphoid compartment. There are several stages in extravasation: **rolling, firm adhesion, and diapedesis**, as shown in Figure 5. Cytokines, such as tumor necrosis factor-alpha (TNF-α), are released during inflammation and stimulate the endothelium of veins to express the surface adhesion molecule P-selectin (also E-selectin). E- and P-selectins bind reversibly to glycoproteins on leukocytes causing them to **roll** along the endothelial surface. Intercellular adhesion molecules (eg, ICAM-1) are up-regulated and bind to the leukocyte integrins, lymphocyte function-associated antigen 1 (LFA)-1 and complement receptor type 3 (CR3). Adhesion of leukocytes results in arrest of leukocyte motion, allowing

TABLE 11. CONNECTIVE TISSUE CELLS

Cell Type	Origin	Function
Fibroblast	Mesenchyme	Synthesis of fibers (collagen, elastic, reticular) and ground substance (proteoglycans and glycoproteins of connective tissue matrix)
Macrophages (eg, Kupffer cells, Langerhans cells, and microglia)	Monocyte (bone marrow)	Phagocytosis, antigen presentation, produce and respond to cytokines
Lymphocytes		
T lymphocytes	Bone marrow (thymus-educated)	Cell-mediated immunity (CD_8^+) and helper T cells (CD_4^+)
B lymphocytes	Bone marrow (bone marrow-educated)	Humoral immunity
Plasma cell	B lymphocyte	Immunoglobulin secretion
Neutrophils (PMNs)	Bone marrow	First cells to enter a site of inflammation, secrete myeloperoxidase, phagocytose bacteria, and die (forming pus)
Eosinophils	Bone marrow	Source of major basic protein, histaminase (breakdown of histamine), arylsulfatases (degradation of leukotrienes), phagocytosis of antigen-antibody complexes and parasites
Basophils	Bone marrow (different stem cell from mast cell)	Blood source of histamine
Mast cells, connective tissue mast cells (CTMC), and mucosal mast cells (MMC)	Bone marrow	CTMC are T-lymphocyte independent, MMC are T-lymphocyte dependent, secrete histamine and slow-reacting substance of anaphylaxis ([SRS-A] increase vascular permeability), heparin (anticoagulant), eosinophil chemoattractant factor of anaphylaxis ([ECF-A], chemoattraction of eosinophils), leukotrienes (smooth muscle contraction)

secreted proteases to disrupt endothelial tight junctions and the basement membrane, subsequently resulting in **diapedesis**. L-selectins expressed by leukocytes are also involved in the process (Fig. 5).

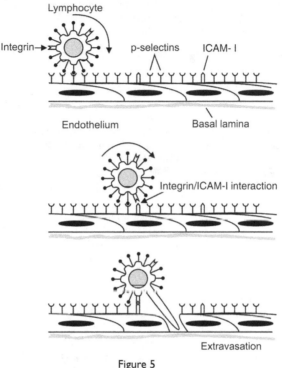

Figure 5
Leukocyte extravasation.

Type I collagen and elastin make up the predominant fibers found in connective tissue, including bone and fibrocartilage. Ground substance includes proteoglycans and glycoproteins that organize and stabilize the fibrillar network. **Type II collagen** is associated with hyaline cartilage. **Type III collagen** forms the collagenous component of reticular connective tissue found in highly cellular organs, such as the liver and lymphoid organs. **Type IV collagen** forms a **sheet-like meshwork** or **insoluble scaffolding** of the basal lamina. Other types of collagen exist and include the **fibril-associated collagens** with interrupted triple helices **(FACIT)**. Collagen fibrils are connected to other extracellular matrix molecules by the FACIT collagens. Table 12 lists the location of the major types of collagen.

TABLE 12. MAJOR COLLAGEN TYPES		
Type	**Location**	**Function and Other Information**
*I	General connective tissue, bone, and fibrocartilage	Most abundant type of collagen, 67-nm periodicity, tensile strength
*II	Hyaline and elastic cartilage	Thinner fibrils than type I, tensile strength, electrostatic interactions between type II collagen and proteoglycan aggregates form the molecular basis for the rigidity of hyaline cartilage.
*III	Spleen, bone marrow, and lymph nodes, skin and blood vessels (elasticity)	Reticular framework in highly cellular organs, stains with silver. Also found in skin and blood vessels where elasticity is required. It is abundant during embryogenesis and is also crucial for collagen I fibrillogenesis.
*IV	Basement membrane	Filtration, support, meshwork scaffolding, interacts with heparan sulfate proteoglycan to produce a polyanionic charge distribution that facilitates selective filtration; synthesized by epithelia; it retains propeptides that are used to form a meshwork; also interacts with fibronectin
V	Placental basement membrane, muscle basal lamina	Linkage function in basement membrane
VII	Basement membrane of skin and amnion	Anchoring fibers
VIII	Endothelium	Angiogenesis, bridging ECM components
IX-XII	Cartilage	Fibril-associated collagens with interrupted triple helices (FACIT) regulate orientation and function of fibrillar collagens

*Most common collagen types and most testable

SPECIALIZED CONNECTIVE TISSUES: BONE AND CARTILAGE

Bone contains three major cell types: **osteoblasts** that secrete **type I collagen** and noncollagenous proteins; **osteocytes,** which maintain mature bone; and **osteoclasts** that resorb bone by acidification. Osteoclastic activity uses **protons**

(H^+) derived from carbonic acid formed by the enzyme **carbonic anhydrase.** Carbonic anhydrases are zinc-containing enzymes that catalyze the reversible reaction between carbon dioxide hydration and bicarbonate dehydration:

$$H_2O + CO_2 \leftrightarrow H^+ + HCO_3^-$$

In the region of the **ruffled border, protons and lysosomal enzymes,** such as acid phosphatase, are released into a sealed zone (Howship lacuna). Breakdown of bone occurs due to the **acidification of this extracellular compartment** that is analogous to an intracellular secondary lysosome. Bone deposition is regulated primarily by **parathyroid hormone (PTH),** which is secreted in response to low serum calcium levels. PTH increases serum calcium, as summarized below (Fig. 6). The increased serum calcium inhibits PTH secretion by negative feedback. PTH stimulates:

- **Osteoclasts** to resorb bone (through PTH receptors on osteoblasts)
- Renal synthesis of **1,25-dihydroxycholecalciferol,** which in turn increases intestinal absorption of Ca^{++}
- **Intestinal absorption of Ca^{++}**

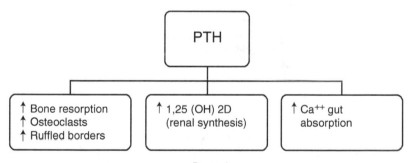

Figure 6
Systemic effects of parathyroid hormone.

PTH regulates osteoclasts by an indirect mechanism through **PTH receptors** on osteoblasts (Fig. 7). There are *no* PTH receptors on osteoclasts. PTH stimulation of osteoblasts releases **macrophage colony-stimulating factor (M-CSF)** and **RANK-L.** M-CSF stimulates differentiation of **monocytes into osteoclasts.** RANK-L is found in both membrane and soluble forms and binds to **RANK (receptor for activation of nuclear factor kappa B)** on osteoclasts and osteoclast

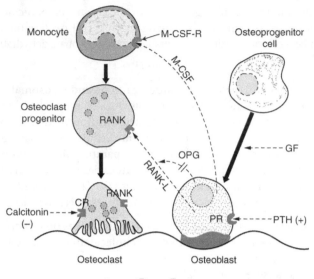

Figure 7
Molecular interactions between bone cells.
GF = growth factors, OPG = osteoprotegerin, PR = parathyroid hormone receptor,
PTH = parathyroid hormone, RANK = receptor for activation of nuclear factor kappa
B, RANK-L = ligand for RANK, M-CSF = macrophage colony-stimulating factor,
M-CSF-R = MCSF receptor

precursors, stimulating osteoclastic activation/ruffled border formation. **Osteoprotegerin (OPG), from osteoblasts, is a decoy receptor for RANK-L,** binds RANK-L, and leads to inhibition of osteoclastic activity. Those molecules create the link between osteoblasts and osteoclasts, known as the **ARF (activation-resorption-formation)** cycle, in which activation of osteoclasts is inextricably linked to osteoblasts. This has been one of the problems in treating **osteoporosis**, in which osteoclastic activity dominates osteoblastic activity. Growth factors such as transforming growth factor-beta (TGF-β) and insulin-like growth factors also play a role in differentiation of osteoblasts and osteoclasts. TGF-β is found in an inactive form in the bone matrix and is activated by acid produced by osteoclasts. TGF-β then inhibits osteoclast differentiation and stimulates osteoblastic activity.

Calcitonin opposes the actions of PTH, but plays a lesser role overall. Bone is highly vascular and mineralized with **hydroxyapatite**. In contrast, the three types of cartilage are avascular and contain chondrocytes that synthesize fibers and ground substance. **Hyaline cartilage** covers articular surfaces and forms the cartilage model in long bone development. **Elastic cartilage** is found in the pinna of the ear and in the epiglottis, while **fibrocartilage** is an intermediate form found in the intervertebral discs, pubic symphysis, and connecting tendon and bone. Hyaline cartilage contains matrix comprised of type II collagen electrostatically bound to proteoglycans. Elastic cartilage contains type II collagen and elastic fibers, and fibrocartilage, like bone, contains type I collagen.

MUSCLE AND CELL MOTILITY

Skeletal and cardiac (striated) muscles contract by sliding **myosin** and **actin** filaments past each other in a process facilitated by ATP. Myosin contains a motor that interacts with the actin filament and allows myosin to ratchet along the actin. The filaments are arranged in a banded pattern in individual sarcomeres, which act in series. Specialized invaginations of the plasma membrane (**T tubules**) spread the surface depolarization to the interior of the cell to release calcium from the **sarcoplasmic reticulum,** initiating contraction. **Troponin** and **tropomyosin** are specialized proteins that permit contraction of skeletal and cardiac muscle to be regulated by calcium. Skeletal muscle is a syncytium, while cardiac muscle consists of individual cells connected by intercalated disks. The organization of striated muscle is shown Figure 8 below:

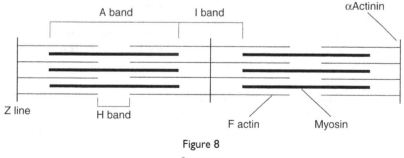

Figure 8

Sarcomere

The average length of a sarcomere is 2.5 μm. This distance is measured from one Z line to the next Z line. If the resting length of the A band is 1.5 μm and the length of the I band is 1.0 μm, then the resting length of the sarcomere is determined by adding the length of the I band to the length of the A band. If there is a 20% contraction of the muscle (contraction to 80% of its length), then the sarcomere is reduced in length from 2.5 to 2.0 μm. The size of the A band remains unchanged, therefore the length of the I band is reduced from 1.0 to 0.5 μm and "makes up" for the 0.5 μm reduction in length during the muscle contraction. The processes of skeletal muscle contraction and relaxation are shown in Figure 9.

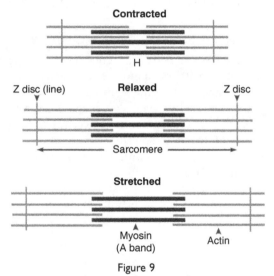

Figure 9
Muscle contraction and relaxation.
The sarcomere extends from Z disc (line) to Z disc. The H band is located between the ends of the thin actin filaments. The A band is defined by the width of the thick (myosin) filaments. The I bands are not shown completely on the figure because they are found between adjacent A bands.

Extrafusal muscle fibers generate the force of contraction while intra-fusal fibers (both IA and II-type fibers [receptors]) serve as sensory detectors signaling muscle location (proprioception) and the rate of contraction.

Smooth muscle contraction closely resembles cell motility exhibited in other cell types. It also occurs through the action of actin and myosin, which are arranged in a lattice-like pattern. Troponin is *not* present in smooth muscle.

NERVOUS SYSTEM

Myelin, which insulates neuronal projections and permits rapid (saltatory) conduction, is produced by **oligodendroglia (oligodendrocytes)** in the central nervous system (CNS) and by **Schwann cells** in the **peripheral nervous system (PNS). Microglia** are brain macrophages. **Astrocytes** provide physical and metabolic support of neurons. Astrocytes **induce and maintain the blood-brain barrier,** but they *do not* constitute the **barrier function,** which is established by **endothelial tight junctions (zonula occludentes).** Neurons conduct electrochemical impulses and move neurotransmitters to their synaptic termini by **axoplasmic transport.** Axonal transport occurs by several different mechanisms. Slow axonal transport/dendritic transport (1-5 mm/day) involves the movement of cytoskeletal elements such as actin, tubulin, and neurofilaments from the perikaryon down the axon. Rapid anterograde (away from the perikaryon) and retrograde (toward the perikaryon) transport (200-300 mm/day) moves membrane-bound organelles, for example, newly formed secretory vesicles and mitochondria anterogradely. Receptors, recycled membranes, and worn-out organelles are transported retrogradely.

Transneuronal transmission is accomplished by calcium-regulated release of **synaptic vesicles.** Neurons also synapse with muscle cells. A typical contact between a myelinated neuron and skeletal muscle **(neuromuscular junction)** is shown in Figure 10.

In the **cerebral** and **cerebellar** cortices, **gray matter** (neuronal cell bodies and immediately adjacent processes) is located peripherally and white matter centrally; this pattern is reversed in the **spinal cord.** The cerebellar cortex consists of **molecular, Purkinje,** and **granular** layers **(mnemonic: miles per gallon [MPG])** with extensive arborization of the neuronal processes. The **cerebral cortex** consists of a homogenous layer I with multiple deeper layers of large **pyramidal** and other types of **neurons.** The number of layers varies, depending on the cortical region. Neuronal cell bodies **(perikarya)** are also localized in **ganglia** in the peripheral nervous system and the **autonomic nervous system (ANS).**

Myelination is a critical process in normal neural function. Myelination in the CNS and PNS occurs by similar methods, although there are differences in the supportive cells responsible. In the CNS, the oligodendrocytes myelinate axons, whereas Schwann cells myelinate axons in the PNS. In the PNS, formation of myelin is initiated by the invagination of an axon into a Schwann cell. A mesaxon is formed as the outer leaflets of the

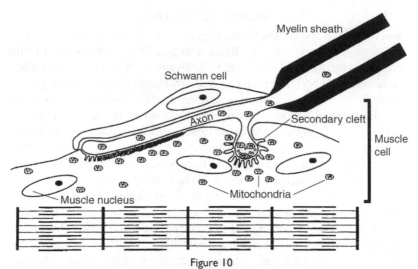

Figure 10
Neuromuscular junction: Axonal terminals (telodendria) rest in shallow depressions (primary clefts) on the surface of the striated muscle fiber. Secondary clefts increase the surface area for interaction with a neurotransmitter (acetylcholine). Muscle cell nuclei and mitochondria are abundant near the junction.

cell membrane fuse. Subsequently, the mesaxon of the Schwann cell wraps itself around the fiber. In the CNS, oligodendrocytes form myelin around multiple axon segments compared with the 1:1 relationship between Schwann cells and axon segments in the PNS. Myelination occurs in both pre- and postnatal development. CNS myelin is the target for attack by components of the immune system in multiple sclerosis, and PNS myelin is the target in Guillain-Barré syndrome (GBS), also called acute inflammatory demyelinating polyneuropathy or Landry ascending paralysis. GBS is an inflammatory disorder of the PNS characterized by rapid onset of weakness and, often, paralysis of the legs, arms, respiratory muscles, and muscles of facial expression.

CARDIOVASCULAR SYSTEM, BLOOD, AND BONE MARROW

Blood vessels are comprised of three layers or tunics: intima, media, and adventitia. In large arteries close to the heart, the *tunica media* contains high amounts of elastin to buffer the heart's pulsatile output. Smaller muscular arteries distribute blood to organs and capillary beds; their contractions are mediated by both the **sympathetic nervous system (SNS)** and by humoral factors. **Endothelial cells**, found in the tunica intima, line the vascular lumen in contact with the blood, and secrete **vasoactive substances** that regulate relaxation and contraction of the underlying smooth muscle. For example, **endothelin 1** is a **potent vasoconstrictor**; **nitric oxide** is **synthesized** from **L-arginine** and induces relaxation of the smooth muscle through a **cGMP-dependent** mechanism. **Prostacyclin**, also synthesized by endothelial cells, is a smooth muscle relaxant that functions through a **cAMP-dependent** mechanism. Prostacyclin **inhibits platelet adhesion** and **prevents intravascular clot formation**. Endothelial cells produce molecules that regulate fibrinolysis and thrombogenesis. Endothelial cell-derived factors are stored in intracellular granules and released into the blood stream upon stimulation. There are two contrasting factors, **fibrinolytic tissue-type plasminogen activator (tPA)** and **von Willebrand factor (vWF)**. In contrast to tPA, vWF induces **coagulation and thrombus formation**. Endothelial cells also produce **tissue factor**, the only non-plasma protein in the clotting cascade, which initiates the common blood clotting pathway. **E-selectin** expression on endothelial cells modulates **extravasation** of **monocytes** and **neutrophils**. **Chemokines (chemo**attractant cyto**kines)** induce expression of E-selectins on the endothelium under normal conditions and following inflammation. **Smooth muscle cells** undergo **hyperplasia** and **hypertrophy** in hypertension. The heart contains specialized cardiomyocytes that function as impulse-generating and conducting cells regulated by the ANS. The **heart** also functions as an **endocrine organ**, releasing **atrial natriuretic factor** (peptide [ANP or ANF]) in response to **increased plasma volume**. ANP reduces plasma volume by (1) increasing urinary sodium (**natriuretic**) and water excretion (**diuretic**), (2) inhibiting **aldosterone** synthesis and **angiotensin II** production, and (3) inhibiting **vasopressin** release from the neurohypophysis.

Blood cells include **erythrocytes**, which are specialized for oxygen transport; **lymphocytes** that function in cellular and humoral immune responses; **neutrophils**, which are early responders to acute inflammation; **monocytes** that are the precursors of tissue macrophages; **eosinophils**, which respond to parasitic infection and release histaminases to counteract basophils and mast cells; and **basophils**, which contain histamine and heparin and assist mast cell function.

Bone marrow is the site of blood cell development in adults. The erythrocyte lineage includes the following stages: proerythroblasts → basophilic erythroblasts (early normoblasts) → polychromatophilic (polychromatic) erythroblasts (intermediate normoblasts) → orthochromatophilic (orthochromatic) erythroblasts (late normoblasts) → reticulocytes → erythrocytes. The white cell series includes myeloblasts → promyelocytes → myelocytes → metamyelocytes → mature granular leukocytes. Specificity of granules occurs at the myelocyte stage.

LYMPHOID SYSTEM AND CELLULAR IMMUNOLOGY

Functional cells include B lymphocytes (humoral immunity), T lymphocytes (cellular immunity), macrophages (phagocytic and one of several types of antigen-presenting cells), and mast cells.

Immunity and T and B cells

There are two types of immunity:

- **Innate immunity** is the first-line of defense and comprises basic mechanisms of host defense including **barriers** (eg, skin, **zonulae occludentes/ tight junctions**) and **phagocytic cells**, such as **macrophages** and **neutrophils**. Innate immunity is *not* specific for particular pathogens or individuals of the species.
- **Adaptive immunity** is a response **to antigenic challenge** and possesses four essential characteristics that are *not* part of innate immunity:

  - Specificity of response to antigen
  - Memory
  - Diversity
  - Recognition of self versus nonself

Lymphocytes display the four attributes listed above. There are two types of lymphocytes: B cells and T cells. B cells are involved in humoral immunity. On first exposure to an antigen it recognizes on its surface, a naïve B cell proliferates to produce a memory B cell and a plasma cell that is the effector, synthesizing antibodies for release. T cells are unable to recognize antigen on their own. They require antigen-presenting cells (**macrophages, dendritic cells,** and **B cells**) to process antigen and bind it to membrane proteins known as **major histocompatibility molecules (MHC). Class I MHC** is found on virtually all cells of the body, while **Class II MHC** is specific for **antigen-presenting cells (APCs).** On first encounter with a specific antigen-MHC II complex, the T cell proliferates, resulting in a memory T cell and an effector T cell. There are several subtypes of T cells:

- **T_H cells,** which express the specific glycoprotein, CD4, are called CD4⁺
- **T_C cells,** which express the specific glycoprotein, CD8, are called CD8⁺

- T_{reg} cells, (suppressor T cells) are critical for maintenance of **immunological tolerance**

The T_H cell secretes cytokines (small protein or peptide intercellular communication molecules) that activate T_C cells, B cells, and macrophages. Release of cytokines by T_H cells induces T_C cells to proliferate and differentiate into effector cells. In that case the effectors are **cytotoxic T lymphocytes (CTLs)** that recognize Class I MHC-antigen complex on the surface of altered self-cells (eg, cells of a foreign tissue graft or self-cells infected with virus). CTLs recognize altered self-cells and form a conjugate with them; the target cell is killed by release of **perforins** (pore-forming proteins) and serine proteases **(granzymes)**, leading to **apoptosis** of the target.

T_H cells are regulated by APCs that internalize antigen and then process it through the secretory pathway to a membrane-bound MHC II-antigen complex. The T_H cell is activated by a co-stimulatory signal from the APC. Cytokines from T_H cells are required for B cells to proliferate and differentiate into a memory B cell and an antibody-producing plasma cell. Two of the key cytokines involved in the interaction of those cells are IL-1 produced by activated macrophages and IL-2 that regulates T cell, but also B-cell proliferation. Another critical cytokine is **interferon-gamma (IFN-γ)** that activates macrophages and is secreted by activated T_H cells. There are two types of T_H cells expressing different cytokine profiles:

- T_H1 response is primarily directed toward macrophages and T cells and the support of the inflammatory response.
- T_H2 response is primarily directed toward B cells and, therefore, antibody responses.

T_{reg} cells are CD4$^+$, express CD25 and produce IL-10 and TGF-β, lymphokines that are both strong immunosuppressants inhibiting T_H1 and T_H2 cells.

NK cells are not T cells, but kill cellular targets such as tumor cells in a nonspecific manner.

Lymphoid Organs

Lymphoid organs may be either **primary (bone marrow** and **thymus)** or **secondary (lymph nodes** and **dispersed lymphatic nodules, spleen,** and **tonsils)**. The B lymphocytes are educated in the bone marrow (differentiation of antigen-binding receptors [antibodies]) and are seeded to specific B-cell regions of the secondary lymphoid organs, while T lymphocytes are educated in the thymus (differentiation of T-cell receptors [TcR]) and are seeded to **T-cell-dependent regions** of the secondary lymphoid organs.

The thymus is recognized by lobulation, separate cortex and medulla in each lobule, the absence of germinal centers, and the presence of Hassall corpuscles. The lymph nodes, which filter lymph and blood, are characterized by a central medulla consisting of cords with many plasma cells and a cortex containing primary and secondary follicles. The spleen, which filters blood, is characterized by red and white pulp. The tonsils are characterized by crypts with an epithelial lining on one side. That lining is stratified squamous epithelium in palatine tonsils and pseudostratified epithelium on pharyngeal tonsils.

RESPIRATORY SYSTEM

The respiratory epithelium consists of **conducting pathways** (nasal cavities, naso- and oropharynx, larynx, trachea, bronchi, and bronchioles) and **respiratory portions** (respiratory bronchioles and alveoli). The nasal epithelium includes a region of specialized olfactory receptors. Ciliated cells appear in all portions of the respiratory system except the respiratory epithelium and move mucus and particulates toward the oropharynx **(mucociliary escalator)**. Gas exchange in the lungs takes place across a **minimal barrier** consisting of the **capillary endothelium**, a **joint basal lamina**, and an **exceedingly thin alveolar epithelium** consisting **primarily of type I pneumocytes**. **Type II pneumocytes** are responsible for the secretion of surfactant, a primarily lipid substance that facilitates respiration by reducing alveolar surface tension. The type II pneumocyte is recognizable at the EM level by the presence of **lamellar bodies** that contain surfactant, comprised primarily of **lecithin (dipalmitoyl phosphatidylcholine, DPPC)**, as well as some cholesterol and sphingomyelin. Although surfactant is produced beginning at about the 28th week, premature births before 30 weeks are likely to result in **respiratory distress syndrome (RDS)** because of the absence of surfactant. There are a variety of treatments for RDS, including glucocorticoid administration to the mother before delivery and the administration of artificial surfactant and ventilation for the premature infant. In cystic fibrosis, mutations in the cystic fibrosis transmembrane conductance regulator (CFTR) result in defective Cl^- transport and increased Na^+ absorption. HCO_3^- transport through the CFTR is also defective. The result is thick, more viscous (less watery) mucus in the airways that promotes bacterial infections and reduces the effectiveness of the mucociliary escalator.

Emphysema and chronic bronchitis are the obstructive pulmonary diseases (COPD). Emphysema is characterized by irreversible dilation of the airspaces distal to the terminal bronchiole. It occurs in several forms; the two major forms are centriacinar (centrilobular) emphysema in which the target is the central part of the acinus formed by the respiratory bronchiole and panacinar (panlobular) emphysema in which the initial target is the alveolar duct and alveolus. In emphysema, the balance between proteases (especially elastases) produced by neutrophils and antiprotease activity is disturbed. It occurs in an inherited form caused by a deficiency in alpha (α)-1-antitrypsin (protease) deficiency and a second form related to chronic inhalation of foreign particles such as tobacco smoke and/or air pollution.

INTEGUMENTARY SYSTEM

The epidermis of thick skin consists of five layers of cells **(keratinocytes)**: *stratum basale* (proliferative layer), *stratum spinosum* (characterized by tonofibrils and associated desmosomes), *stratum granulosum* (characterized by keratohyalin granules), *stratum lucidum* (a translucent layer *not* obvious in thin skin), and *stratum corneum* (characterized by dead and dying cells with compacted keratin). Specialized structures of the skin include hair follicles (found only in thin skin), nails, and sweat glands and ducts. Nonkeratinocyte epidermal cells include **melanocytes** (derived from **neural crest**), **Langerhans cells** (antigen-presenting cells derived from monocytes), and **Merkel cells** (sensory mechanoreceptors). Various sensory receptors and extensive capillary networks are found in the underlying dermis. There are skin diseases with a cell biological etiology. Psoriasis is a disease characterized by dermal and epidermal infiltration of inflammatory cells. Those cells release cytokines, which cause hyperplasia of the epidermis. Proliferation occurs throughout the epidermis and is *no* longer restricted to the basal layer and there is a thickening of the stratum corneum with nucleated keratinocytes present. **Pemphigus** is an autoimmune disease in which **autoantibodies** are produced to the **desmogleins,** members of the cadherin family. The desmosomes break apart, resulting in blistering of the skin. The basal layer remains intact and attached to the basal lamina because the hemidesmosomes link epithelial cells to the basal lamina through integrins and *not* cadherins. In contrast, **bullous pemphigoid** is a disease in which the antigen recognized by the autoantibodies is **BPAG (bullous pemphigoid antigen)**, involved in the linkage of the basal layer to the basal lamina. Bullous pemphigoid is also a blistering disease, but the blistering occurs at the epidermal-dermal junction.

GASTROINTESTINAL TRACT AND GLANDS

The epithelium of the gastrointestinal (GI) tract is simple and columnar throughout, except for the stratified squamous epithelia in regions of maximal friction (esophagus and anus). The **stomach** is a grinding organ with glands in the fundus and body, which produce mucus (surface and neck cells), pepsinogen (chief cells), and hydrochloric acid (HCl) and intrinsic factor (parietal cells). Intrinsic factor binds to vitamin B_{12} and is required for its uptake from the ileum (distal small intestine). The parietal cell functions in a similar fashion to the osteoclast in using carbonic anhydrase to produce protons that are pumped into the **intracellular canaliculi**, which are lined by **microvilli** in the **active parietal cell**. In the **inactive parietal cell, the proton pumps are sequestered in tubulovesicles in the cytosol.**

The **small intestine** is an absorptive organ with folds at several levels (**plicae, villi,** and **microvilli**) that increase surface area for more efficient absorption. The microvilli also contain specific enzymes for the breakdown of **sugars (disaccharidases), lipids (lipases),** and **peptides (peptidases).** The major digestive processes in the small intestine occur through the action of the **pancreatic juice,** which contains **trypsinogen, chymotrypsinogen, procarboxypeptidases, amylase, lipase,** and other enzymes. **Trypsinogen** is activated by **enterokinase** found on the microvilli and trypsin activates the other pancreatic protease proenzymes. Lipids are broken down to **triglycerides** in the small intestinal lumen which are subsequently degraded to **glycerol, fatty acids,** and **monoglycerides** that are transported into the enterocyte. Once in the cytosol of the enterocyte, the **SER** resynthesizes the **triglycerides,** which are coupled with protein to form **chylomicra.** The chylomicra are exocytosed into the **lacteals** and travel to the cisterna chyli and through the thoracic duct to the venous system. They return to the liver through the arterial system (hepatic artery). In the liver the lipid processing is similar, but reversed to form **very low density lipoprotein (VLDL)** from chylomicra. Other digested materials travel through the **hepatic portal vein** to the liver where hepatocytes process the digested nutrients.

Cell types in the small intestine include **enterocytes (absorption), Paneth cells (production of lysozyme, defensins, and cryptidins),** goblet cells (mucus), and **enteroendocrine cells (secretion of peptide hormones).** All of those cells originate from a single **stem cell** in the **crypt.** New cells are born in the crypt, move up the villus, die by **apoptosis,** and are sloughed off at the tip. The primary function of the **colon,** which appears histologically as **crypts with prominent goblet cells** and no villi, is water resorption.

The major salivary glands (**parotid, submandibular,** and **sublingual**) are exocrine glands that secrete **amylase** and mucus, primarily **regulated** by the autonomic nervous system. In contrast, the **pancreas** has both exocrine (**acinar cells**) and endocrine (**islet cells**) components that synthesize pancreatic juice and blood sugar–regulating hormones, respectively. The exocrine pancreas is primarily regulated by the hormones cholecystokinin (CCK) and secretin, which are also the main regulators of acinar and ductal secretion, respectively.

The **liver** is also a dual-function gland whose exocrine product is **bile**, synthesized by hepatocytes, and transported by a duct system to the gallbladder for storage and concentration. Bile **emulsifies lipids** for more efficient enzymatic access. The endocrine products include **glucose** and **major blood proteins (albumin, fibrinogen, coagulation proteins)**. The liver subserves numerous other functions including synthesis of cholesterol and **detoxification of lipid-soluble drugs**, such as **phenobarbital** by the **SER** (using the **P450 enzyme system**). **Alcohol detoxification** is one of the major processes carried out in the hepatocyte. Alcohol detoxification involves alcohol dehydrogenase **(ADH), MEOS** (microsomal ethanol oxidation system, P450 enzymes in the SER), and catalase in peroxisomes. The primary metabolic pathway is ADH. At higher alcohol levels the MEOS and even catalase systems are activated. The **bile canaliculus** is defined as **apical**, the **junctional complexes** as **lateral**, and the blood surface with the **space of Disse** and **hepatic sinusoids** is considered **basal**. The sinusoids are lined by **hepatic stellate cells**, endothelial cells, and **Kupffer cells**. The **hepatic stellate cells** are affected following chronic alcohol toxicity and are converted into **myofibroblasts** during the onset of **cirrhosis**. Those cells synthesize large quantities of collagen and are responsible for the fibrotic changes observed in cirrhosis. The **Kupffer cells** are the **antigen-presenting cells** of the liver and are derived from monocytes. Hepatocytes are arranged in interlocking cords and plates so there are several ways of analyzing the histological organization of the liver. The **classic lobule** emphasizes the **endocrine** function of the liver; the **portal lobule** emphasizes the **exocrine** function of the liver, and the **liver acinus** focuses on actual **blood supply** and regeneration.

ENDOCRINE GLANDS

The **pituitary (hypophysis)** is formed from two embryonic sources. The **adenohypophysis** is derived from the **oral ectoderm** of Rathke pouch and is regulated through the **hypophyseal portal system** carrying factors that stimulate or inhibit secretion. The **anterior pituitary** contains **acidophils**, which produce **prolactin** and **growth hormone (GH)**, and **basophils** that produce **luteinizing hormone (LH)**, **follicle-stimulating hormone (FSH)**, **thyroid-stimulating hormone (TSH)**, **adrenocorticotropic hormone (ACTH)**, and **melanocyte-stimulating hormone (MSH)**. The **neurohypophysis** is derived from the floor of the diencephalon and consists of astrocyte-like glial cells **(pituicytes)** and expanded terminals of nerve fibers originating in the hypothalamus. The neurohypophysis contains the hormones **vasopressin** and **oxytocin**, which are synthesized in the **supraoptic** and **paraventricular** nuclei.

The **adrenal (suprarenal) gland** consists of two parts. The **adrenal cortex**, derived from **intermediate mesoderm**, and covered by a connective tissue capsule, consists of three zones: the *zona glomerulosa* produces **aldosterone** (a mineralocorticoid) and is regulated primarily by **angiotensin II**; the *zona fasciculata* and *zona reticularis* produce glucocorticoids (eg, cortisol) and weak androgens and are regulated primarily by **ACTH**. The **adrenal medulla**, derived from the **neural crest**, synthesizes **epinephrine** and **norepinephrine** (Fig. 11). Most of the blood that reaches the adrenal medulla

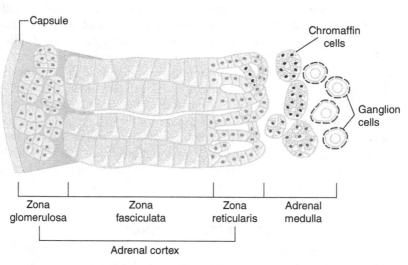

Figure 11

Adrenal (suprarenal) gland. The gland is covered by a connective tissue capsule and divided into a cortex containing steroid-producing cells with prominent lipid droplets and a medulla containing chromaffin cells that secrete catecholamines and neuropeptides.

has passed through the adrenal cortex and contains glucocorticoids that regulate the norepinephrine/epinephrine balance in the adrenal medulla through the action of phenylethanolamine-N-methyltransferase. The **fetal adrenal cortex** functions to produce **dehydroepiandrosterone**, an androgen that is transported to the placenta where it serves as a precursor of estrogen. The hormones of the adrenal gland are summarized in Table 13.

TABLE 13. HORMONES OF THE ADRENAL (SUPRARENAL) GLAND			
Zone	**Secretion**	**Target**	**Regulatory Factors**
Zona glomerulosa	Mineralocorticoids (aldosterone)	Collecting tubules	Angiotensin II
Zona fasciculata	Glucocorticoids (cortisol, hydrocortisone) and weak androgens	Gluconeogenesis by the liver	ACTH (adrenocorti cotropic hormone)
Zona reticularis	Glucocorticoids and weak androgens	Androgens are precursors of estradiol in the fetus	ACTH
Medulla	Norepinephrine and epinephrine	Preparation for "flight or fight"	Preganglionic sympathetic fibers from the splanchnic nerves

There are a number of adrenal hormonal disorders. Adrenogenital syndrome **(congenital virilizing adrenal hyperplasia)** results from the deficiency of an enzyme required for cortisol production. The result is elevated ACTH and secretion of dehydroepiandrosterone from the fetal cortex causing masculinization (virilizing) of the female genitalia. The fetal adrenal cortex is a key component of the fetal-placental unit. **Hypercortisolism** or **Cushing syndrome** is five times more common in women than men. Cushing syndrome may be caused by a tumor in the corticotrophs of the anterior pituitary (Cushing disease), an adrenal adenoma, or administration of exogenous glucocorticoids. **Addison disease** is **primary chronic adrenal insufficiency** and is most often caused by **autoimmune mechanisms** leading to atrophy of the adrenal cortex. Elevated ACTH levels lead to hyperpigmentation, especially in exposed areas of the skin or at pressure points such as the elbows and knuckles.

The **thyroid gland** is characterized by an extracellular hormone precursor (iodinated thyroglobulin) stored in its follicles. The follicular cells endocytose the storage product to form the thyroid hormones (triiodothyronine [T_3] and thyroxine [T_4]). Scattered between the follicular cells are "C" cells (parafollicular cells), which secrete **calcitonin**, a hormone that reduces blood calcium levels. Diseases of the thyroid include **Hashimoto thyroiditis**, an autoimmune disease, in which autoantibodies to thyroglobulin and thyroid peroxidase (antimicrosomal antibodies) are produced. Binding of antibodies to those molecules interferes with their uptake and function, respectively. Infiltrating T cells and autoantibodies destroy the **thyroid follicular cells**, resulting in **hypothyroidism**. In Hashimoto thyroiditis, autoantibodies are also produced to the **thyroid-stimulating hormone (TSH) receptor**. In that case, the autoantibody recognizes an epitope, which results in **blocking the activity of TSH**. In contrast, in **Graves disease** autoantibodies are produced to the **TSH receptor**, but they are **long-acting thyroid stimulating (LATS) antibodies**. The result is unregulated activation of the receptor and overproduction of thyroid hormones (**hyperthyroidism**).

The **parathyroid gland** consists primarily of chief cells that secrete **parathyroid hormone (PTH)**, which increases blood calcium levels by stimulating ruffled border activity in osteoclasts, decreases renal Ca^{++} excretion and increases intestinal Ca^{++} absorption.

The pineal gland contains pinealocytes that secrete melatonin and is innervated by postganglionic sympathetic fibers. Darkness stimulates the production of melatonin in the pineal gland.

The **pancreas** is both an exocrine and endocrine gland. Endocrine cells of the pancreatic islets primarily secrete **insulin** and **glucagon**, hormones that **regulate blood sugar by lowering and raising glucose, respectively**. Blood entering the islets bypasses the peripherally located glucagon-secreting cells to reach the more centrally located insulin-producing **β-cells**. Blood leaving the beta cells contains insulin that influences glucagon secretion from the **α-cells**. Blood leaving the islets travels to the surrounding exocrine pancreas and influences secretion from the acini. In **type I diabetes mellitus**, formerly known as insulin-dependent diabetes mellitus (IDDM), an autoimmune reaction results in **destruction of β-cells** and thus the absence of insulin. Type II diabetes, formerly known as non-insulin-dependent diabetes, is the most common form of diabetes mellitus. Type II diabetes can occur at any age and is reaching epidemic proportions in the United States. **Type II diabetes** begins with insulin resistance, a condition in which adipocytes, muscle cells, and hepatocytes *cannot* efficiently use insulin because of a decrease in insulin receptors or defective glucose transporter function. The β-cells are overworked and eventually lose their ability to secrete enough insulin in response to meals. Individuals who are overweight and inactive have an increased chance of developing type II diabetes.

Scattered through several organ systems (eg, digestive and respiratory systems) are **enteroendocrine cells,** which synthesize peptide hormones for local regulation.

URINARY SYSTEM

The **filtration apparatus** of the renal glomeruli consists of an expanded basement membrane and slit pore associated with **podocytes.** Epithelial cells of the **proximal tubule** are specialized for absorption and ion transport. They remove most of the **sodium** and **water** from urine, as well as virtually all of the amino acids, proteins, and glucose. The **brush border** of the proximal tubule cells contains proteases. The cells of the **distal tubule,** under the influence of **aldosterone, resorb sodium and acidify the urine.** Specialized cells of the distal tubule (the **macula densa**) monitor ion levels in the urine and stimulate the **juxtaglomerular (JG) cells** of the **afferent arteriole** to secrete **renin,** an enzyme that cleaves **angiotensinogen** to a precursor of **angiotensin II. Collecting ducts** contain light and dark (intercalated) cells; they are sensitive to **antidiuretic hormone (ADH)** and are the **final mechanism for concentrating urine.** Transitional epithelium (allowing for stretch) is found lining the calyces, renal pelvis, ureters, and urinary bladder.

MALE REPRODUCTIVE SYSTEM

The **testes** produce **sperm** and **testosterone** under the influence of **luteinizing hormone (LH)** and follicle-stimulating hormone **(FSH),** secreted by **gonadotrophs** of the **anterior pituitary.** The testicular epithelium contains **Sertoli cells** and precursors of sperm. **Spermatogenesis** involves the following lineage: spermatogonia (germ cells) → (spermatocytogenesis) → primary spermatocytes → secondary spermatocytes → (completion of meiosis) → spermatids (spermiogenesis) → mature sperm. Sertoli cells perform several functions: (1) **maintenance of the blood-testis barrier,** (2) **phagocytosis,** and (3) **secretion of androgen-binding protein** and **inhibin,** as well as **Müllerian inhibiting hormone** in the fetus.

The **epididymis**, like most of the male duct system, is lined by a pseudostratified columnar epithelium characterized by modified microvilli (**stereocilia**). The **seminal vesicles** produce **fructose** and other molecules that **activate spermatozoa.**

The **prostate** is a **fibromuscular** organ that produces the **enzymes** responsible for the liquefaction of the **ejaculate.** Virtually all males over 70 show some form of **prostatic hypertrophy. Prostatic malignancies are the second most common form of cancer in males.**

FEMALE REPRODUCTIVE SYSTEM

The ovaries produce ova, estrogen, and progesterone under the influence of LH and FSH. Oocyte (germ cell) maturation involves several stages of follicular development (granulosa cells plus the oocyte): primordial follicle → primary follicle → secondary follicle → mature, or Graafian, follicle. In the secondary follicle, the stroma differentiates into a theca. The *theca interna* synthesizes androgens, which are converted into estradiol by granulosa cells. After ovulation, these thecal cells form the *theca lutein;* the granulosa cells become the *granulosa lutein,* which produces progesterone (Fig. 12). Human chorionic gonadotropin (hCG) in the placenta maintains the corpus luteum of pregnancy.

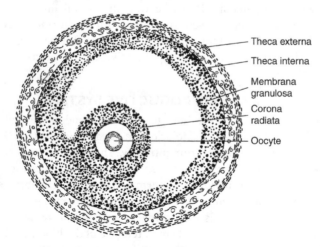

Theca externa

Theca interna

Membrana granulosa

Corona radiata

Oocyte

Figure 12
Mature follicle.

The **uterine endometrium** goes through a monthly cycle during which the **functionalis** is lost and replaced from the **basalis**. The **menstrual phase** occupies the first 4 days of the cycle (in the absence of hCG), followed by the **proliferative phase** under the influence of FSH (days 5-14), and then the **secretory phase** under the influence of LH (days 15-28). During this phase, endometrial cells accumulate glycogen preliminary to the synthesis and secretion of glycoproteins.

Figure 13 summarizes the events of the menstrual cycle.

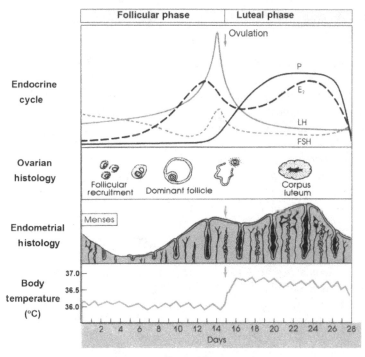

Figure 13

(Reproduced, with permission, from Kasper DL, et al (eds). Harrison's Principles of Internal Medicine. 16th ed. New York, NY: McGraw-Hill; 2005: 2201.)

The **vaginal epithelium** is made up of stratified squamous cells and varies with maturity, phase of the menstrual cycle, pregnancy, and cancer (detected by vaginal Pap smear).

When fertilization and implantation occur, the placenta, consisting of the **chorion (fetal part)** and **decidua basalis (maternal part)**, is established for O_2/CO_2 exchange, as well as its endocrine role (eg, conversion of androgens to estradiol, placental lactogen secretion). During parturition, oxytocin secreted by the neurohypophysis stimulates the contraction of uterine smooth muscle.

The **breast (mammary gland)** is a resting alveolar gland except during pregnancy, when the **lactiferous ducts** proliferate and **milk** production is initiated. Milk synthesis and ejection are under the influence of **prolactin** and **oxytocin.**

EYE

The photosensitive layer of the retina is derived from the inner layer of the **optic cup** and contains the **rod** and **cone** cells involved in visual signal transduction. **Rhodopsin** is a visual pigment found within lamellar disks of the outer segment of the rod cell. Rhodopsin consists of **retinal** and **opsin;** photons induce an isomeric change in retinal, leading to dissociation of the retinal/opsin complex. The resulting decrease in the intracellular second messenger, cyclic guanosine $3',5'$-monophosphate **(cGMP)**, directs closure of membrane sodium channels and leads to **hyperpolarization** of the photoreceptor cell. This signal is transmitted to interneurons within the retina and finally to ganglion cells. The fovea defines the center of the retina, and is the point of sharpest visual acuity. The **fovea** contains all cones and is directed toward whatever object you wish to see or read, for example, these PreTest words at this very moment.

The **lens** arises from **surface ectoderm** during development. Production of lens fibers (elongated, protein-filled cells) continues throughout life without replacement. Increased opacity of the lens **(cataract)** may be caused by congenital factors, excess ultraviolet (UV) radiation, or by diabetes.

The **choroid** and **sclera** are the supportive, protective coats of the eye. The **aqueous humor,** produced by processes of the ciliary body, flows between the lens and iris to the anterior chamber of the eye toward the **iridocorneal angle,** where it is drained into the **canal of Schlemm.** Blockage of the canal of Schlemm or associated structures leads to **increased intraocular pressure** and **glaucoma.**

EAR

The ear functions in two separate but related signal transduction systems, audition and **equilibrium**. The **external ear**, largely formed from the **first two branchial arches**, funnels sound to the **tympanic membrane**. The middle ear is made up of the **malleus, incus, and stapes** formed from the first two arch cartilages. The **internal ear** consists of a **membranous** and a **bony labyrinth** filled with **endolymph** and **perilymph**, respectively. The **saccule (ventral)** and **utricle (dorsal)**, parts of the membranous labyrinth, form from the **otic vesicle** (an ectodermal invagination). The **cochlea** contains three spaces, the *scala vestibuli, scala media* (**cochlear duct**, which extends from the **saccule**), and *scala tympani*. The **semicircular canals** (which extend from the **utricle**) contain the *cristae ampulares*, made up of **cupulae** with **hair cells** embedded in a gelatinous matrix that respond to **changes in direction** and **rate of angular acceleration**. The hair cells are located within the **organ of Corti** and respond to **different frequencies**. In the **saccule** and **utricle**, the **maculae**, along with **stereocilia, kinocilia**, and **otoconia** (crystals of protein and calcium carbonate), detect **changes in position** with reference to gravity.

High-Yield Facts

Anatomy

UPPER EXTREMITY

- **Axillary nerve injury** often results from shoulder joint dislocation or fractures at the surgical neck of the humerus. The injury causes deltoid muscle paralysis and skin anesthesia over the lateral deltoid region. Shoulder contour may be lost with time as the deltoid atrophies. Arm abduction is lost when the arm is abducted beyond the first 15 degrees.
- **Midhumeral fracture** may involve the deep brachial artery and the radial nerve as they wind about the posterior aspect of the humerus. Arterial injury produces ischemic contracture; nerve injury paralyzes the wrist extensors and extrinsic extensors of the hand ("wrist-drop"). Except on the ulnar side (flexor carpi ulnaris and 4-5 flexor digitorum profundus), the **forearm flexor compartment** is innervated by the median nerve.
- **Scaphoid fracture** is the most common hand bone break because it transmits forces from the extended hand directly to the radius. Because the blood supply enters distally, the **proximal portion** of the scaphoid is especially **prone to avascular necrosis.**
- **Lunate dislocation** is most common in falls on the out-stretched hand, compressing the median nerve within the carpal tunnel and producing carpal tunnel syndrome.
- **Extension** of the medial four digits at the **metacarpophalangeal joints** and **interphalangeal joints** is accomplished by the extensor digitorum in the forearm, innervated by the radial nerve. In addition, extension of the interphalangeal joints of the medial four digits is carried out by the lumbricals, which are innervated by both the median nerve (lumbricals 1-2 on the lateral side) and ulnar nerve (lumbricals 3-4 on the medial side). Lumbricals also flex the metacarpophalangeal joints of the medial four digits.
- **Proximal phalangeal flexion** at the metacarpophalangeal joint is by: (a) the interossei (ulnar nerve) and lumbricals muscles; (b) the flexor digitorum superficialis (median nerve) muscle; (c) the flexor digitorum profundus (medial and ulnar nerves) muscles. **Middle phalangeal flexion** at the

proximal interphalangeal joint is by (b) and (c). **Distal phalangeal flexion** at the distal interphalangeal joint is by (c).

- **Digital abduction** is a function of the dorsal interossei ("DAB"—dorsal abduction); digital adduction is a function of palmar interossei ("PAD"—palmar adduct).
- The **ulnar artery** is the principal vascular supply to the superficial palmar arch. The radial artery is the principal blood supply to the deep palmar arch (**mnemonic: USDR, ulnar is superficial and radial is deep**).
- **Lymphatic drainage** from the palmar hand and digits is toward the dorsal subcutaneous space of the hand, explaining the extreme swelling of this region that accompanies infections of the digits or volar surface.
- **Radial sensory function** is tested in the web space of the thumb; **ulnar sensory function** is tested along the fifth digit. The **digital branches** of the median and ulnar nerves lie along the sides of the fingers where they may be anesthetized (Fig. 14 and Table 14).

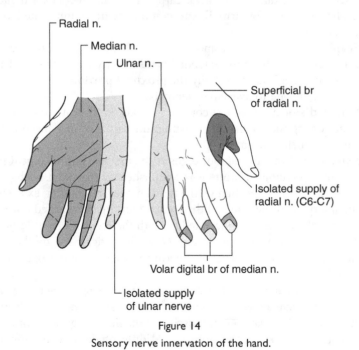

Figure 14
Sensory nerve innervation of the hand.

TABLE 14. NERVE FUNCTION, TESTS, AND DYSFUNCTION

Nerve	Muscle Group	Reflex Test	Sign or Functional Deficit
Long thoracic	Serratus anterior		Winged scapula
Suprascapular	Supraspinatus, infraspinatus		Difficulty initiating arm abduction
Axillary	Deltoid		Inability to fully abduct arm
Radial	Extensors of forearm, wrist, proximal phalanges, and thumb	Triceps and wrist extension reflexes	Loss of arm extension; loss of forearm extension, supination, abduction; loss of wrist extension (**wrist-drop**); loss of proximal phalangeal extension and thumb extension
Musculo-cutaneous	Flexors of arm, forearm	Biceps reflex	Weak arm flexion, weak forearm flexion, weak forearm supination
Median	Wrist and hand flexors	Wrist flexion reflex	Paralysis of flexor, pronator, and thenar muscles; inability to fully flex the index and middle fingers (**sign of benediction**)
Ulnar	Wrist and hand flexors, phalangeal extensors		Inability to flex the fourth and fifth fingers (**clawhand**); loss of thumb adduction

BACK

- **Fracture of the dens** of the axis with posterior dislocation may crush the spinal cord at the level of the first cervical vertebra with terminal paralysis of respiratory musculature.
- The **cruciform ligament** is the principal structure preventing subluxation at the atlantoaxial joint because the articular surfaces between the axis and atlas are nearly horizontal and there is no intervertebral disk.

• **Herniation** occurs in the L4/L5 or L5/S1 **intervertebral disks**, 90% of the time, because of the pronounced lumbar curvature and the considerable body mass superior to this region.
• The **anterior** and **posterior longitudinal ligaments** reinforce the underlying annulus fibrosus but do not meet posterolaterally, resulting in a weak area predisposed to intervertebral disk herniation.
• **Lumbar puncture** and intrathecal anesthesia should be introduced below the third lumbar vertebra as the spinal cord usually terminates between the first and second lumbar vertebrae.
• **Posterolateral disk prolapse** impinges on the spinal nerve of the next lower vertebral level, causing symptoms associated with the dermatomic and myotomal distributions of this nerve (Table 15).

TABLE 15. HERNIATED DISK INVOLVEMENT, SIGNS, AND REFLEX TEST

Hernia	Involvement	Signs	Reflex Test
C3-C4	C4 (Phrenic, C3-C5)	Weak diaphragmatic respiration	
C4-C5	C5 (Suprascapular, C4-C6)	Weak arm abduction	
C5-C6	C6 (Musculocutaneous, C5-C6)	Weak forearm flexion	Biceps
C6-C7	C7 (Radial, C6-C8)	Weak forearm extension	Triceps
C7-C8	C8 (Ulnar, C7-T1)	Weak thumb adduction	
L1-L2	L2 (Genitofemoral, L1-L2)	Weak hip flexion	Cremaster
L2-L3	L3 (Obturator, L2-L4)	Weak hip adduction	
L3-L4	L4 (Femoral, L1-L4)	Weak leg extension	Knee jerk
L4-L5	L5 (Fibular, L4-S1)	Weak dorsiflexion	
L5-S1	S1 (Tibial, L5-S2)	Weak plantar flexion	Ankle jerk

LOWER EXTREMITY

• **Intracapsular fractures** of the femoral neck dislocations tear the retinacular arteries that supply the proximal fragment; avascular necrosis may result (Table 16).
• The **femoral triangle** is bounded by the inguinal ligament, the sartorius muscle, and the adductor longus muscle. A **femoral pulse** is palpable high within the femoral triangle, just inferior to the inguinal ligament. The femoral vein, lying just medial to the femoral pulse, is a preferred site for insertion of venous lines. The mnemonic NAVEL (moving lateral

| TABLE 16. NEUROVASCULAR CONTENTS OF THE BUTTOCK |||
Quadrant	Contents	Symptoms
Upper lateral	No major vessels or nerves; a preferred location for intramuscular injection	
Upper medial	Superior gluteal neurovascular bundle	Abductor lurch
Lower lateral	Inferior gluteal neurovascular bundle	Difficulty climbing stairs or rising from a chair
Lower medial	Sciatic nerve	Foot-drop

to medial) is N = femoral Nerve, femoral Artery, femoral Vein, E = empty (lymphatics), and L = Lacunar ligament.

- The **anterior cruciate ligament** is a key stabilizer of the knee joint, preventing posterior movement of the femur on the tibial plateau.
- The **medial meniscus,** being less mobile and attached to the medial collateral ligament, is most likely to be injured. Twisting movements that combine lateral displacement with lateral rotation pull the medial meniscus toward the center of the joint where it may be trapped and crushed by the medial femoral condyle.
- The **adductor canal,** the location of popliteal aneurysms, contains the femoral artery, femoral vein, and saphenous nerve.
- The **deep fibular (peroneal) nerve** innervates the muscles of the anterior compartment (dorsiflexors of the foot and pedal digits). The **superficial fibular nerve** innervates the lateral crural compartment (plantar flexors and everters of the foot). The **tibial nerve** innervates the posterior crural muscles, which plantarflex and invert the foot.
- The **posterior tibial artery** descends posteriorly to the medial malleolus where the **posterior tibial pulse** is normally palpable.
- **Inversion sprains,** the most common ankle injury, involve the **lateral collateral ligaments**—most frequently the anterior talofibular ligament.
- The **plantar calcaneonavicular (spring) ligament** supports the head of the talus and thereby maintains the longitudinal plantar arch. Laxity of this ligament results in fallen arches or **"flat feet."**
- **Sensory distribution of the anterior leg:** The web space between the first and second toes is specific for the deep fibular nerve (L5) (Fig. 15 and Table 17).

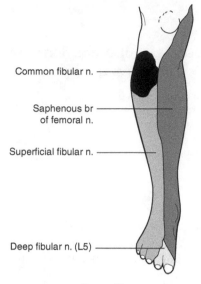

Common fibular n.

Saphenous br
of femoral n.

Superficial fibular n.

Deep fibular n. (L5)

Figure 15
Sensory nerve innervation of the leg.

TABLE 17. NERVE FUNCTION, TESTS, AND DYSFUNCTION

Nerve	Muscle Group	Reflex	Sign or Functional Deficit
Genitofemoral	Cremaster	Cremasteric (L2-L3)	Cremaster paralysis
Femoral	Anterior thigh	Patellar (L4)	Weakness of hip flexion and loss of knee extension
Obturator	Medial thigh		Loss of thigh adduction
Superior gluteal	Gluteus medius and minimus		Abductor lurch (inability to keep pelvis level when contralateral foot is raised = Trendelenburg sign)
Inferior gluteal	Gluteus maximus		Difficulty rising from seated position and difficulty climbing stairs
Sciatic	Hamstrings	Hamstring (L5)	Weakness of hip extension and knee flexion
Fibular	Anterior and lateral crural compartments		Foot slap, inability to stand back on heels
Tibial	Posterior crural compartment	Achilles (S1)	Inability to stand on tip-toes

THORAX

Thoracic Cage and Lungs

- The **anterior border** of the **left pleural cavity** deviates laterally between the fourth and sixth ribs to form the cardiac notch—a preferred route for needle insertion into the pericardial cavity.
- Respiratory musculature is summarized in Table 18.

TABLE 18. RESPIRATORY MUSCULATURE

Function	Muscles
Inspiration	External intercostals, interchondral portion of internal intercostals, and the diaphragm
Expiration	Internal intercostals proper, transverse thoracic, and abdominal muscles

- When upright, excess fluid tends to collect in the **costodiaphragmatic recess.**
- Introduction of air into the pleural space results in **pneumothorax** with loss of lung ventilation. Fluid or blood produces hydrothorax and hemothorax, both of which limit expansion of the lung with reduced ventilation/perfusion ratio.
- The **right mainstem bronchus** is wider, shorter, and more vertical than the left mainstem bronchus, and therefore, is where large aspirated objects commonly lodge.
- The **right lower lobar bronchus** is most vertical, most nearly continues the direction of the trachea, and is larger in diameter than the left, and therefore, is where small aspirated objects commonly lodge, causing segmental atelectasis.
- A **bronchopulmonary segment** is defined by a segmental bronchus and accompanying segmental artery that lie centrally, as well as by intersegmental veins that form a peripheral venous plexus.
- Because the **superior segmental bronchi** of the lower lobes are the most posterior, and therefore dependent, when the patient is supine, they are most frequently involved in gastric acid aspiration pneumonia (Mendelson syndrome).

Heart

- The transverse cardiac diameter varies with inspiration and expiration but normally should not exceed one-half the diameter of the chest.
- An **apical pulse** is palpable at the point of maximal impulse (PMI) in **the fifth intercostal space just beneath the nipple.**
- **Ventricular coronary flow** occurs during ventricular diastole when a pressure differential occurs between the left ventricle and the aorta (Table 19).

TABLE 19. CARDIAC FEATURES		
Landmark	Location	Contents
Coronary sulcus	Between atria and ventricles; nearly vertical behind sternum; marks the annulus fibrosus that supports the valves	Right side contains the right coronary artery and small cardiac vein; crossed by anterior cardiac veins Left side contains circumflex branch of the left coronary artery and coronary sinus
Anterior interventricular sulcus	Between left and right ventricles; marks the interventricular septum	Contains the anterior interventricular branch of the left coronary artery and the great cardiac vein
Posterior interventricular sulcus	Delineates the interventricular septum, posteriorly	Contains the posterior interventricular branch of the right coronary artery and the middle cardiac vein

- The **papillary muscles** take up the slack in the chordae tendineae to maintain the competence of the valvular closure as ventricular volume is reduced during blood ejection. The valves close passively.
- A **ventricular septal defect** (VSD) produces a serious **left-to-right shunt** with cyanosis- "**blue-baby**" syndrome because left ventricular pressure exceeds that in the right ventricle. A large VSD is the principal factor in **tetralogy of Fallot** (Table 20).

TABLE 20. HEART VALVES		
Valve	Auscultation	Comment
Aortic	Right of sternum over second intercostal space	Stenosis will tend to be auscultated as a high-pitched systolic murmur with possible radiation to the carotid arteries
Pulmonary	Left of sternum over second intercostal space	
Tricuspid	Left of sternum in fifth intercostal space	
Mitral	Apex of heart in fifth intercostal space at left midclavicular line	Insufficiency produces a low-pitched, late systolic blowing murmur

Note: Left and right are the patient's left and right. As you "read" from left to right and down the patient's chest the valves order is the same as the mnemonic (APTM): "All Professors enjoy Teaching Medicine."

- The **atrioventricular bundle** passes through the annulus fibrosus and descends along the posterior border of the membranous part of the interventricular septum to enter the muscular portion of the septum. It transmits electrical activity to the ventricles (Table 21).
- **Autonomic pathways** consist of two motor neurons, a myelinated preganglionic (presynaptic) neuron and an unmyelinated postganglionic (postsynaptic) neuron (Tables 22 and 23).

TABLE 21. CARDIAC NODAL TISSUE			
Node	**Location**	**Function**	**Vasculature**
Sinoatrial	In myocardium between crista terminalis and opening of superior vena cava	Initiates contractile event with electrical depolarization spreading throughout atrial musculature	Nodal branch of the right coronary artery (60% occurrence)
Atrioventricular	In right atrial floor in the interatrial septum near the opening of the coronary sinus	Stimulated by atrial depolarization; it leads into the atrioventricular (AV) bundle to synchronize ventricular depolarization	Branch of right coronary artery near the posterior interventricular branch

TABLE 22. SUMMARY OF AUTONOMIC PATHWAYS			
Division	**Presynaptic Pathway**	**Postsynaptic Pathway**	**Effect**
Sympathetic	From spinal levels T1-L2 along the ventral root; reach the chain of sympathetic ganglia via white rami communicantes	1. Fibers that synapse return to the spinal nerve via a gray ramus to mediate cutaneous piloerection, vasoconstriction, and sudomotor (sweat gland) activity	Adrenergic neurotransmission increases heart rate, increases stroke volume, dilates coronary and pulmonary arteries

(Continued)

TABLE 22. SUMMARY OF AUTONOMIC PATHWAYS (Continued)			
Division	Presynaptic Pathway	Postsynaptic Pathway	Effect
		2. Fibers that do not synapse pass through the chain as splanchnic nerves to synapse in prevertebral ganglia; from these ganglia, postsynaptic neurons run in perivascular plexuses to innervate visceral target tissues	
Parasympathetic	Presynaptic cell bodies are located in the dorsal vagal nuclei of the brain; the myelinated synaptic axons form cranial nerve X, the vagus nerve	Postganglionic cell bodies lie in numerous ganglia close to the target organ	Cholinergic neurotransmission decreases heart rate, decreases stroke volume, and produces bronchoconstriction

TABLE 23. PAIN REFERRAL FROM THORACIC VISCERA		
Organ	Referral Area	Pathway
Pericardial cavity	T1-T5: upper and midthorax	Intercostal nerves T1-T5
Heart	T1-T4: upper thorax, postaxial brachium	Cervical and thoracic splanchnic nerves
Thoracic esophagus	T1-T5: thorax and epigastric region	Thoracic splanchnic nerves
Diaphragm central	C3-C5: neck and shoulder	Phrenic nerve
marginal	T7-T10: thorax	Intercostal nerves

ABDOMEN

Abdominal Wall

- The **abdominal musculature** has three distinct layers that take three different directions. The external oblique muscle, internal oblique muscle, and transverse abdominis muscle may be sequentially split and retracted so that extensive suturing is unnecessary to provide a strong repair (McBurney incision). (Abdominal dermatomal landmarks, Table 24).

TABLE 24. DERMATOMAL LANDMARKS	
Dermatome	Region
T4	Nipple
T7	Xiphoid process
T10	Umbilicus
L1	Inguinal ligament

- Because the **linea alba** is relatively avascular, this is a preferred site for incisions.
- **Above the arcuate line,** the anterior leaf of the **rectus sheath** is formed by fusion of the external oblique and internal oblique aponeuroses; the posterior leaf is formed by fusion of the internal oblique and transverse abdominis aponeuroses.
- **Below the arcuate line,** the anterior leaf of the rectus sheath is formed by fusion of all three aponeuroses and there is no posterior leaf.
- The **inferior epigastric artery** passes into the rectus sheath at the arcuate line. This is a potential site for Spigelian herniation (lateral ventral) into the rectus sheath (Fig. 16 and Table 25).

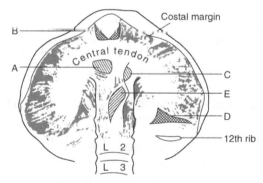

Diaphragm–inferior surface

Figure 16

A = T8 = inferior vena cava
C = T10 = esophageal hiatus, left and right vagus nerves
E = T12 = aorta, azygous vein, and sympathetic chain
B = pathological foramen of Morgagni
D = pathological foramen of Bochdalek

TABLE 25. HERNIA CHARACTERISTICS	
Hernia	**Pathway**
Direct inguinal	Through the inguinal triangle bounded by inguinal ligament, inferior epigastric artery, and rectus abdominis; therefore, **medial** to the inferior epigastric artery. Exits through the superficial inguinal ring generally adjacent to the spermatic cord. Usually acquired.
Indirect inguinal	Through the deep inguinal ring and along the inguinal canal; therefore, **lateral** to the inferior epigastric artery. Exits through the superficial ring within the spermatic cord. Usually congenital.
Femoral	Passes inferior to the inguinal ligament through the femoral ring into the thigh. More prevalent in women.

GI Tract (see Table 26 for structures and locations)

- **Peptic ulceration** of the lower esophagus, stomach, or superior duodenum is referred along the greater splanchnic nerve to the fifth and sixth dermatomes, which include the epigastric region.
- The **hepatic triangle,** bounded by the cystic duct, gallbladder, and common hepatic duct, contains the cystic arteries and right hepatic artery with potential for extensive variation.
- The **duodenal papilla** usually contains the hepatopancreatic ampulla, formed by the joining of the common bile duct and the pancreatic duct. If blocked by a stone, pancreatitis may develop.

TABLE 26. CHARACTERIZATION OF ABDOMINAL STRUCTURES BY LOCATION AND SUPPORT	
Characterization	**Organ**
Peritoneal (supported by mesentery)	Abdominal esophagus, stomach, superior duodenum, liver, pancreatic tail, jejunum, ileum, a variable portion of the cecum, appendix, transverse colon, and sigmoid colon
Secondarily retroperitoneal (adherent)	Descending and inferior duodenum, pancreatic head and body, ascending colon, and descending colon. These may be surgically mobilized with an intact blood supply.
Extra/retroperitoneal	Thoracic esophagus, rectum, kidneys, ureters, and adrenal glands

- The **tail of the pancreas** contains most of the pancreatic islets (of Langerhans), a consideration in pancreatic resection.
- **Ileal (Meckel) diverticulum**, found in about 2% of the population, is located within 2 ft of the ileocecal junction (on the anti-mesenteric side of the ileum), and is usually about 2 in long. Often contain two types of ectopic tissue (gastric and pancreatic). Peptic ulceration of adjacent ileal mucosa and volvulus are complications.
- The **hepatic portal vein** directs venous return from the gastrointestinal tract to the liver (Table 27).

Because the **hepatic portal system has no valves**, blood need not flow toward the liver. Liver disease (such as cirrhosis) or compression of a

TABLE 27. ABDOMINAL ORGANIZATION BASED ON EMBRYOLOGY			
Structures	**Foregut**	**Midgut**	**Hindgut**
Organs	Esophagus, stomach, liver, gall bladder, pancreas, 1/2 of duodenum	1/2 of duodenum, jejunum, ileum, cecum, ascending colon, 2/3 of transverse colon	1/3 of transverse colon, descending and sigmoid colon, rectum, and 2/3 of anal canal
Arteries and branches	**Celiac** splenic, left gastric, short gastric, common hepatic, right gastric, gastroduodenal	**Superior Mesenteric** inferior pancreatico-duodenal, intestinal middle colic, right colic, ileocolic	**Inferior Mesenteric** left colic, superior rectal
Veins	Portal vein	Portal vein	Portal vein
Lymph	Celiac nodes (supracolic compartment)	Superior mesenteric nodes (infracolic compartment)	Inferior mesenteric nodes (infracolic compartment)
Nerves:			
Parasympathetic	Vagus	Vagus	Pelvic splanchnic, (S2-S4)
Sympathetic	Greater thoracic splanchnic (T5-T9)	Lesser thoracic splanchnic (T 10, T11)	Least thoracic splanchnic (T12), upper lumbar splanchnic (L1, L2)
Pain refers to:	**Epigastric region**	**Umbilical region**	**Suprapubic region**

Modified, with permission, after a table by Joseph D. Bast, PhD. Professor of Anatomy and Cell Biology, University of Kansas Medical Center.

vein (as in pregnancy or constipation) results in blood shunting through the anastomotic connections to the systemic venous system (Table 28).

Location	**TABLE 28. PORTAL-SYSTEMIC ANASTOMOSES OCCUR IN SEVERAL AREAS** Anastomotic Connections	Signs and Symptoms
Esophagus	Azygos veins with left gastric and short gastric veins	Esophageal varices, intractable hematemesis
Umbilicus	Paraumbilical veins with superior and inferior epigastric veins	Caput medusae
Rectum	Superior rectal vein with middle and inferior rectal veins	Internal and external hemorrhoids

Kidneys, Ureters, and Adrenal Glands

• The **renal fascia** (the false capsule or **Gerota fascia**) is a discrete fascial layer that surrounds each kidney. Paranephric fat outside this capsule and perinephric fat inside this fascial layer support the kidney.
• **Minor calyces** receive one or two pyramids before fusing into major calyces. Two to four minor calyces join to form **major calyces** that coalesce to form the renal pelvis.
• The **ureters** narrow at three points—at the renal pelvis, at the pelvic brim, and at the bladder wall. Kidney stones may lodge at these locations with pain referred, respectively, to the subcostal, inguinal, and perineal regions. (Referred pain from the abdomen, Table 29).
• **Adrenal arteries** arise from the inferior phrenic arteries, the aorta, and the renal arteries. The right adrenal vein usually drains medially into the inferior vena cava; the left adrenal vein usually drains inferiorly into the left renal vein.

PELVIS

Perineum

• The **external anal sphincter,** innervated by the pudendal nerve, provides the brief voluntary contraction necessary to counter the passage of a peristaltic wave.
• The **rectal submucosal venous plexus** forms anastomotic connections between the middle rectal veins that drain directly into the internal iliac veins and the superior rectal veins that drain into the hepatic portal system. This is a site for varices (hemorrhoids).

TABLE 29. PAIN REFERRAL FROM ABDOMINAL VISCERA		
Organ	**Referral Area**	**Pathway**
Diaphragm:		
Central	C3-C5: neck and shoulder	Phrenic nerve
Marginal	T5-T10: thorax	Intercostal nerves
Foregut:		
Stomach, gallbladder, liver, bile duct, superior duodenum	T5-T9: lower thorax, **epigastric region**	Celiac plexus to greater splanchnic nerve
Midgut:		
Inferior duodenum, jejunum, ileum, appendix, ascending colon, transverse colon	T10-T11: **umbilical region**	Superior mesenteric plexus to lesser splanchnic nerve
(Kidney, upper ureters, gonads)	T12-L1: lumbar and ipsilateral inguinal	Aorticorenal plexus to least splanchnic nerve regions
Hindgut:		
Descending colon, sigmoid colon, mid-ureters	L1-L2: **suprapubic** and inguinal regions, anterior scrotum or labia, anterior thigh	Aortic plexus to lumbar splanchnic nerves

- The **internal pudendal arteries** are the sole vascular supply of both male and female erectile tissue.
- The **deep dorsal vein** provides venous return from the penis or clitoris by passing through the urogenital diaphragm and draining into the prostatic or vesicle venous plexus, respectively.
- The **cremaster muscle** of the spermatic cord is innervated by the genital branch of the genitofemoral nerve. This provides the efferent limb for the cremaster reflex (L1-L2), the elevation of the testes within the scrotum when the inner thigh is touched.
- The cavity of **tunica vaginalis** is a potential space that represents the detached portion of the peritoneal cavity that surrounds the testis except posteriorly. The testis is "retroperitoneal" even in the scrotum.
- Because the superficial perineal space is limited by superficial fascial attachment to the deep transverse perineal muscle, extravasations of blood or urine will not pass into the anal triangle.

- The superficial perineal space contains "sexually pleasurable structures" (thanks to Dr L. Wetzel MD for the mnemonic) and is superficial to the perineal membrane (Table 30). and limited by Scarpa and Colles superficial fascia in females and Scarpa, dartos, and Colles superficial fascia in males. Scarpa superficial fascials attached to deep investing fascia of external oblique and rectus abdominis half way up to the umbilicus and laterally at the inguinal ligament. Colles superficial fascials attached to ischiopubic ramus and inferior edge of perineal membrane (Table 30).

TABLE 30. CONTENTS OF THE PERINEAL SPACES ARE GENDER SPECIFIC

Gender	Superficial Perineal Space	Deep Perineal Space
Male	Testes, crura of penis, bulb of penis, penile urethra, superficial transverse perineal muscles	Deep transverse perineal external urethral sphincter, bulbourethral glands, membranous urethra
Female	Crura of the clitoris, vestibular bulbs, superficial transverse perineal muscles, greater vestibular glands	Deep transverse perineal muscle, external urethral sphincter, urethra

- The **male external urethral sphincter** is formed by two muscles: sphincter urethra and compressor urethrae muscles, both in the deep perineal space. The female external urethral sphincter is formed by three muscles: sphincter urethra, compressor urethrae, and urethrovaginalis muscles.
- A **pudendal block** can be carried out by injecting an anesthetic into the vicinity of the pudendal nerve in the pudendal (Alcock) canal close to the ischial spine. (Pelvic autonomic function, Table 31).

TABLE 31. PELVIC AUTONOMIC FUNCTION

Function	Sympathetic	Parasympathetic	Somatic
Erection		Hypogastric plexus, pelvic plexus, cavernous plexus (S2-S4)	
Emission	L1-L2: lumbar splanchnic nerves		
Ejaculation	(some pelvic splanchnic nerves)		Pudendal nerve, S2-S4

Pelvic Viscera

- The **female pelvis** is less massive, the subpubic angle is greater (almost 90°), and the pelvic inlet more ovoid than the male pelvis.
- The **obstetric conjugate** is the least anteroposterior diameter of the pelvic inlet from the sacral promontory to a point a few millimeters below the superior margin of the pubic symphysis.
- The **transverse midplane diameter**, measured between the ischial spines, is the smallest dimension of the pelvic outlet.
- The **levator ani muscle** forms most of the pelvic floor and its puborectalis portion (rectal sling) is the principal mechanism for maintenance of fecal continence when the rectum is full.
- The **rectum** is usually empty because feces are stored in the sigmoid colon. Movement of feces into the rectal ampulla generates the urge to defecate.
- **Metastatic carcinoma of the rectum** may be widely disseminated within the abdomen, pelvis, and inguinal region. The upper rectum drains along the superior rectal lymphatics. The mid-rectum drains along middle rectal lymphatics. The lower rectum drains along the inferior rectal lymphatics and then along both internal and external pudendal lymphatic channels. The lower part of the anus drains to superficial inguinal nodes.
- **Urinary continence** of the partially full to full urinary bladder is a function of the external urethral sphincter (Table 32).

TABLE 32. URINARY BLADDER INNERVATION IS BY BOTH SYMPATHETIC AND PARASYMPATHETIC ROUTES

Function	Pathway
Afferent limb of the detrusor (bladder-emptying) reflex	Pelvic plexus and pelvic splanchnic nerves (parasympathetic pathways) to spinal segments S2-S4
Efferent limb of the detrusor reflex	Pelvic splanchnic nerves (parasympathetic pathways) from S2-S4

- A **patent urachus** (rare) allows reflux of urine through the umbilicus.
- The **testes** develop as retroperitoneal structures and remain so in the scrotum. Testicular torsion has high potential for testicular ischemia and necrosis.
- The testicular **pampiniform plexus** functions as a countercurrent heat exchanger that maintains testicular temperature a few degrees below core body temperature.

- The superior mesenteric artery may compress the left renal vein, which receives the left testicular vein. The result may be **varices of the pampiniform plexus** on the left side with reduced fertility.
- In the **male**, palpable during a **digital rectal examination** are posterior and lateral lobes of the **prostate gland**, seminal vesicles if enlarged, and bladder when filling.
- Each **uterine artery** crosses immediately **superior to a ureter** in the transverse cervical ligament—an important surgical consideration.
- Normal uterine position is anteflexed (uterus bent forward on itself at the level of the internal os [orifice of uterus]) and anteverted (angled approximately 90° anterior to the vagina), lying on the urinary bladder.
- In the **female, palpable per vagina** are the cervix and ostium of the uterus, the body of the uterus if retroverted, the rectouterine fossa, and variably the ovary.
- The **lymphatic drainage from the vagina** is by three routes: the external and internal iliac nodes from the upper portion of the vagina and the internal iliac nodes as well as the superficial inguinal nodes from the lowest third (Tables 33 and 34).

TABLE 33. PAIN REFERRAL FROM PELVIC VISCERA		
Organ	**Referral Areas**	**Pathway**
Testes and ovaries	T10-T12: umbilical and pubic regions	Gonadal nerves to aortic plexus and then to lesser and least splanchnic nerves
Middle ureters, urinary bladder, uterine body, uterine tubes	L1-L2: pubic and inguinal regions, anterior scrotum or labia, anterior thigh	Hypogastric plexus to aortic plexus and then to lumbar splanchnic nerves
Rectum, superior anal canal, pelvic ureters, cervix, epididymis, vas deferens, seminal vesicles, prostate gland	S3-S5: perineum and posterior thigh	Pelvic plexus to pelvic splanchnic nerves

TABLE 34. PELVIC VISCERAL AFFERENT INNERVATION			
Organ	Afferent Pathway	Level	Referral Areas
Kidneys Renal pelvis Upper ureters	Aorticorenal plexus, least splanchnic nerve, white ramus of T12, subcostal nerve	T12	Subcostal and pubic regions
Descending colon Sigmoid colon Mid-ureters Urinary bladder Oviducts Uterine body	Aortic plexus, lumbar splanchnic nerves, white rami of L1-L2, spinal nerves L1-L2	L1-L2	Lumbar and inguinal regions, ante- rior mons and labia, anterior scrotum, ante- rior thigh
None	No white rami between L3-S1	L3-S1	No visceral pain refers to dermatomes L3-S1
Cervix Pelvic ureters Epididymis Vas deferens Seminal vesicles Prostate gland Rectum Proximal anal canal	Pelvic plexus, pelvic splanchnic nerves, spinal nerves S2-S4	S2-S4	Perineum, thigh, lateral leg and foot

HEAD AND NECK

Somatic Portions

- **The scalp includes a layer of loose connective tissue** between the epicranial aponeurosis and the periosteum forms the subaponeurotic or "danger" space. Emissary veins connect with the dural sinuses with potential for vascular spread of infection through the calvaria. There is a valuable **SCALP** mnemonic: **S** = skin, **C** = connective tissue, **A** = aponeurosis, **L** = loose (areolar) connective tissue, and **P** = periosteum.
- **Cranial fractures** preferentially pass through cranial foramina injuring the contained nerves (Tables 35-39).

TABLE 35. PRINCIPAL FORAMINA OF THE ANTERIOR CRANIAL FOSSA

Foramen	Contents	Result of Injury
Olfactory	Olfactory nerves	Anosmia
Foramen cecum	An emissary vein	

TABLE 36. PRINCIPAL FORAMINA OF THE MIDDLE CRANIAL FOSSA

Foramen	Contents	Results of Injury
Optic canal	Cranial nerve (CN) II	Unilateral blindness
	Ophthalmic artery	Ischemic unilateral blindness
Superior orbital	CN III	Ophthalmoplegia
	CN IV	Inability to look down and out
	CN V$_1$	Unilateral loss of blink reflex
	CN VI	Inability to abduct eye
	Superior ophthalmic vein	Retinal engorgement
Foramen rotundum	CN V$_2$	Loss of sensation under eye
Foramen ovale	CN V$_3$	Masticatory paralysis, loss of jaw-jerk reflex
Foramen spinosum	Middle meningeal artery	
Foramen lacerum	Nothing (except occasionally the greater superficial petrosal nerve)	
Hiatus of the Gr.sup.p.n.	Greater superficial petrosal nerve	Dry eye, loss of submandibular, and sublingual secretion

TABLE 37. PRINCIPAL FORAMINA OF THE POSTERIOR CRANIAL FOSSA

Foramen	Contents	Results of Injury
Internal auditory meatus	CN VII	Facial paralysis
	CN VIII	Auditory and vestibular deficits
Jugular foramen	CN IX	Loss of gag and carotid reflexes
	CN X	Loss of cough reflex; paralysis of laryngeal muscles and some palatine muscles
	CN XI	Inability to shrug shoulders
	Internal jugular vein	
Hypoglossal canal	CN XII	Paralysis of tongue muscles; lingual deviation toward side of injury upon protrusion

TABLE 38. GANGLIA ASSOCIATED WITH CRANIAL NERVES

Nerve (Classification)	Ganglion	Function
Optic (SSA)	Bipolar cells	Vision
Oculomotor (GVE)	Ciliary	Pupillary constriction, accommodation
Trigeminal (GSA)	Semilunar (trigeminal)	General sensation from the face, nasal and oral cavities, including afferent limbs of blink, sneeze, and jaw-jerk reflexes
Facial (GSA)	Geniculate	General sensation from external ear
(SVA)	Geniculate	Taste from anterior 2/3 of tongue
(GVE)	Pterygopalatine	Secretomotor for lacrimal, nasal, and palatine glands
(GVE)	Submandibular	Secretomotor for sublingual and submandibular glands
Vestibulocochlear (SSA)	Vestibular and spiral	Balance, audition
Glossopharyngeal (GSA)	Jugular (superior)	General sensation from external auditory meatus
(GVA)	Petrosal (inferior)	Visceral sensation from posterior 1/3 of tongue and pharynx; afferent limb of gag and carotid reflexes
(SVA)	Petrosal (inferior)	Taste from posterior 1/3 of tongue
(GVE)	Otic	Secretomotor for parotid gland
Vagus (GSA)	Jugular (superior)	General sensation from external auditory meatus
(GVA)	Petrosal (inferior)	Visceral sensation from larynx; afferent limb of cough and aortic body reflexes
(SVA)	Nodose (inferior)	Taste from epiglottis
(GVE)	Distal ganglia	Visceral smooth muscle and gland control

GSA: general somatic afferent; GVA: general visceral afferent; GVE: general visceral efferent; SSA: special somatic afferent; SVA: special visceral afferent.

TABLE 39. COURSE, DISTRIBUTION, AND PRINCIPAL FUNCTION OF CRANIAL NERVES

CN	Foramen	Distribution	Function
I	Cribriform plate	Nasal mucosa	Olfaction
II	Optic canal	Retina	Vision
III	Superior orbital fissure	Levator palpebrae superioris, superior rectus, medial rectus, inferior rectus, inferior oblique muscles	Ocular elevation, depression, adduction, pupillary constriction, accommodation
IV		Superior oblique muscle	Ocular depression and abduction
V_1	Superior orbital fissure	Forehead, conjunctiva	Sensation, afferent limb of blink reflex
V_2	Foramen rotundum, infraorbital foramen	Mid-face	Sensation, afferent limb of sneeze reflex
V_3	Foramen ovale, mandibular foramen, mental foramen	Jaw, lateral face, anterior tongue	Sensation, afferent limb of jaw-jerk reflex, anterior tongue sensation Motor to muscles of mastication
VI	Superior orbital fissure	Lateral rectus muscle	Ocular abduction
VII	Internal acoustic meatus, facial canal, stylomastoid foramen	Face, lacrimal, nasal, sublingual, and submaxillary glands	Motor to muscles of facial expression and efferent limb of blink reflex; secretomotor for lacrimation, nasal and anterior oral secretion Taste from anterior part of tongue
VIII	Internal acoustic meatus	Cochlear and vestibular apparatus	Audition and balance
IX	Jugular foramen	Oropharynx	Sensation to posterior tongue and pharynx, afferent limb of gag reflex; taste from posterior part of tongue, carotid reflex Motor to stylopharyngeus muscle
X	Jugular foramen	Pharynx, larynx	Laryngeal sensation, afferent limb of cough reflex; epiglottic taste Motor to palatine and laryngeal muscles
XI	Foramen magnum, jugular foramen	Sternomastoid and trapezius muscles	Motor to sternomastoid and trapezius muscles
XII	Hypoglossal canal	Tongue	Motor to all intrinsic and most extrinsic tongue muscles

- The cerebral aqueduct is prone to occlusion, leading to hydrocephalus (Table 40).
- **Regions of the orbit** that are prone to fracture include the ethmoid lamina papyracea and the maxilla near the infraorbital groove (Table 41).

TABLE 40. CSF IS PRODUCED BY THE CHOROID PLEXUSES THAT PROJECT INTO THE VENTRICLES OF THE BRAIN

CSF Production	Through	Into
Lateral ventricles	Foramina of Monro	Third ventricle (interventricular)
Third ventricle	Cerebral aqueduct	Fourth ventricle
Fourth ventricle	Foramina of Magendie and Luschka	Cisterna magna of subarachnoid space
From	**Through**	**CSF Uptake**
Subarachnoid space	Arachnoid villi	Superior sagittal venous sinus

TABLE 41. CRANIAL AND CEREBRAL HEMATOMAS

Hematoma	Prognosis	Location	Cause
Epicranial	Resolves	Subaponeurotic space	Superficial vessels
Epidural	Life-threatening	Epidural space	Torn middle meningeal artery
Subdural	Serious	Subdural space	Torn cerebral vein (usually)
Subarachnoid	Lethal	Subarachnoid space	Torn cerebral artery, cerebral aneurysm
Subpial	Usually resolves	Cerebrum	Cerebral contusion

- Contraction of the **orbicularis oculi muscle, innervated by the facial nerve,** produces the blink (Tables 42).
- Clinically the function of the extraocular eye muscles is tested using the "H" test with the medial rectus tested by horizontally crossing one's eyes and the lateral rectus tested by moving the eye laterally (abducing). From either full adduction or abduction the eye is then moved in a second direction. When fully adducted, gazing below the horizon tests the superior oblique muscle. (Remember "SO" look like the edge of the nose "S" forming the ala and "O" the nostril.) When fully adducted, raising the eye above the horizon tests the inferior oblique muscle. When

TABLE 42. ORBITAL MUSCLE FUNCTION AND INNERVATION			
Muscle	**Primary Function**	**Secondary Functions (normally balance)**	**Innervation**
Pupil	Constriction		CN III parasympathetic
	Dilation		Sympathetic chain
Ciliary muscle	Accommodation		CN III parasympathetic
Superior tarsal muscle	Augment levator palpebrae superioris		Sympathetic chain
Levator palpebrae superioris	Elevate eyelid		CN III (oculomotor)
Medial rectus	Adduction		CN III (oculomotor)
Superior rectus	Elevation	Adduction, intorsion	CN III (oculomotor)
Inferior oblique	Elevation	Abduction, extorsion	CN III (oculomotor)
Inferior rectus	Depression	Adduction, extorsion	CN III (oculomotor)
Superior oblique	Depression	Abduction, intorsion	CN IV (trochlear)
Lateral rectus	Abduction		CN VI (abducens)

fully abduced, gazing below the horizon tests the inferior rectus muscles. When fully abduced, raising the eye above the horizon tests the superior rectus muscle. See the "H" below patient's left eye (Fig. 17).

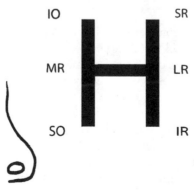

Figure 17

- **Parasympathetic innervation** to the pupil originates in the Edinger-Westphal nucleus and travels with the oculomotor nerve. Temporal lobe herniation (from tumor, hematoma, or edema) compresses the oculomotor nerve within the tentorial notch, causing a dilated pupil that is unresponsive to light.

  Common disruptions of the visual pathway are summarized in Figure 18.

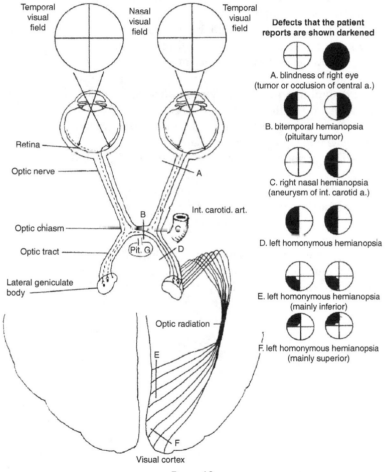

Figure 18
Visual fields and pathways.

- Paralysis of the stapedius muscle, as a result of facial nerve palsy, produces hyperacusis.

Visceral Portions

- The **infrahyoid muscles,** innervated by the ansa cervicalis (C1-C3), stabilize the hyoid bone and larynx during deglutition and phonation.
- The **pretracheal space,** deep to the pretracheal fascia, surrounds the trachea and thyroid gland. Infection in this space may migrate into the superior mediastinum.
- The **retropharyngeal (retrovisceral) space** lies posterior to the oropharynx and esophagus and is defined by septa from the pretracheal fascia. Infection within this space may migrate into the posterior mediastinum.
- The **mandibular neurovascular bundle** enters the mandibular foramen adjacent to the lingula, the point of minimal movement. It may be anesthetized by directing a needle posteriorly through the buccal wall just lateral to the pterygomandibular raphe.
- The **deep cervical nodes** receive lymph from the anteroinferior portion of the face, the nasal cavities, and the oral cavity.
- The **nasal vestibule** (the most common site for nosebleeds) receives vascular branches from internal and external carotid arteries.
- The **palatine tonsil** receives vascular branches from the maxillary, facial, and lingual arteries.
- **Abduction of the vocal cords** is a function of the posterior cricoarytenoid muscle only, innervated by the recurrent laryngeal nerve (Table 43).
- **Sensory innervation of the face** is by the trigeminal nerve (Fig. 19).

TABLE 43. CRANIAL NERVE FUNCTIONS AND TESTS				
Nerve	**Foramen**	**Sensory**	**Motor**	**Test**
CN V (trigeminal)				
V1 reflex	Superior orbital fissure, supraorbital notch	Forehead	None	Blink (afferent)
V2	Foramen rotundum, maxillary foramen	Mid-face	None	Sneeze reflex
V3	Foramen ovale, mandibular foramen, mental foramen	Anterior pinna, jaw 2/3 of tongue	Muscles of mylohyoid, anterior belly of digastric, tensor palatini and tensor tympani	Jaw jerk
CN VII (facial)	Internal auditory meatus, facial canal, stylomastoid foramen	Concha of ear, taste anterior 2/3 of tongue via chorda tympani	Muscles of facial expression, stylohyoid, posterior belly of digastric, tensor tympani, tensor palati parasympathetic to lacrimal, nasal, palatine, lingual, and submandibular glands via greater superficial petrosal nerve	Blink reflex (efferent)
CN IX (glosso-pharyngeal)	Jugular foramen	External auditory, meatus, oropharynx, carotid body and sinus, taste posterior 1/3 of tongue	Stylopharyngeus muscle, parasympathetic to parotid gland via tympanic and lesser superficial s petrosal nerve	Gag reflex, carotid reflex

(Continued)

| TABLE 43. CRANIAL NERVE FUNCTIONS AND TESTS *(Continued)* | | | | |
Nerve	Course	Sensory	Motor	Test
CN X (vagus)	Jugular foramen	External auditory meatus, larynx, taste from epiglottis, aortic body	Palatine muscles, pharyngeal muscles, laryngeal muscles	Phonation
CN XI (spinal accessory)	Foramen magnum, jugular foramen	None	Sternocleidomastoid, upper trapezius	Turn head to opposite side
CN XII (hypoglossal)	Hypoglossal canal	None	Intrinsic and 3/4 of extrinsic tongue muscles	Protrudes straight

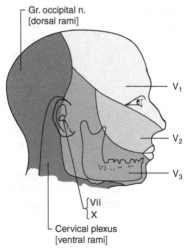

Figure 19

High-Yield Facts

Neural Pathways

ASCENDING PATHWAYS

Cells in the spinal cord receive inputs from ipsilateral structures. Pathways to the thalamus cross to terminate on the contralateral side.

The major ascending pathways are the dorsal (posterior) columns and the anterolateral system.

Pain, Temperature, and Tactile
- Simple receptors, unmyelinated, or poorly myelinated fibers.
- Enter via dorsal root and may ascend or descend a few segments.
- Secondary fibers cross the midline in the ventral commissure and ascend in ventral and lateral funiculi (ventral and lateral spinothalamic tracts).
- Terminate in ventral posterior lateral nucleus of thalamus.
- Tertiary fibers project via the internal capsule to terminate in the post-central gyrus.
- Injury to the spinothalamic tracts results in loss of pain and temperature sensation on the opposite side of the body.
- Syringomyelia interrupts pain and temperature fibers crossing in the ventral white commissure and thus results in bilateral sensory deficit.

Proprioception, Tactile Discrimination, and Stereognosis
- Primary fibers arising from more complicated receptors are generally well myelinated.
- Afferents enter the spinal cord via the dorsal root and ascend in the dorsal funiculus. The dorsal funiculus divides into a medial fasciculus gracilis (sacral, lumbar, and lower thoracic inputs) and a lateral fasciculus cuneatus (upper thoracic and cervical inputs). Both fasciculi terminate in corresponding nuclei in the medulla.
- Secondary fibers from the nucleus gracilis and nucleus cuneatus cross the midline and ascend in the medial lemniscus to terminate in the ventral posterior lateral nucleus of the thalamus.
- Tertiary fibers terminate in the postcentral gyrus.

- Muscle spindle information is sent to the cerebellum via two major pathways. The dorsal spinocerebellar tract originates from the Clarke nucleus in the thoracic cord and enters the cerebellum via the inferior cerebellar peduncle. The ventral spinocerebellar tract originates from spinal cord gray matter and enters the cerebellum via the superior cerebellar peduncle.
- Interruption of primary fibers in the dorsal funiculus will cause loss of proprioception, and so forth, on the same side of the body as the lesion.
- Interruption of secondary fibers in the medial lemniscus will give rise to contralateral deficits.
- Tabes dorsalis and pernicious anemia attack the dorsal funiculi.

Trigeminal Pathways
- Primary trigeminal fibers enter at the level of the pons.
- Primary afferents of the descending root terminate in the spinal trigeminal nucleus.
- Secondary fibers ascend through the medulla and pons as the trigeminal lemniscus to terminate in the ventral posterior medial (VPM) nucleus of the thalamus.
- The ascending root primary tactile afferents terminate in the main sensory nucleus of CN V.
- Secondary fibers ascend in the trigeminal lemniscus to the VPM.
- The cell bodies of the primary proprioceptive afferents from the muscles of mastication are located in mesencephalic nucleus of CN V, and thus are "like" dorsal root ganglion cells embedded in the brain. They project to the motor nucleus of CN V for a monosynaptic jaw-jerk reflex.
- Lesion of the descending root of CN V and the adjacent lateral spinothalamic tract on one side of the medulla will result in pain and temperature deficits on the contralateral side of the body and the ipsilateral side of the head.

Vestibular Pathways
- Primary afferents terminate in the vestibular nuclei and in the cerebellum on the same side.
- Secondary fibers ascend or descend in the medial longitudinal fasciculus or the ventral funiculus of the spinal cord.
- Unilateral lesions of the vestibular system result in movement of the head, body, and eyes (nystagmus) to the affected (ipsilateral) side. Symptoms include vertigo, nausea, and a tendency to fall to the affected side.

Visceral Afferents

- Primary general visceral afferents have cell bodies in the dorsal root ganglia and terminate in the dorsal horn. Ascending secondary neurons make abundant reflex connections with autonomic and somatic pathways and terminate in the reticular formation and intralaminar thalamic nuclei.
- Central processes of primary general visceral afferents associated with cranial nerves VII, IX, and X enter the solitary fasciculus and terminate in the nucleus of the solitary tract. Secondary fibers make reflex connections with visceral motor nuclei. Taste is represented in the thalamus in a region medial to the VPM nucleus.

DESCENDING (MOTOR) PATHWAYS

- In the brain, the cell bodies of general somatic efferent neurons are located in columns ventral to the cerebral aqueduct and fourth ventricle and ventrolateral to the central canal. Special visceral efferents (associated with branchial arch-derived muscle) are located lateral and ventral to the general somatic efferents. In the spinal cord, they originate in the ventral horn.
- These are lower motor neurons, or the "final common pathway." Total, or flaccid, paralysis results from destruction of peripheral nerves or motor nuclei. Destruction of upper motor neurons (from higher centers) results in spastic paralysis: initially hyporeflexia and later hyperreflexia.

Cerebellar Pathways

- The dentate nucleus receives fibers from the Purkinje neurons of the cerebellum and projects via the superior peduncle to the reticular formation (descending limb) and to the basal ganglia/thalamus-motor cortex (ascending limb).
- The cerebellum is involved with coordination of fine movements.
- Lesions to the cerebellum or superior peduncle result in ataxia, hypotonia, hyporeflexia, and/or intention tremor on the same side as the lesion.

CORTICOSPINAL (PYRAMIDAL) PATHWAYS

- Fibers arise from pyramidal neurons in layer 5 of the precentral gyrus and premotor areas and descend through the internal capsule and basis pedunculi, cross at the spinomedullary junction and form the lateral corticospinal tract in the lateral funiculus of the spinal cord. They terminate on lower motor neurons in the ventral horn or on interneurons.

- Most muscles are represented in the contralateral motor cortex. However, some (such as the muscles of the upper face, the muscles of mastication, and muscles of the larynx) are represented bilaterally.
- With the noted bilateral exceptions, lesion of the pyramidal tract above the decussation results in spastic paralysis, loss of fine movements, and hyperreflexia on the contralateral side.
- Lesion of the corticospinal tract in the cord results in ipsilateral deficits.

The Extrapyramidal (Basal Ganglia) System
- The basal ganglia (caudate, putamen, globus pallidus) and associated nuclei (eg, substantia nigra) do not project directly to medullary or spinal lower motor neurons, but to the motor cortex.
- The system controls coarse, stereotyped movements. Lesions result in altered muscle tone (usually rigidity), paucity of movement, and the appearance of rhythmic tremors and writhing or jerky movements.

Reticular Pathways
- Nuclei of the reticular system send ascending projections to the hypothalamus and thalamus as well as descending projections to the motor nuclei of cranial nerves, and the intermediate gray of the spinal cord.
- The reticular formation has reciprocal connections with most other areas of the CNS and produces both facilitatory and inhibitory effects on motor systems, receptors, and sensory conduction pathways.

Embryology: Early and General

Questions

1. A 29-year-old woman (gravida 3, para 2) gave birth to a healthy baby after 38 weeks of gestation and delivered the intact placenta spontaneously. The pregnancy was complicated by preeclampsia, but fetal monitoring and ultrasound were normal throughout gestation. The predominant structures shown in the accompanying photomicrograph of the placenta are derived from which one of the following?

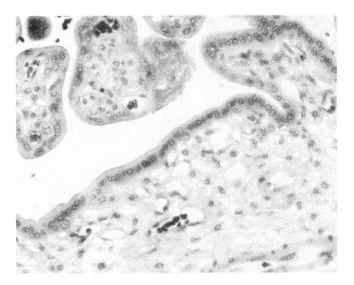

   a. A combination of fetal and maternal tissues
   b. Endometrial glands
   c. Endometrial stroma
   d. Fetal tissues
   e. Maternal blood vessels

2. A married couple, with diagnosed 6-year-long infertility, presents to the fertility clinic. A spermocytogram, confirmed by electron microscopy, reveals that the husband produces all spermatozoa with rounded heads, a condition known as globozoospermia. The missing sperm structure is associated with which one of the following?

a. Loss of decapacitation factors
b. Retention of the developing spermatids from Sertoli cells
c. Maturation of lytic enzymes
d. Mitotic activity
e. Meiotic divisions

3. A 38-year-old (gravida 0, para 0) woman is recently married and pregnant. The zygote is a result of a haploid ovum fertilized by her husband's sperm. Which of the following is required for continuation of the second meiotic division to produce the haploid ovum?

a. Elevation of progesterone titers
b. Expulsion from the mature follicle
c. The environment of the oviduct and uterus
d. Fertilization by a spermatozoon
e. The presence of human chorionic gonadotropin (hCG)

4. A married couple, diagnosed with infertility presents to the fertility clinic. The husband's semen contains only 40 million sperm total with a forward motility index slightly below normal. A hamster egg penetration assay (SPA) was performed in which hamster eggs are collected and their zona pellucidae are enzymatically removed prior to mixing with sperm. The husband's sperm have normal morphology, but his penetration assay results are 3.7% (normal 10%). Sperm penetration in SPA requires which one of the following?

a. Resumption of the second meiotic division
b. Formation of the male pronucleus
c. Initiation of cleavage
d. Addition of cholesterol to the sperm plasma membrane
e. A decrease in the fluidity of the sperm plasma membrane
f. Sequestration of acrosomal enzymes
g. Capacitation and the acrosome reaction

5. A 23-year-old woman with a natural menstrual cycle is nearing ovulation. The oocyte of a mature follicle will be induced to undergo the first meiotic division as a result of which one of the following hormonal stimuli?

a. The cessation of progesterone secretion
b. The gradual elevation of follicle-stimulating hormone (FSH) titers
c. The low estrogen titers associated with the maturing follicle
d. The slow elevation of progesterone produced by luteal cells
e. The surge of luteinizing hormone (LH) initiated by high estrogen titers

6. A couple is trying to conceive a child. Following intercourse, which one of the following is responsible for the prevention of polyspermy?

a. Resumption of the first meiotic division
b. Resumption of the second meiotic division
c. Capacitation
d. The cortical reaction
e. The release of enzymes from the sperm acrosome

7. Oogonia reach their maximum number at which one of the following stages of human development?

a. Five months of fetal life
b. Birth
c. Puberty (12-14 years of age)
d. Adolescence (16-20 years of age)
e. Early adulthood (21-26 years of age)

8. A 26-year-old man contracted viral influenza with an unremitting fever of 39.5°C (103°F) for 3 days. Because spermatogenesis cannot occur above a scrotal temperature of 35.5°C (96°F), he was left with no viable sperm after his recovery. Approximately how much time is required for the return of viable sperm to the epididymis?

a. 3 days
b. 1 week
c. 5 weeks
d. 2 months
e. 4 months

9. Implantation of the conceptus at which site in the accompanying diagram of the female reproductive system is most likely to result in excessive, perhaps fatal, vaginal bleeding immediately prior to parturition?

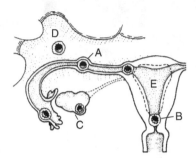

a. A
b. B
c. C
d. D
e. E

10. A 36-year-old woman (para 2, gravida 2) undergoes routine ultrasound during the third trimester of her pregnancy. Her obstetrician diagnoses an external sacrococcygeal teratoma (SCT). A Cesarean section is performed and the tissue sent to the pathologist. Which one of the following is the embryological source of the tissues found in the SCT?

a. Cytotrophoblast
b. Epiblast
c. Syncytiotrophoblast
d. Hypoblast
e. Yolk sac

11. A 23-year-old woman with a positive home pregnancy test smokes a pack of cigarettes and drinks a six pack of beer each day. She is advised by her obstetrician to drastically reduce or eliminate both activities. Her obstetrician is concerned because in the developing human embryo/fetus, most of the internal organs begin to form in which month?

a. First
b. Second
c. Fourth
d. Sixth
e. Ninth

12. A 28-year-old woman (gravida 2, para 2) and her 27-year-old husband have been trying to have a third child. The couple has successfully conceived and normal embryonic development is progressing. Which one of the following events occurs in the second week of embryonic development?

a. Formation of the blastomeres.
b. Segregation of blastomeres into embryoblast and trophoblast.
c. Formation of the inner cell mass.
d. The formation of the epiblast and hypoblast from the embryoblast.
e. Morula develops a fluid-filled cavity and is transformed into a blastocyst.
f. The decidual reaction.
g. The corpus luteum discontinues secretion of progesterone.
h. Neurulation.
i. The heart begins to beat.
j. Gastrulation begins.
k. Formation of the primordial of the major organ systems.

13. The ectoderm is derived directly from which one of the following?

a. Hypoblast
b. Epiblastic cells that undergo gastrulation
c. Mesoderm
d. Endoderm
e. Nongastrulated epiblast

14. Fetal blood from the placenta is about 80% oxygenated. However, mixture with unoxygenated blood at various points reduces the oxygen content. Which one of the following fetal vessels contains blood with the highest oxygen content?

a. Abdominal aorta
b. Common carotid arteries
c. Ductus arteriosus
d. Pulmonary artery
e. Pulmonary vein

15. A female infant is born approximately 10 weeks prematurely (at 30 weeks) and weighs 1710 g. She has respiratory distress syndrome and is treated with endogenous surfactant. She is intubated endotracheally with mechanical ventilation immediately after birth. Over the first 4 days after birth the ventilator pressure and the fraction of inspired oxygen are reduced. Beginning on the fifth day after birth, she has brief desaturations that become more persistent. She needs increased ventilator and oxygen support on the seventh day after birth. She becomes cyanotic. Further examination, echocardiogram, and x-rays reveal left atrial enlargement, an enlarged pulmonary artery, increased pulmonary vasculature, and a continuous machine-like murmur. Which one of the following is the most likely diagnosis?

a. Persistent foramen ovale
b. Patent ductus arteriosus
c. Ventricular septal defect
d. Pulmonary stenosis
e. Coarctation of the aorta

16. Which one of the following hematopoietic tissues or organs develops from endoderm?

a. Thymus
b. Tonsils
c. Bone marrow
d. Spleen
e. Blood islands

17. Which one of the following processes places the developing heart in the presumptive thoracic region cranial to the septum transversum?

a. Gastrulation
b. Lateral folding
c. Cranial folding
d. Neurulation
e. Fusion of the endocardial heart tubes

18. Which one of the following is in direct contact with maternal blood in lacunae of the placenta?

a. Cells of the cytotrophoblast
b. Extraembryonic mesoderm
c. Fetal blood vessels
d. Cells of the syncytiotrophoblast
e. Amniotic cells

19. A dental hygienist is concerned about the effects of radiation on the in utero development of her baby. During which one of the following periods is the embryo most susceptible to environmental influences that could induce the formation of nonlethal congenital malformations?

a. Fertilization to 1 week of fetal life
b. The second week of fetal life
c. The third through eighth weeks of fetal life
d. The third month of fetal life
e. The third trimester of fetal life

20. During a visit to her gynecologist, a patient reports that she received vitamin A treatment for her acne unknowingly during the first 2 months of an undetected pregnancy. Which one of the following organ systems in the developing fetus is most likely to be affected?

a. The digestive system
b. The endocrine organs
c. The respiratory system
d. The urinary and reproductive systems
e. The skeletal and central nervous systems

21. A 32-year-old (gravida 2, para 1) woman presents to her obstetrician with abdominal discomfort, increased back pain, shortness of breath, and swelling in her feet and ankles. Ultrasound reveals an amniotic fluid index (AFI) of 27 cm (normal 5-24 cm). The condition is caused by which one of the following?

a. Duodenal or esophageal atresia
b. Bilateral agenesis of the kidneys
c. Precocious development of the swallowing reflex in the fetus
d. Hypoplasia of the lungs
e. Obstructive uropathy

22. A newborn child is born with lumbar spina bifida myeloschisis (rachischisis) resulting in a flattened, plate-like mass of nervous tissue with no overlying epidermis or meninges. The mass of neural plate in this congenital dysmorphology forms directly from which one of the following structures?

a. Ectoderm
b. Endoderm
c. Somatopleuric mesoderm
d. Splanchnopleuric mesoderm
e. Hypoblast

23. In experiments in mice, deficiency of the *FGFR1* gene results in expansion of axial mesoderm (notochord) at the expense of the paraxial mesoderm. Formation of which one of the following is most likely to be affected by a deficiency in paraxial mesoderm?

a. Adrenal cortex
b. Adrenal medulla
c. Humerus
d. Biceps brachii
e. Masseter

24. A 1-month-old boy who appears normal and healthy at birth presents with very slow development, difficulty swallowing, spasticity, hypotonia, and seizures including severe "infantile spasms." He is diagnosed with lissencephaly based on the symptoms, magnetic resonance imaging, and computed tomography. The corpus callosum is absent and the cerebral cortices are smooth with scarce sulci and gyri. The syndrome is hypothesized to originate from a maternal infection or hypoxia affecting the development of the cerebral cortex from which one of the following neural embryonic structures?

a. Telencephalon
b. Myelencephalon
c. Metencephalon
d. Mesencephalon
e. Diencephalon

25. A 2-year-old boy presents with a testicular tumor of soft consistency with a microcystic appearance on cross section. The tumor is removed and the histopathology indicates that it is derived from the structure labeled "F" in the accompanying diagram. Which one of the following best describes the importance of that structure in human embryonic development?

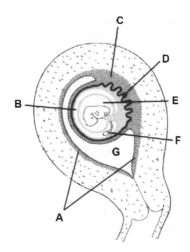

(Modified, with permission, from Sweeney L. Basic Concepts in Embryology. New York, NY: McGraw-Hill; 1998.)

a. The major site of yolk storage
b. Transfer of nutrients after the uteroplacental circulation has been established
c. The origin of the ligamentum teres hepatis
d. The source of the amniotic fluid
e. The initial site of hematopoiesis

26. A 32-year-old man presents with a complaint of a painless left testicular mass. That testis was cryptorchid at birth and descended by 6 postnatal months without treatment. He is diagnosed with a seminoma originating from primordial germ cells. The primordial germ cells that eventually form the oogonia and spermatogonia originate in which one of the following?

a. Dorsal mesentery of the hindgut
b. Gonadal ridge
c. Endodermal lining of the yolk sac
d. Primary sex cords of the developing gonad
e. Chorion

27. A 32-year-old woman (gravida 1, para 1) has an ultrasound done as part of her obstetrician visit in the fifth week of her pregnancy. The ultrasound reveals the presence of one gestational sac with two yolk sacs visible inside it. This condition arises from which one of the following events?

a. Fusion of the embryonic blastomeres from two zygotes
b. Fertilization of two oocytes by two sperm
c. Fertilization of one oocyte by two sperm
d. Division of the inner cell mass (embryoblast) into two embryonic primordia
e. Extra cleavage divisions of the zygote induced by the presence of separate chorions

28. A subcutaneous nodule is found in the skin overlying the bregma of a newborn boy. It is a 2 cm in diameter, asymptomatic, rubbery mass that is nonpulsatile, noncompressible, not tender, and appears tinged with blue. The skin overlying the cyst appears normal. The mass is removed and found to include hair follicles, sweat glands, hair, teeth, and nerves. Which one of the following best describes the embryological origin of the mass?

a. Endoderm
b. Myotome
c. Sclerotome
d. Intermediate mesoderm
e. Somatic mesoderm
f. Ectoderm

29. A 4-year-old girl presents with severe proximal bilateral claudication, headache, fatigue, and hypertension. Digital subtraction aortography shows localized occlusion of the abdominal aorta ascribed to a developmental anomaly in the fusion and maturation of the paired dorsal aortae. Which one of the following processes is responsible for fusion of the paired dorsal aortae?

a. Lateral folding
b. Craniocaudal folding
c. Looping of the heart tube
d. Gastrulation
e. Neurulation

Embryology: Early and General

Answers

1. The answer is d. (*Sadler, pp 95-101. Moore and Persaud, pp 37-38, 111-112, 117-118.*) The placental structures shown in the photomicrograph are chorionic villi that are fetal tissues. The mother's contribution to the placenta **(answers a and e)** is the blood that flows past the chorionic villi (a few maternal RBCs are visible, top left of photomicrograph). A fertilized ovum reaches the uterus about 4 days after fertilization as a multicellular, hollow sphere referred to as a blastocyst. The blastocyst adheres to the secretory endometrium and differentiates into an inner cell mass that develops into the embryo and a layer of primitive trophoblast. The expanding trophoblast penetrates the surface endometrium **(answers b and c)** and erodes into maternal blood vessels. Eventually, it develops two layers, an inner cytotrophoblast and an outer syncytiotrophoblast. Solid cords of trophoblast form the chorionic villi, which then are invaded by fetal blood vessels.

2. The answer is c. (*Alberts, pp 1297-1299. Sadler, pp 37-38. Mescher, pp 378-379. Moore and Persaud, pp 29-31.*) The husband in the scenario has sperm, which lack the acrosome (globozoospermia) and therefore the enzymes necessary for penetration of the ovum are missing. The formation of the acrosome, a specialized secretory granule, is one of many maturation events occurring during spermiogenesis (the process by which mature sperm are formed from the spermatids). Acrosome formation involves lytic enzyme maturation and occurs after division of secondary spermatocytes. It involves no mitotic or meiotic activity **(answers d and e)**. The acrosome develops from Golgi vesicles just like other secretory granules. It contains acrosin, a serine protease, hyaluronidase, and neuraminidase, responsible for the penetration ability of the sperm. The developing cells are in contact with Sertoli cells for all of the stages of spermiogenesis. At the end of spermiogenesis, spermatids are released by Sertoli cells in a process called spermiation **(answer b)**. Decapacitation factors are not involved in acrosomal maturation **(answer a)**.

3. **The answer is d.** (*Alberts, pp 1287-1292. Sadler, pp 24-27. Mescher, pp 388-392.*) The secondary oocyte enters the second meiotic division at the time of ovulation and arrests at metaphase. Fertilization by a spermatozoon provides the stimulation for the division of chromatin to the haploid number. By the time the fertilized ovum reaches the uterus, the progesterone (**answer a**) produced by the corpus luteum has initiated the secretory phase in the endometrium. Once implantation occurs and the chorion develops, human chorionic gonadotropin (hCG) is synthesized and the corpus luteum is maintained (**answer e**). Expulsion from the follicle (**answer b**) and the environment of the oviduct and uterus (**answer c**) do not induce the second meiotic division.

4. **The answer is g.** (*Mescher, pp 378-379. Moore and Persaud, pp 29-30. Gilbert, pp 194-195. Sadler, pp 37-38.*) Capacitation and the acrosome reaction are required for sperm penetration in the hamster egg penetration assay (SPA) also known as the hamster egg penetration test (HEPT). SPA is a complex sperm function assay that is based on the capacity of the human spermatozoa to fuse with zona pellucida-free golden hamster oocytes, leading to subsequent decondensation of the sperm nuclei. Capacitation prepares the sperm for fertilization and requires an increase in fluidity of the sperm plasma membrane. Sperm must reside in the female reproductive tract or under appropriate in vitro conditions for about 1 hour for capacitation to occur. During capacitation there is a loss of decapacitation factors that have been added to the sperm by epididymal cells and accessory male reproductive organs. Resumption of the second meiotic division (**answer a**), formation of the male pronucleus (**answer b**), and initiation of cleavage divisions (**answer c**) occur after sperm penetration of the egg and thus are not directly tested in a hamster egg penetration assay. Cholesterol is removed (not added, **answer d**) from the sperm plasma membrane during this period, which results in the increased fluidity (not a decrease, **answer e**) of this membrane that is required for the fusion of the acrosomal membrane with the sperm plasma membrane. Next, there is release of the acrosomal enzymes (not sequestration, **answer f**), which are required for the breakdown of the corona radiata and the zona pellucida of the oocyte to facilitate sperm penetration.

5. **The answer is e.** (*Sadler, pp 24-27. Ross, p 774.*) Primary oocytes have developed by the time of birth. From puberty to menopause, these germ

cells remain suspended in meiotic prophase I (diplotene or dictyate stage). A midcycle surge of LH triggers the resumption of meiosis and causes the FSH-primed follicle to rupture and discharge the ovum. Under the influence of LH, the ruptured follicle is transformed into a corpus luteum, which produces progesterone **(answers a and d)**. FSH and LH produced in the adenohypophysis result in growth and maturation of the ovarian follicle. Under FSH stimulation **(answer b)**, the theca cells proliferate, hypertrophy, and begin to produce estrogen **(answer c)**.

6. The answer is d. *(Sadler, pp 36-39.)* On fusion of the first sperm with the oocyte cell membrane, the contents of secretory granules stored just beneath the oocyte membrane (cortical granules) are released (the cortical or zona reaction). Enzymes stored in those granules cause biochemical changes in the zona pellucida and electrical changes in the oocyte membrane that prevent the binding of additional sperm. Primitive female germ cells (oogonia) enter the first meiotic division during fetal development **(answer a)**. This process becomes arrested in prophase I until individual primary oocytes are hormonally induced to resume the first meiotic division during ovulation. Fusion of the sperm and oocyte membranes initiates the resumption of the second meiotic division, resulting in the formation of a haploid pronucleus in the oocyte and extrusion of the second polar body **(answer b)**. Capacitation **(answer c)** is a process by which enzymatic secretions of the uterus and oviducts strip glycoproteins from the sperm cell membrane. This is required for penetration of the layer of cells surrounding the oocyte (corona radiata). The release of enzymes **(answer e)** from the sperm acrosomal cap (an enlarged secretory granule) results in digestion of the zona pellucida surrounding the oocyte, allowing penetration by sperm.

7. The answer is a. *(Moore and Persaud, pp 16, 18, 20. Sadler, pp 24-27.)* The maximum number of oogonia occurs at about the fifth month of development. Primordial germ cells arrive in the embryonic gonad of a genetic female during the 7th to 12th week where they differentiate into oogonia. After undergoing a number of mitotic divisions, those fetal cells form clusters in the cortical part of the ovary. Some of those oogonia differentiate into the larger primary oocytes (not to be confused with primary follicles). The primary oocytes begin meiosis. At the same time, the number of oogonia continues to increase to about 6,000,000 by the fifth month. At this time, most of the surviving oogonia and some of the oocytes become atretic (**answers b and c**). However, the surviving primary oocytes (400,000-1,000,000) become surrounded by epithelial cells and form the primordial follicles by the seventh month. During childhood (**answers d and e**) there is continued atresia, so that by puberty only about 40,000 primary oocytes remain.

8. The answer is d. *(Sadler, pp 27-30. Moore and Persaud, pp 15, 17, 19, 20.)* In men, the time required for the progression from spermatogonium to motile spermatozoon is between 61 and 64 days—about 2 months (**answers a → c, e**). Spermatogenesis, the process by which spermatogonia undergo mitotic division to produce primary spermatocytes, occurs at 1°C (34°F) below normal body temperature. Subsequent meiotic divisions produce secondary spermatocytes with a bivalent haploid chromosome number and then spermatids with a monovalent haploid chromosome number. Spermiogenesis, the maturation of the spermatid, results in spermatozoa. Spermatozoa are moved to the epididymis, where they become fully motile.

9. The answer is b. *(Moore and Persaud, pp 45-48, 52. Sadler, pp 51-54.)* Implantation of the conceptus low on the uterine wall near the cervical opening (os) could result in growth of the placenta between the embryo and the cervical os (placenta previa). The placenta could become dislodged from the uterine wall before, as well as during delivery, resulting in rapidly fatal hemorrhage. Implantation at site **A** (the uterine tube or oviduct) results in rupture of the oviduct wall, whereas implantation on the ovary (**C**) would result in destruction of that organ. Implantation could also occur in the wall of the peritoneal cavity (**D**). Implantation normally occurs in the superior, posterior, or posterolateral walls of the uterus (**E**).

10. The answer is b. *(Moore and Persaud, pp 57-59. Sadler, pp 47-51, 55, 63.)* Teratomas include tissues from all three germ layers: ectoderm, endoderm, and mesoderm, are associated with gastrulation, and may arise from remnants of the primitive streak or from primordial germ cells that fail to migrate to the gonadal ridge. Cells of the inner cell mass (embryoblast) of the blastocyst differentiate into the epiblast and hypoblast. Cells of the epiblast migrate toward the primitive streak during the second week and become internalized, forming the mesodermal and endodermal germ layers.

Remaining cells of the epiblast become the ectodermal germ layer. Cells of the hypoblast (**answer d**) will contribute to the yolk sac. Cells of the outer cell mass of the blastocyst will differentiate into the cytotrophoblast and syncytiotrophoblast (**answers a and c**), which will contribute to formation of the placenta. The yolk sac (**answer e**) is incorporated into the embryo as the primitive gut during embryonic folding.

11. The answer is b. *(Sadler, p 87. Moore and Persaud, p 73.)* Formation of most internal organs occurs during the second month, the period of organogenesis. The first month (**answer a**) of embryonic development generally is concerned with cleavage, formation of the germ layers, and establishment of the embryonic body. The period from the ninth week to the end of intrauterine life (**answers c, d, and e**), known as the fetal period, is characterized by maturation of tissues and rapid growth of the fetal body.

12. The answer is f. *(Schoenwolf, pp 41-44, 51-53, 69, 101. Moore and Persaud, pp 44, 116-118, 128. Sadler, pp 47, 48, 50, 63-65.)* The second week of development follows the "rule of twos." In the second week, many critical developmental events occur in "twos": the embryoblast forms the epiblast and hypoblast; the trophoblast forms the syncytiotrophoblast and the cytotrophoblast; two new cavities, the amniotic and yolk sac cavities are formed; the extraembryonic tissue forms two layers, the parietal and visceral layers. In addition, implantation is completed and the uteroplacental circulation is established during the second week when maternal blood flows through the trophoblast system. First week events include: the formation of the blastomeres, segregation of blastomeres to form the embryoblast (inner cell mass) and trophoblast, the development of the blastocyst, and the decidual reaction by which endometrial stromal cells respond to progesterone and the adherent blastocyst by becoming active secretory cells (**answers a → e**). The corpus luteum discontinues secretion of progesterone and degenerates in the absence of an implanted embryo (**answer g**). The heart begins to beat on day 22 (**answer h**), and gastrulation and neurulation (**answer i**) occur during week 3 of development. The formation of the primordia of the major organ systems and embryonic folding occur during week 4 (**answer j**).

13. The answer is e. *(Sadler, pp 47, 55, 57, 58, 60. Moore and Persaud, pp 43, 55-57.)* The nongastrulating cells of the epiblast form the ectoderm (epidermis, epidermal appendages, and the nervous system [see figure below]). During the second week of development, the embryoblast gives rise to two primitive germ layers, the epiblast and the underlying hypoblast **(answer a)**. At the beginning of the third week, cells from the epiblast **(answer b)** migrate toward the midline (primitive streak) and move inward (gastrulation). The migrating epiblast cells displace the hypoblast cells to the periphery to form the endodermal lining **(answer d)** of the digestive tract and form an intermediate layer of mesoderm **(answer c)** that will give rise to muscle, bone, and cartilaginous structures.

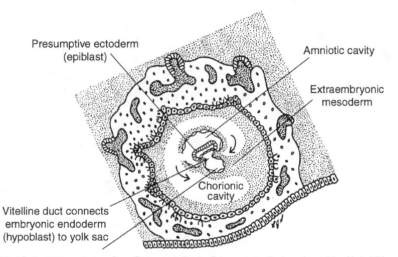

(Modified, with permission, from Sweeney L. Basic Concepts in Embryology. New York, NY: McGraw-Hill; 1998.)

14. The answer is b. *(Moore and Persaud, pp 328-330. Sadler, pp 196-199.)* Blood from the placenta in the umbilical cord is about 80% oxygenated. Mixture with unoxygenated blood from the vitelline veins and the inferior vena cava reduces the oxygen content somewhat. However, this stream with relatively high oxygen content is directed by the valve of the inferior vena cava directly through the foramen ovale into the left atrium. This prevents admixture with oxygen-depleted blood entering the right atrium from the superior vena cava. Thus, the oxygen-saturated blood entering the left ventricle and pumped into the aortic arch, subclavian arteries, and common carotid arteries has the highest oxygen content. The oxygen-depleted blood from the superior vena cava is directed into the right ventricle and then to the pulmonary trunk. Although a small portion of this flow passes through the lungs (where any residual oxygen is extracted by the tissue of the nonrespiring lung), most is shunted into the thoracic aorta via the ductus arteriosus and thereby lowers the oxygen content of that vessel. This occurs distal to the origins of the carotid arteries and ensures that the rapidly developing brain has the best oxygen supply. The pattern of blood supply in the fetus and the changes that occur at birth are shown in High-Yield Facts, Figures 2 and 3.

15. The answer is b. (*Sadler, pp 196-199. Moore and Persaud, pp 327, 330-333. See High-Yield Facts, Figures 2 and 3.*) The presence of a murmur could be indicative of any of the conditions. The presence of a continuous machine-like murmur is indicative of a patent ductus arteriosus (PDA). Usually, as in this case, the premature baby with PDA does not acutely become cyanotic and ill, although brief desaturations can occur that become more persistent. The ventilator requirements are increased due to increasing pCO_2 (as the lungs become "wet," the pCO_2 increases). The diastolic blood pressure usually drops and there is a widened pulse pressure (usually greater than 20). The PDA was always there, it is just that her pulmonary vascular resistance relaxed enough to allow more left-to-right shunting and more blood flow to the lungs (less to the body). An atrial septal defect (ASD), such as a persistent foramen ovale, could be eliminated from the diagnosis because the murmur would be heard as an abnormal splitting of the second sound during expiration **(answer a)**. A patent foramen ovale is a common echo finding in premature babies and is usually not followed up unless it appears remarkable to the pediatric cardiologist or there is a persistent murmur. A patent foramen ovale might result in only minimal or intermittent cyanosis during crying or straining to pass stool. A murmur caused by a ventricular septal defect (VSD, **answer c**), occurs between the first and second heart sounds (S_1 and S_2) and is described as holosystolic (pansystolic) because the amplitude is high throughout systole. Pulmonary stenosis would be heard as a harsh systolic ejection murmur **(answer d)**. Coarctation of the aorta **(answer e)** would result in a systolic murmur. PDA refers to the maintenance of the ductus arteriosus, a normal fetal structure. In the fetus, the ductus arteriosus allows blood to bypass the pulmonary circulation, since the lungs are not involved in CO_2/O_2 exchange until after birth. The placenta subserves the function of gas exchange during fetal development. The ductus arteriosus shunts flow from the left pulmonary artery to the aorta. High oxygen levels after birth and the absence of prostaglandins from the placenta cause the ductus arteriosus to close in most cases within 24 hours. A PDA most often corrects itself within several months of birth, but may require infusion of indomethacin (a prostaglandin inhibitor) as a treatment, insertion of surgical plugs during catheterization, or actual surgical ligation.

16. The answer is a. *(Moore and Persaud, pp 67, 167, 334, 339. Sadler, pp 81, 215, 272.)* The thymic parenchyma (epithelial cells) develops from endoderm of the third pharyngeal (branchial) pouches. The thymic rudiment is invaded by bone marrow–derived lymphocyte precursors early in the third month of development. The tonsils **(answer b)** develop as partially encapsulated lymphatic nodules. Their parenchymal framework is derived from pharyngeal mesoderm. Bones, whether formed by intramembranous or endochondral ossification, are derived from mesoderm. Their forming marrow cavities are populated by hematopoietic stem cells **(answer c)** beginning in the second month of fetal life. The connective tissue capsule and skeletal framework of the spleen develop from splanchnic lateral plate mesoderm during the fifth week and are quickly invaded by hematopoietic cells of the myeloid lineage **(answer d)**. The spleen remains an active hematopoietic organ until at least the seventh month in utero. Blood islands develop by differentiation of mesodermal cells in the extraembryonic mesoderm lining the yolk sac during the third week of fetal development **(answer e)**. They give rise to vitelline vessels and are the major site of red blood cell formation in the early embryo.

17. The answer is c. *(Moore and Persaud, pp 73-75. Sadler, pp 82-83, 165-167.)* Cranial folding is responsible for the placement of the developing heart in the presumptive thoracic region of the embryo. Initially, the developing cranial portion of the neural tube lies dorsal and caudal to the oropharyngeal membrane. However, overgrowth of the forebrain causes it to extend past the oropharyngeal membrane and overhang the cardiogenic area. Subsequent growth of the forebrain pushes the developing heart ventrally and caudally to a position in the presumptive thoracic region caudal to the oropharyngeal membrane and cranial to the septum transversum that will form the central tendon of the diaphragm. Gastrulation **(answer a)** is the process by which epiblast cells migrate to the primitive streak and become internalized to form the mesodermal and endodermal germ layers. Lateral folding **(answer b)** of the embryo forms the endodermal tube and surrounding concentric layering of mesoderm and ectoderm. Neurulation refers to formation of the neural tube from surface ectoderm **(answer d)**. The fusion of the two endocardial heart tubes **(answer e)** occurs as lateral folding occurs. The fused tube will form the endocardium surrounded by the primordial myocardium derived from splanchnic mesoderm that will form the heart muscle (myocardium).

18. The answer is d. *(Moore and Persaud, pp 38, 43, 111-118. Sadler, pp 63-65.)* In the developing fetus, the maternal blood is in direct contact with the syncytiotrophoblast. During implantation, the syncytiotrophoblast invades the endometrium and erodes the maternal blood vessels. Maternal blood and nutrient glandular secretions fill the lacunae and bathe the projections of syncytiotrophoblast. Primary villi consist of syncytiotrophoblast with a core of cytotrophoblast cells **(answer a)**. In secondary villi, the cytotrophoblast core is invaded by mesoderm and subsequently by umbilical blood vessels in tertiary villi. Extraembryonic mesoderm **(answer b)**, fetal blood vessels **(answer c)**, and amniotic cells **(answer e)** are not in direct contact with maternal blood.

19. The answer is c. *(Sadler, pp 95, 114-116. Moore and Persaud, pp 472-476.)* Exposure of the embryo to harmful environmental factors (teratogens), such as chemicals, viruses, and/or radiation, can occur at any time. During the third through eighth weeks of embryonic life, organ systems are developing and are most susceptible to teratogens. During that time, each organ system has its own specific period of peak susceptibility. Exposure of the embryo to teratogens during the first 2 weeks of fetal life **(answers a and b)** generally induces spontaneous abortion and is, therefore, lethal. After the eighth week of intrauterine development **(answers d and e)**, teratogenic exposure generally results in retardation of organ growth rather than in new structural or functional changes.

20. The answer is e. *(Sadler, pp 67, 75, 135, 136, 305. Moore and Persaud, pp 472, 479.)* Vitamin A is a member of the retinoic acid family. Retinoic acid directs the polarity of development in the central nervous system, the axial skeleton (vertebral column), and probably the appendicular skeleton. Retinoic acid induces transcription of various combinations of homeobox genes, depending on tissue type and location (distance and direction from the source of retinoic acid). Exogenous sources of retinoic acid may induce the wrong sequence or combination of homeobox genes, leading to structural abnormalities in nervous and skeletal systems. The other organ systems listed are not as susceptible to vitamin A (answers a, b, c, and d).

21. The answer is a. (*Sadler, pp 104, 195, 206. Moore and Persaud, pp 128-133.*) An amniotic fluid index of 27 cm is indicative of polyhydramnios. Duodenal and/or esophageal atresia results in an inability of the fetus to swallow amniotic fluid (answer c). The result is that normal recirculation of amniotic fluid through the embryo is greatly reduced or eliminated, causing an excess of amniotic fluid. Excess amniotic fluid is defined as greater than 2000 mL in the third trimester. Low volumes of amniotic fluid (oligohydramnios) are caused by rupture of the fetal membranes, bilateral agenesis of the kidneys (answer b), or obstructive uropathy (answer e, blockage of the calyces or ureters), which prevents urine from being added to the amniotic fluid. Hypoplasia of the lungs (answer d) and compression of the umbilical cord are associated with oligohydramnios, but do not cause it. The presence of adequate fluid in the uninflated lungs is essential for lung maturation, and growth factors in the amniotic fluid may also be important. Low levels of amniotic fluid severely inhibit lung development. The formula for understanding the relationship between urine and amniotic fluid is:

Less urine output = less amniotic fluid; less swallowing = more amniotic fluid.

22. The answer is a. (*Sadler, pp 67-71, 267. Moore and Persaud, pp 62-64. Alberts, pp 1140-1141, 1370-1371, 1385.*) The first stage of neural tube formation is the induction by notochord and prechordal plate mesoderm of the neural plate that forms from ectoderm. This is known as primary induction and is accompanied by molecular changes in cell adhesion molecules. This first stage of neural tube development is followed by a reshaping phase, neurulation, and neural tube closure. Spina bifida with myeloschisis (rachischisis) is the most severe form of spina bifida in which the neural tube fails to close leaving a plate-like mass of neural tissue.

Endoderm **(answer b)** is responsible for the formation of the GI tract and respiratory system. The somatopleuric mesoderm **(answer c)** makes important contributions to the skin (dermis) and nonmuscle portions of the limbs. The splanchnopleuric mesoderm **(answer d)** forms the heart and the muscles of the GI tract and urinary system. The hypoblast **(answer e)** is the thin layer of cells ventral to the epiblast; it is displaced by the epiblast cells, which form endoderm.

23. The answer is d. (*Sadler, pp 74-79.*) The muscles of the extremities form from the somites that are derived from paraxial mesoderm; the bones, tendons, and connective tissue of the extremities are derived from somatopleuric mesoderm. The fibroblast growth factor receptor genes (*FGFR*) play a key role in differentiation of the paraxial mesoderm. The intermediate mesoderm is the origin of the urogenital systems and the adrenal cortex **(answer a)**. The adrenal medulla **(answer b)** forms from the neural crest. The humerus **(answer c)** forms from somatopleuric mesoderm, but the muscles attached to it are of somite origin. The masseter **(answer e)** is a muscle of mastication formed from the first branchial arch and innervated by special visceral efferent (SVE) fibers from the nucleus ambiguus compared with the general somatic efferent (GSE) innervation of the biceps and other muscles, not of branchial arch origin.

24. The answer is a. (*Sadler, pp 310, 312, 323. Moore and Persaud, pp 401-405, 408, Waxman, pp 2, 7-8.*) The cerebral cortex forms from the telencephalon. The cortex develops in waves of proliferation, forming layers I to VI with the innermost layers forming first and the more superficial layers later. The wall of the developing CNS contains three layers: ventricular, mantle (intermediate), and marginal zones. The cortex, a peripheral area of gray matter, is formed through the migration of cells from the mantle zone to the marginal zone. The derivatives of the other brain vesicles **(answers b → e)** are listed in the High-Yield Facts (Table 4).

25. The answer is e. (*Sadler, pp 12, 55-56, 58-59, 101, 203-206. Moore and Persaud, pp 44, 45, 133-134.*) The yolk sac is important as a source of blood until the fetal liver replaces this function in about the sixth week of development. The yolk sac produces predominantly hematocytoblasts (stem cells) and primitive erythroblasts. Vasculogenesis is also initiated in the yolk sac. The endoderm of the yolk sac is incorporated into the embryo as part of the primitive gut during embryonic folding and is home to the primordial germ cells before they migrate to the hindgut. The tumor in the vignette is an endodermal sinus tumor ([EST], also known as a yolk sac tumor, or infantile embryonal carcinoma) and is a member of the germ cell tumor group. It is the most common testicular tumor in children under the age of 3. There is no yolk storage in human embryos **(answer a)**. The transfer of nutrients is an important function of the yolk sac early in development, but once the uteroplacental circulation is established, the placenta takes over that role **(answer b)**. The umbilical vein forms the ligamentum teres hepatis **(answer c)**. The cells of the amnion **(answer d)** form the amniotic fluid with eventual addition of urine from the developing kidneys. The figure below illustrates the location of the yolk sac and other embryonic structures and provides answers to the labels in the figure for Question 25.

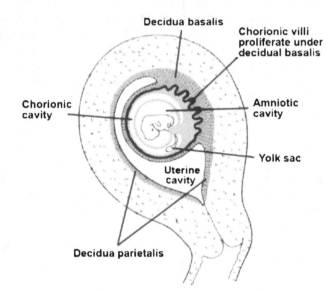

(Modified, with permission, from Sweeney L. Basic Concepts in Embryology. New York, NY: McGraw-Hill; 1998.)

26. The answer is c. *(Sadler, pp 11-12. Moore and Persaud, pp 133-134, 263.)* The primordial germ cells are first seen in the endodermal lining of the wall of the yolk sac (derived from the hypoblast) in the region of the allantois at the end of the third or beginning of the fourth week. During embryonic folding, the dorsal part of the yolk sac is incorporated into the embryo as the primitive gut. The primordial germ cells subsequently migrate along the dorsal mesentery of the hindgut **(answer a)** and into the gonadal (genital) ridge by week 6 **(answer b)**. The primary sex cords grow into the mesenchyme underlying the ridge, and the primordial germ cells become incorporated into the primary sex cords **(answer d)**. The chorion **(answer e)** is the outermost fetal membrane and is composed of extraembryonic somatic mesoderm, cytotrophoblast, and the syncytiotrophoblast. It is divided into the chorion frondosum, where the villi form and proliferate, and the smooth chorion, also known as the chorion laevae. The figure in Answer 25 illustrates the arrangement of the fetal membranes. Germ cell tumors originate from primordial germ cells during embryonic development, although the progression and eventual detection of the disease occurs decades later.

27. The answer is d. (*Sadler, pp 104-107. Moore and Persaud, pp 134-138. Alberts, p 1153. Schoenwolf, p 181.*) The presence of one gestational sac with two yolk sacs is indicative of the presence of monozygotic twins (MZ). MZ twins arise from divisions of the embryoblast to form two embryos. Splitting that occurs at the two-cell stage results in separate amnions, chorions, and placenta as occurs in dizygotic twins (DZ). MZ twins can arise anywhere from the two-cell (blastomere) to the blastocyst stage. Splitting early in the blastocyst stage results in splitting of the inner cell mass (separate amnions, with common chorion and placenta). Splitting later in the blastocyst stage results in a common amnion, chorion, and placenta. MZ twins may have fused or separate placentae, separate or fused dichorionic sacs or one chorionic sac, and diamniotic sacs. Dizygotic (DZ) twins arise from fertilization of two oocytes by two sperm **(answer b)** and are merely "womb mates." They differ in genotype and, therefore, may be different sexes. Fertilization of one oocyte by two sperm **(answer c)** cannot occur because of the Ca^{2+}-dependent block to polyspermy (see Question 6). That egg cortical reaction affects the zona pellucida in two ways: (1) hydrolysis of carbohydrate prevents sperm binding and (2) proteolytic activity hardens it. Fusion of blastomeres would lead to polyploid embryos or mosaics **(answer a)**. Cleavage divisions are not induced by the chorion and fetal membranes form after twinning has been determined **(answer e)**.

28. The answer is f. (*Kumar, p 262.*) The child in the vignette has a dermoid cyst caused when skin and skin structures become trapped during fetal development. The cyst walls are epidermal and may contain multiple structures such as hair follicles, sweat glands, and sometimes teeth, or nerves. Dermoid cysts are almost always present at birth, although subtle lesions may not be noticed until, for example, trauma causes inflammation. The most common locations are overlying the bregma (junction of the coronal and sagittal sutures), anterior fontanelle, upper lateral region of the forehead, lateral upper eyelid, and sub-mental region, although lesions can occur anywhere on the scalp, face, or spinal axis. The gastrointestinal and respiratory systems develop from endoderm (**answer a**). The myotomes form the skeletal muscle of the trunk and extremities (**answer b**). The sclerotomes form cartilage and bone (**answer c**, also see Question 23). The intermediate mesoderm is the origin of the urogenital systems and the adrenal (suprarenal) gland (**answer d**). The somatic mesoderm (**answer e**) contributes to the non-muscular components of the extremities and the dermis.

29. The answer is a. (*Sadler, pp 155-157. Moore and Persaud, pp 73-75, 292.*) The fusion of the dorsal aortae occurs through lateral folding. Fusion of the endocardial heart tube and incorporation of the yolk sac into the primitive gut also occurs as a result of lateral folding. Middle aortic syndrome (MAS) is generated by segmental narrowing of the abdominal or distal descending thoracic aorta. In this case, MAS is congenital, ascribed to failure in the fusion and maturation of the paired embryonic dorsal aortas. Craniocaudal folding (**answer b**) establishes the definitive head and tail regions of the embryo. Fusion is already complete at the time that looping of the heart tube occurs (**answer c**). Gastrulation (**answer d**) establishes the three germ layers (trilaminar disk), and neurulation establishes the neural groove with two neural folds. Neurulation is the formation of the neural tube (**answer e**).

Cell Biology: Membranes

Questions

30. The region labeled with the arrow in the accompanying electron micrograph of the plasma membrane is primarily responsible for which one of the following functions?

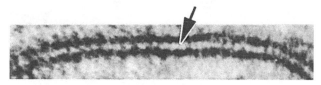

a. Creation of a barrier to water-soluble molecules
b. Specific cellular receptors for ligands
c. Catalyzing membrane-associated activities
d. Transport of small ions
e. Connections to the cytoskeleton

31. A 14-month-old boy presents with a fever of 102°F. The child has a long-standing history of recurrent lower respiratory tract infections including bronchitis and pneumonia. Chronic diarrhea is a long-standing problem. His mother reports that she had numerous upper respiratory infections and chronic diarrhea as a young child. A complete blood count, lung function tests, and urinalysis values are all within normal range. Serum immunoglobulin levels are normal for IgG and IgM, but IgA is 25 mg/dL (normal = 40-60 mg/dL). There are numerous neutrophils and other white cells in the stool sample and the stool is cultured for specific bacteria. IgA coats pathogens facilitating repulsion of the negative charge on the cell membrane. That negative charge on the cell membrane is primarily caused by which one of the following?

a. Free saccharide groups
b. Glycoproteins
c. Cholesterol
d. Peripheral membrane protein
e. Integrins

32. The face labeled by asterisks in the freeze-fracture preparation of the eukaryotic cell membrane shown below may be characterized as which one of the following?

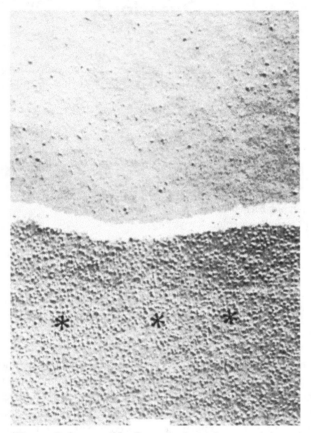

(Micrograph Courtesy of Dr. Giuseppina Raviola.)

a. Containing primarily glycoproteins and glycolipids
b. Facing away from the cytoplasm
c. In direct contact with the cytoplasm
d. Backed by the extracellular space
e. Generally possessing a paucity of intramembranous particles

33. Band 3 protein exists as a 95-kDa multipass membrane protein that functions as the primary anion exchanger in erythrocytes. Within the red blood cell (RBC) membrane, band 3 binds to spectrin dimers and tetramers indirectly through ankyrin. The spectrin tetramers are bound together by actin and band 4.1 protein, which also binds to band 3 and glycophorin. Null mutations in band 3 occur in the human population. Which one of the following is most likely to decrease in the absence of band 3 protein?

a. Osmotic fragility
b. Destruction of RBCs in the spleen
c. Bile production
d. Erythroid production in the bone marrow
e. Blood pH

34. A 56-year-old man who drinks a six pack of beer a day, with higher alcoholic intake on weekends, holidays, and "special days," presents to the internal medicine clinic. He has an abnormal plasma lipoprotein profile. It is known that erythrocyte fluidity is altered in liver disease. Which one of the following would increase membrane fluidity in the hepatocytes of this patient's liver?

a. Restriction of rotational movement of proteins and lipids in the membrane
b. Transbilayer movement of phospholipids in the plasma membrane
c. Increased cholesterol/phospholipids ratio in the plasma membrane
d. Binding of integral membrane proteins with cytoskeletal elements
e. Binding of an antibody to a cell-surface receptor

35. The asymmetry of the cell membrane is established primarily by which one of the following?

a. Membrane synthesis in the endoplasmic reticulum
b. Membrane modification in the Golgi apparatus
c. Presence of carbohydrates on the cytoplasmic surface
d. The distribution of cholesterol
e. Flipping proteins between the leaflets of the lipid bilayer ("filp-flop")

36. A 44-year-old African American woman calls 911. When the MedAct unit arrives they find a patient with acute shortness of breath and audible wheezing. A physical examination reveals pulse 115 (normal 60-100), respiratory rate 42 (normal 15-20) with signs of accessory muscle use. She is coughing up mucus. Auscultation reveals decreased breath sounds with wheezing on inspiration and expiration. The patient has taken her prescribed medications with no relief of symptoms prior to her 911 call. Her current medication is albuterol, a moderately selective β_2-receptor agonist. Which one of the following is true regarding those receptors?

a. They possess a single hydrophobic transmembrane segment in the form of an α-helix.

b. They can activate plasma membrane-bound enzymes or ion channels.

c. They possess an intracellular ligand-binding domain.

d. They possess intrinsic enzyme activity.

e. They are arranged so that both the amino- and the carboxy-terminals are located intracellularly.

Cell Biology: Membranes

Answers

30. The answer is a. (*Ross, pp 28, 30. Alberts, pp 617-620.*) The hydrophobic layer of the cell (plasma) membrane is labeled with the arrow. It is responsible for the fundamental structure of the membrane and provides the barrier to water-soluble molecules in the external milieu. It also provides a two-dimensional solvent for membrane proteins. Other membrane functions are performed primarily by proteins that function as receptors, enzymes (catalysis of membrane-associated activities), and transporters (**answers b, c, and d**). Connection to the cytoskeleton (**answer e**) is performed by members of the spectrin family of proteins reinforcing the membrane on the cytosolic side.

The membrane consists of a bilayer of phospholipids with the nonpolar, hydrophobic layer in the central portion of the membrane and the hydrophilic polar regions of the phospholipids in contact with the aqueous components at the intra- or extracellular surfaces of the membrane. Proteins are generally dispersed within the lipid bilayer. The polar head groups of the lipid bilayer react with osmium to create the trilaminar appearance observed in electron micrographs of the plasma membrane. Cell membranes range in thickness from 7 to 10 nm (1 nm = 10^{-9}m, 1 μm = 10^{-6}m; the diameter of a RBC [erythrocyte] is 7 μm).

31. The answer is b. (*Alberts, pp 622-624, 628-629, 635-637. Mescher, pp 18-21. Ross, pp 23-25. Fauci, pp 2058-2059.*) The child in the scenario suffers from IgA deficiency, the most common immunoglobulin deficiency. IgA functions in several ways, one of which is to coat pathogens with a negative charge that repels the polyanionic charge on the cell surface. In IgA deficiency, pathogens can more easily attach to the cell surface leading to persistent infections. The carbohydrate of biological membranes is found in the form of glycoproteins and glycolipids rather than as free saccharide groups (**answer a**). The polyanionic charge of the membrane is produced by the sugar side chains on the glycoproteins and glycolipids. Glycoproteins often terminate in sialic acid side chains, which impart a negative (polyanionic) charge to the membrane. Similarly, the glycolipids (also called glycosphingolipids), particularly the gangliosides, terminate in sialic acid residues with a strong negative charge. Cholesterol (answer c) alters membrane fluidity (see Question 34) and is amphipathic (hydrophilic and hydrophobic properties). It reduces the packing of lipid acyl groups through its steroid ring structure and hydrocarbon tail and cements hydrophilic regions of the membrane through interactions with its hydroxyl (OH^-) region. Peripheral membrane proteins (answer d) are found primarily on the cytosolic leaflet of the membrane bilayer. Integrins (answer e) are heterodimeric receptors that bind with extracellular matrix molecules such as laminin and fibronectin. The structure of the cell membrane is shown in High-Yield Facts, Figure 4.

32. The answer is b. (*Alberts, p 609. Ross, p 30.*) The P face of a cell-membrane freeze fracture is labeled with the asterisks and faces away from the cytoplasm (answers a, c, and d). Freeze fracture is a procedure in which the tissue is rapidly frozen and fractured with a knife. The fracture plane occurs through the hydrophobic central plane of membranes, the plane of least resistance to the cleavage force. The two faces are essentially the two interior faces of the membrane—the extracellular face (E face) and the protoplasmic face (P face). The cytoplasm is the backing for the P face, which in general contains numerous intramembranous particles composed mostly of protein (answer e). The E face is backed by the extracellular space and in general contains a paucity of intramembranous particles (see upper part of figure) compared with the P face (labeled with asterisks).

33. The answer is e. (*Alberts, pp 646-648. Rubin, p 1039. Kumar, pp 642-643. Fauci, pp 653-655.*) In its anion exchanger role, band 3 protein exchanges bicarbonate ion for chloride ion. Bicarbonate is transported by band 3 out of the RBC in exchange for chloride, permitting the highly efficient transport of CO_2 to the lungs as bicarbonate. In the absence of band 3 protein, the bicarbonate buffering of the blood is reduced, leading to acidosis or lowering of blood pH. The result is reduced capacity to carry CO_2. In addition to its functional, bidirectional anion exchanger role, band 3 plays a key membrane structural role, since the cytoplasmic domain of the protein interacts with spectrin through an ankyrin bridge. Spectrin exists as dimers and trimers; the trimers are bound together by actin, thus providing a connection to the cytoskeleton maintaining the shape and stability of the RBC. The result of a null mutation in band 3 is the formation of erythrocytes that are small and round instead of biconcave (spherocytosis). Spherocytes are osmotically fragile because of their decreased surface area per unit volume (**answer a**). The defective RBCs do not readily pass through the small sinusoids of the spleen, resulting in destruction and further membrane conditioning, which leads to accelerated destruction (**answer b**) and, eventually, enlargement of the spleen (splenomegaly). The accelerated hemolysis leads to increased bile production (**answer c**) and jaundice. Hemoglobin production is also increased, as exemplified by an increase in mean corpuscular hemoglobin concentration (MCHC) by about 35% to 40%. The bone marrow compensates for the increased destruction of RBCs with hyperplasia of erythroid precursors in the bone marrow (**answer d**) and increase in the number of reticulocytes (polychromasia).

34. The answer is e. *(Alberts, pp 622-624.)* The patient in the scenario is suffering from cirrhosis in which there are alterations in plasma lipoproteins. Binding of an antibody to a cell-surface receptor leads to lateral diffusion of protein in the lipid bilayer, resulting in increased membrane fluidity—patching and capping. Rotational and lateral movements of both proteins and lipids contribute to membrane fluidity. Restriction reduces membrane fluidity (**answer a**). Phospholipids are capable of lateral diffusion, rapid rotation around their long axes, and flexion of their hydrocarbon (fatty acyl) tails. They undergo transbilayer movement (**answer b**), known as "flip-flop," between bilayers in the endoplasmic reticulum; however, in general this does not occur in the plasma membrane. Other factors reduce membrane fluidity. An increase in the amount of cholesterol relative to phospholipid (**answer c**) has been shown by a variety of physicochemical techniques to decrease fluidity in both biological and artificial membranes by interacting with the hydrophobic regions near the polar head groups and stiffening this region of the membrane. Association or binding of integral membrane proteins with cytoskeletal elements (**answer d**) on the interior of the cell and peripheral membrane proteins on the extracellular surface limit membrane mobility and fluidity.

35. The answer is a. *(Alberts, pp 743-745.)* Asymmetry of the lipid bilayer is established during membrane synthesis in the endoplasmic reticulum (**answer a**) before reaching the Golgi apparatus (**answer b**). Carbohydrates are associated with the N-terminals of transmembrane proteins that extend from the extracellular surface, not the cytoplasmic surface (**answer c**). Cholesterol is different from proteins and phospholipids that are asymmetrically distributed within the bilayer (**answer d**). Cholesterol is found on both sides of the bilayer. The small polar head group structure of cholesterol allows it to flip-flop from leaflet to leaflet and respond to changes in shape. In contrast to cholesterol, most proteins and phospholipids are capable of only rare flip-flop (**answer e**). For example, transbilayer movement of phospholipid is limited mostly to the endoplasmic reticulum.

36. The answer is b. (*Alberts, pp 904-906. Mescher, pp 18-20.*) Albuterol binds to β-receptors, which are multipass G-protein-linked receptors. Binding to G-protein-linked receptors activates or inactivates enzymes bound to the plasma membrane (adenylyl cyclase or phospholipase C) or opens or closes ion channels using G proteins. See High-Yield Facts, Table 6, for G proteins and their functions. The β-receptors, as well as muscarinic cholinergic receptors and rhodopsin, are multipass transmembrane (**answer a**) proteins consisting specifically of seven hydrophobic spanning segments of the single polypeptide chain. The peptide bonds of the spanning segments are polar. In the hydrophobic environment of the lipid bilayer, in the absence of water, they form hydrogen bonds with each other. There is a remarkable homology between the cell-surface receptors linked to the G proteins. Ligand binding occurs on the extracellular surface (**answer c**). Receptors with intrinsic enzyme activity belong to a separate class of single-pass transmembrane proteins (**answer d**). Multipass G-protein-linked receptors are transmembrane proteins that possess a carboxyl terminus on the cytosolic side and N-linked glycosylation sites on the extracellular surface (**answer e**).

Cell Biology: Cytoplasm

Questions

37. A patient is diagnosed with a pleomorphic adenoma of the submandibular gland. The pathologist uses anti-vimentin antibodies with immunocytochemistry to stain the biopsy tissue. One would expect to find vimentin staining in which one of the following structures?

a. Fibrous stromal connective tissue
b. Parasympathetic ganglia
c. Serous acini
d. Mucous acini
e. Striated ducts

38. Which one of the following is the function of the large subunit of the ribosome?

a. Bind messenger RNA (mRNA)
b. Bind transfer RNA (tRNA)
c. Catalyze peptide bond formation
d. Initiate protein synthesis
e. Link adjacent ribosomes in a polyribosome

39. The stability and arrangement of actin filaments as well as their properties and functions depend on which one of the following?

a. The structure of the actin filaments
b. Microtubules
c. Intermediate filament proteins
d. Actin-binding proteins
e. Motor molecules, such as kinesin

40. A 47-year-old man presents with fatigue and over the next few years becomes progressively weaker, eventually becoming paralyzed. He encounters severe problems with speech and swallowing. Weakness and paralysis of the thoracic muscles leads to progressive respiratory insufficiency and death. An autopsy transmission electron microscopy reveals fragmentation of the structures delineated by the arrows within motoneurons. Which one of the following correctly characterizes those structures?

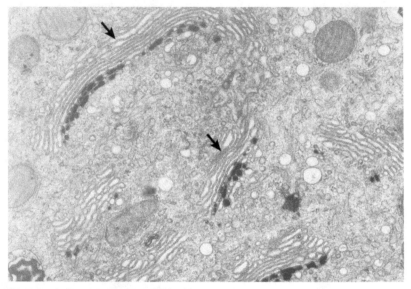

(Micrograph Courtesy of Dr. Daniel Friend.)

a. There is no functional, topological specialization within the stacks.
b. They present an entry face associated with granule formation.
c. They present a *trans* face associated with COat Protein (COP)-II-coated transport vesicles.
d. They are biochemically compartmentalized.
e. They receive proteins but not lipids.

41. A 14-year-old adolescent is diagnosed with epidermolysis bullosa simplex (EBS). His skin blisters easily with rubbing or scratching. Blisters occur primarily on his hands and feet and heal without leaving scars. Mutations in the *KRT5* and *KRT14* genes are identified by genetic analysis. Those genes code for the proteins keratin 5 and keratin 14, respectively. What is the primary function of those proteins?

a. Generate movement
b. Provide mechanical stability
c. Carry out nucleation of microtubules
d. Stabilize microtubules against disassembly
e. Transport organelles within the cell

42. A 20-year-old man arrives in the emergency room by ambulance. He has taken an overdose of "goofballs" (phenobarbital) which he obtained from a drug dealer on the street. In a hepatocyte from this patient, what is occurring in the organelle labeled with arrows in the accompanying transmission electron micrograph?

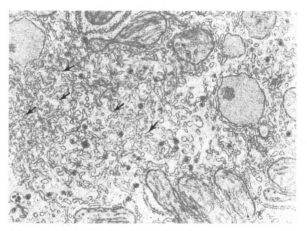

(Micrograph Courtesy of Dr. Robert Bolender.)

a. Oxidative demethylation
b. Decreased P450 expression
c. Decreased solubility of the phenobarbital
d. Increased synthesis of enzymes for detoxification
e. Destruction of the phenobarbital by acid hydrolases

43. About 3 years ago, a 39-year-old Caucasian man became increasingly uncoordinated. His wife describes bouts of depression and apathy beginning about a decade ago. Laboratory results are normal. MRI and CT reveal striatal and caudate atrophy with "boxcar ventricles." His mini-mental status examination score is 24/30. The cranial nerve examination shows dysarthria, saccadic extraocular eye movements, and a hyperactive gag reflex. There is increased tone in all extremities. Polymerase chain reaction reveals one normal band with 20 CAG (trinucleotide) repeats and the other with 49 CAG repeats. Modulation of respiration and mitochondrial membrane potential, and bioenergetic failure are associated with the abnormal gene in this disease. Which one of the following mechanisms used to establish the mitochondrial electrochemical gradient may be altered in this disease?

a. The action of ATP synthase
b. Transfer of electrons from NADH to O_2 in the intermembrane space
c. Pumping of protons into the mitochondrial matrix by respiratory chain activity
d. Proton-translocating activity in the inner membrane
e. Transport of ATP out of the matrix compartment by a specific transporter

44. A 15-month-old girl is referred for ophthalmologic and neurologic follow-up by her pediatrician. The child has shown a failure to thrive, is microcephalic, exhibits myoclonic jerks, delayed psychomotor development, visual disturbance, and seizures. Analysis of fibroblasts from the skin by electron microscopy confirms the presence of fingerprint inclusion bodies. Elevated levels of dolichol are found in the urine. Normally, dolichol is associated with which cellular process?

a. Sulfation in the *trans* compartment of the Golgi
b. O-linked glycosylation in the medial compartment of the Golgi
c. O-linked glycosylation in the *cis* compartment of the Golgi
d. N-linked glycosylation in the endoplasmic reticulum (ER)
e. Sorting of proteins to the lysosome from the *trans*-Golgi network (TGN)

45. A boy is born with epicanthal folds, a high forehead, hypoplastic supraorbital ridges, and upslanting palpebral fissures. He shows growth retardation following birth, feels like a rag doll when held, and exhibits neonatal seizures. He also has a ventricular septal defect, glaucoma, cataracts, elevated iron and copper levels in his blood, and hepatomegaly. A liver biopsy is prepared for electron microscopy and shows the presence of empty peroxisomes. The pathologist describes them as peroxisome "ghosts." Which one of the following cellular activities should be decreased in the hepatocytes from this patient?

a. Energy production
b. Plasmalogen synthesis
c. Exocytosis
d. Detoxification by the smooth endoplasmic reticulum (SER)
e. Lysosomal enzyme synthesis

46. Inhibition of actin assembly by cytochalasins would interfere primarily with which one of the following?

a. Separation of chromosomes in anaphase of the cell cycle
b. Vesicular transport between the Golgi apparatus and cell membrane
c. Ciliary movement
d. Phagocytic activity by macrophages
e. The structure of centrioles

47. A 53-year-old man with a body mass index of 30 is diagnosed with type II diabetes. Clinical studies have demonstrated that chloroquine improves glucose metabolism in such patients. Chloroquine is a weak base that neutralizes acidic organelles. In a pancreatic β cell, which one of the following would be a direct effect of chloroquine treatment?

a. Increased proinsulin content in secretory vesicles
b. Increased release of C peptide
c. Increased number of amylase-containing secretory vesicles
d. Reduced translation of glucagon mRNA
e. Increased stability of insulin mRNA

48. A 6-month-old infant is brought to the pediatric neurology clinic as a referral from a pediatrician concerned about the child's developmental delay, ataxia, hyperventilation, and repeated episodes of vomiting. The parents report one "seizure-like event." Examination reveals hypotonia, some spasticity, and deafness. Mild choreoathetosis is noted when the boy is attempting to move. Laboratory results show high lactate in the cerebrospinal fluid, a muscle biopsy shows normal histology, but tests reveal a deficiency in cytochrome c oxidase (COX), complex IV. In the electron micrograph below, where would one expect to find that enzyme localized?

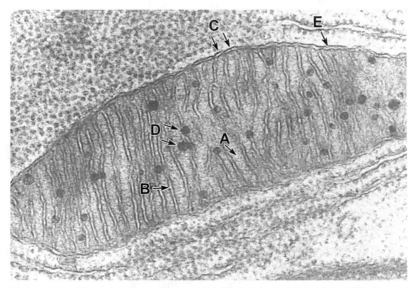

(Reproduced, with permission, from Fawcett DW. The Cell. 2nd ed. Philadelphia, PA: WB Saunders; 1981.)

a. A
b. B
c. C
d. D
e. E

49. A 22-year-old woman presents at the ophthalmology clinic. She describes an initial inability to drive at night because of what she describes as "night blindness." She says that the deterioration of her vision has continued and she is having difficulty seeing objects on the periphery of her vision. Visual acuity, color, visual field, dark adaptation, and electroretinogram (ERG) testing is completed. The tests show rod degeneration with limited peripheral vision. She has pigment deposits in the midperipheral retina known as "bone spicules." She also has attenuated vessels in the retina and paleness of the optic nerves. An ERG is reduced in amplitude. The cause may be related to a failure of opsin and other protein vesicle transport. This transport would occur along which one of the following?

a. Microfilaments (thin filaments)
b. Thick filaments
c. Microtubules
d. Intermediate filaments
e. Spectrin heterodimers

50. A 20-month-old girl presents with very salty-tasting skin; persistent coughing, at times with phlegm; frequent lung infections; wheezing and shortness of breath; poor growth/weight gain in spite of a good appetite; and frequent greasy, bulky stools and straining with bowel movements. She has a positive sweat test. She is diagnosed with the ΔF508 mutation resulting in the absence of the diacidic code regulating exit of a specific molecule from the ER to the Golgi. Which one of the following molecules links to the exit code and coats vesicles transported from the ER to the Golgi apparatus?

a. Clathrin
b. Spectrin
c. Ankyrin
d. Actin
e. Vimentin
f. COP-I
g. COP-II

51. A girl born to parents of eastern Mediterranean Jewish descent is brought to the pediatric neurology clinic. She appeared normal at birth and is now 6 months of age. There is a loss of peripheral vision and an abnormal startle response to auditory stimuli. She has suddenly shown a loss of coordination and has lost some responsiveness to her environment. She has a cherry-red spot on her macula. Treatments to cure this disease might focus on developing therapies that would do which one of the following?

a. Stimulate ganglioside GM2 production
b. Stimulate synthesis of GM2 by the rough endoplasmic reticulum (RER)
c. Stimulate hexosaminidase production
d. Stimulate transport of ganglioside GM2 to the lysosome
e. Remove mannose 6-phosphate from hexosaminidase

52. A 14-year-old adolescent presents with hepatic failure, slurred speech, tremors in the hands and feet, and Kayser-Fleischer rings. A 24-hour urine copper test is 120 µg/24 h (normal below 100 µg/24 h) and ceruloplasmin of 15 mg/dL (normal 25-50 mg/dL). Liver biopsy reveals 295 µg/g (normal <250 µg/g) dry weight of copper with microscopic changes including glycogen nuclei, microvesicular and macrovesicular fatty changes, steatosis and fibrosis. Genetic studies reveal mutations in the *ATP7B* gene which has been localized to the late endosome. Such mutations may alter the transport of cargo within late endosomes to which one of the following?

a. Lysosome for degradation
b. Clathrin-coated pits and vesicles
c. Multivesicular bodies (MVBs)
d. Cell surface to recycle receptors
e. TGN for further processing

53. A 72-year-old woman is brought to the office of her family medicine physician by her daughter. Her daughter indicates that mom has abrupt mood swings and uncharacteristic moments of anger and aggressiveness. She also "gets lost" on travel to routine destinations. The patient has recently been unwilling or unable to bathe or brush her teeth regularly and her hair and clothes are unkempt. She has lost 15 pounds since her last visit to her physician a year ago. While the patient denies any problems with memory or cognitive ability, her daughter reports episodes of forgetfulness and loss of concentration. The pathogenesis of the disease from which this patient suffers, involves the organelles labeled with asterisks in the accompanying electron micrograph. Which one of the following processes occurs abnormally in that structure during the progression of this patient's illness?

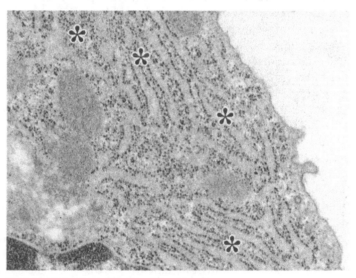

(Micrograph Courtesy of Dr. Kuen-Shan Hung.)

a. *O*-linked glycosylation
b. Sorting of tau proteins
c. Sulfation of amyloid precursor protein
d. Conformational changes and folding
e. Glycogenolysis

Cell Biology: Cytoplasm

Answers

37. The answer is a. (*Alberts, pp 984-987.*) Anti-vimentin is specific for mesenchymal cells such as fibroblasts, macrophages, endothelial cells, and smooth muscle of the vasculature. In the salivary glands, fibrous stromal tissue is derived from mesenchyme. The acini and ducts (**answers c, d, and e**) are epithelial in origin. The parasympathetic ganglia will stain with panneuronal markers such as peripherin (**answer b**). The type of intermediate filament protein is relatively specific for cells derived from the three embryonic germ layers. Antibodies to intermediate filament proteins are used by pathologists to determine the origin of tumors. Intermediate filament proteins have a structural role, but also are involved in the anchorage of the proteins that form ion channels. Cytokeratins (also known as keratins) are specific for epithelial cells. Neurofilament proteins (NFL, NFM, and NFH) are found in neurons. In Alzheimer disease, extensive plaques of neurofilament proteins occur. Desmin is found in striated and most smooth muscle, except vascular smooth muscle. Glial fibrillary acidic protein (GFAP) is specific for astrocytes, not microglia or oligodendrocytes.

38. The answer is c. (*Alberts, pp 373-376. Ross, p 46.*) The large subunit of the ribosome catalyzes peptide bond formation by activation of peptidyl transferase. The small ribosomal subunit contains the peptidyl-tRNA-binding (P) site that binds the tRNA molecule (**answer b**) attached to the carboxyl end of the growing end of the polypeptide chain. The small subunit also contains the aminoacyl-tRNA-binding (A) site that holds the incoming tRNA and amino acid. The initiation factors are loaded on the small ribosomal subunit that must locate the AUG (start) codon to initiate protein synthesis. This occurs before binding of the large subunit. In addition, the initiator tRNA containing methionine provides the amino acid necessary to start protein synthesis. The small ribosomal subunit with the tRNA containing methionine binds to the AUG codon on the mRNA (**answer a**). Therefore, the initiation phase of protein synthesis is regulated by the small subunit of the ribosome (**answer d**). Ribosomes are composed of both protein and RNA (predominantly rRNA, but also mRNA and tRNA). Single ribosomes are involved in synthesis of cytosolic proteins. Polyribosomes, linked by mRNA (**answer e**), synthesize proteins that are translocated into the cisternal space of the RER and destined for export or specific organelles.

39. The answer is d. (*Alberts, pp 1006-1009.*) The stability, arrangement, and functions of actin filaments depend on the actin-binding proteins (**answers a → c, e**). The fundamental structure of the actin molecule is the same no matter what the function or arrangement in a cell. Actin-binding proteins have a variety of functions: (1) tropomyosin strengthens actin filaments, (2) fibrin and villin are actin-bundling proteins, (3) filamin and gelsolin regulate transformation from the sol to the gel state, (4) members of the myosin II family are responsible for sliding filaments, (5) myosin I (minimyosin) is responsible for movement of vesicles on filaments, and (6) spectrin cross-links the sides of actin filaments to the plasma membrane.

40. The answer is d. (*Alberts, pp 751, 754-755. Ross, pp 48-51. Mescher, pp 33-35.*) The biochemically compartmentalized organelle, labeled with the arrows in the electron micrograph, is the Golgi apparatus. There is a specific organization to the Golgi stacks related to the function of specific enzymes. Histochemical stains, such as acid phosphatase and nucleoside diphosphates, show that the Golgi apparatus is topologically compartmentalized (**answer a**). It presents two faces: a *cis* face, which is the point of entry of transport vesicles (COP-II-coated, see Question 50) in transit from the RER to the Golgi (**answer b**), and a *trans* face, which is the exit point associated with granule formation and the maturation of proteins (**answer c**). Both proteins and lipids are transported from the transitional elements of the ER to the Golgi apparatus (**answer e**). Packaging is not the sole function of the Golgi. This organelle is also involved in the processing of proteins (eg, addition and trimming of oligosaccharide chains) that was initiated in the RER as well as sulfation. The patient in the vignette died from amyotrophic lateral sclerosis (ALS, Lou Gehrig disease).

41. The answer is b. (*Alberts, pp 1006-1009, 1010-1011, 1014. Ross, pp 57-58.*) The keratins are intermediate filament proteins. There are differences in the way that intermediate filaments interact with microtubules and microfilaments within the cytoplasm; however, their ropelike arrangement is well suited to provide mechanical stability to the cell and resisting stretch, allowing the cell to respond to tension. The different types of intermediate filaments all have a similar structural pattern: nonhelical head and tail segments with a helical arrangement in the center of the intermediate filament structure. The disease in the vignette is EBS, an inherited skin disorder caused by mutations in keratin 5 and keratin 14, with fragility of basal keratinocytes leading to epidermal cytolysis and blistering. Movement is generated by motor proteins (answer a) such as myosin, dynein, and kinesin. There is a good mnemonic device for remembering the direction of movement directed by kinesin and dynein. Kinesin kicks molecules out; dynein drags them in. The plus end of the microtubule is oriented toward the plasma membrane and the minus end toward the nucleus. This works for fibroblasts as well as neurons, to be discussed in a later chapter. Nucleation of microtubules is conducted by centrosomes (answer c); microtubule-associated proteins stabilize or destabilize microtubules (answer d). Microtubules function in organellar transport—for example, axonal transport (answer e).

42. The answer is a. (*Alberts, pp 723-725. Ross, pp 47-48.*) Oxidative metabolism by cytochrome P450 enzymes in hepatocytes is a primary mechanism for drug metabolism. Barbiturates are modified in the liver by oxidative demethylation through the P450 oxidase system found in the SER (the structure shown in the electron micrograph). The SER in hepatocytes responds to phenobarbital ingestion by increasing its volume. The proliferation (hypertrophy) of the SER facilitates metabolism of drugs. There is a concomitant increase in enzymatic activity (answer b), however, the synthesis of those enzymes occurs in the RER not in the SER (answer d). The purpose of drug metabolism is to make drugs more water soluble (answer c) so they can be more easily excreted from the liver through the bile. Increase in enzymatic activity following phenobarbital ingestion catalyzes reactions that increase the solubility of various xenobiotics including toxins, alcohol, steroids, eicosanoids, carcinogens, insecticides, and other environmental pollutants. Lysosomes, not the SER contain acid hydrolases (answer e). The P450 system and the SER are involved in drug interactions. Hepatocytes adapted to metabolize one drug may develop increased capability to metabolize other drugs. For example, if patients taking phenobarbital for epilepsy increase their alcohol intake, they may be ingesting subtherapeutic levels of the anti-seizure medication because of induction of SER in response to the alcohol.

43. The answer is d. (*Alberts, pp 815-818, 820, 826. Mescher, pp 25-27, 46. Ross, pp 52-54.*) The mitochondrial electrochemical gradient is established by a proton pump located in the inner membrane, associated with the respiratory chain and ATP synthase. The impermeability of the inner membrane to protons causes an osmotic and electrochemical gradient. Mitochondria produce energy that the cell uses in transport and other energy-dependent processes. Cellular energy is stored as ATP, synthesized by the phosphorylation of ADP by ATP synthase **(answer a)**. Mitochondria use the electron-transport (respiratory) chain that transfers energy from NADH to O_2 **(answer b)**. As electrons released by oxidation of substrate in the matrix flow down the respiratory chain, hydrogen ions are pumped into the intermembrane space **(answer c)**. Protons in the matrix drive ATP synthase in a mechanism similar to a waterwheel. ATP synthase, therefore, couples oxidative transport through the electron-transport (respiratory) chain with energy storage (ATP). ATP is not transported out of the matrix compartment by a specific transporter **(answer e)**. Atrophy of the caudate nucleus causes the expansion of the lateral ventricles to form "boxcar ventricles" characteristic of Huntington disease, a fatal, inherited neurodegenerative disorder with loss of memory, cognitive skills, and normal movements. The mutant Huntingtin gene encodes for the huntingtin protein which may cause mitochondrial dysfunction by perturbing transcription of nuclear encoded mitochondrial proteins or by directly modulating mitochondrial respiration, membrane potential, and Ca^{2+} buffering.

44. The answer is d. (*Alberts, pp 737-738, 780-781. Mole, pp 70-76.*) The patient is suffering from the infantile form of Batten disease, neuronal ceroid lipofuscinoses, in which there is a buildup of lipofuscin because of the absence of specific lysosomal enzymes. Dolichol is normally associated with N-linked glycosylation in the RER an en bloc method in which dolichol is added to the protein. O-linked glycosylation occurs in the Golgi, by a mechanism involving oligosaccharide (glycosyl) transferases rather than en bloc with dolichol **(answers b and c).** N-linked oligosaccharides are the most common oligosaccharides found in glycoproteins and contain sugar residues linked to the NH_2 amide nitrogen of asparagine. O-linked oligosaccharides have sugar residues linked to hydroxyl groups on the side chains of serine and threonine. The diversity in oligosaccharides is produced by selective removal of glucose and mannose from the core oligosaccharide. This trimming process begins in the RER before reaching the Golgi, where the final mannose-residue trimming occurs. Sulfation (answer a) and protein sorting (answer e) are carried out in the Golgi apparatus, but do not involve dolichol.

45. The answer is b. (*Alberts, pp 721-723. Ross, p 55. Mescher, p 40.*) The child suffers from Zellweger syndrome, in which peroxisomes are empty. Peroxisomes are the sole site of plasmalogen synthesis. Plasmalogen is a group of glycerol-based phospholipids in which the aliphatic side chains are not attached by ester linkages. They have a widespread distribution with highest concentrations in the brain, spinal cord, liver, and kidney. Energy production (answer a), exocytosis (answer c), detoxification (answer d), and the synthesis of lysosomal enzymes (answer e) would not be as affected in that disease. In Zellweger syndrome, peroxisomes are empty because of the failure of the signal system that sorts protein to the peroxisome. Because the peroxisome lacks a genome (DNA) or synthetic machinery (ribosomes), it must import all proteins. The defect appears to be in the peroxisomal membrane (peroxins), but errors or absence of the peroxisomal signal sequence would result in the same symptoms. Peroxisomes have only a single membrane around them and contain catalase. Peroxisomes carry out oxidation reactions to protect the cell. Those oxidation reactions remove hydrogen atoms from molecules like alcohol and phenols to form hydrogen peroxide. In the peroxidative reaction, catalase breaks down hydrogen peroxide to water and oxygen. Most of the alcohol humans consume is broken down by alcohol dehydrogenase (ADH) and microsomal ethanol-oxidizing system (MEOS, ie, P450 cytochrome) pathways in the hepatocyte (liver cell) cytoplasm. The remaining small percentage is broken down by oxidation in the peroxisomes of hepatocytes using catalase. See High-Yield Facts, Gastrointestinal Tract and Glands, for more information on alcohol metabolism.

46. The answer is d. (*Alberts, pp 988, 1054-1056, 1089-1090, 1092-1094.*) Cytochalasins are potent inhibitors of cell motility and other cellular events that depend on actin assembly: cytokinesis, which is conducted by the actin-containing contractile ring; phagocytosis; and formation of lamellipodia. Cytochalasins bind to the plus end of actin filaments and prevent further polymerization. The movement of chromosomes in anaphase of the cell cycle depends on disassembly of microtubules at the kinetochore in anaphase A and addition at the plus end of the polar microtubules in anaphase B **(answer a)**. Ciliary movement, vesicular transport, and the structure of centrioles depend on microtubules **(answers b, c, and e)**.

47. The answer is a. (*Alberts, pp 151-152, 780, 781.*) Chloroquine neutralizes acidic compartments such as the secretory vesicles. Chloroquine treatment inhibits the conversion of proinsulin to insulin, resulting in decreased formation of insulin within secretory vesicles of the pancreatic β cells. Acidification causes concentration of the contents of secretory vesicles, facilitates breakdown of the contents of phagosomes and lysosomes, and is involved in the cleavage of prohormones to their active forms (eg, proinsulin to insulin). The acidification process functions through a vacuolar H^+ (proton) pump that is present in the membranes of most endocytic and exocytic vesicles, including those of phagosomes, lysosomes, secretory vesicles, and some compartments of the Golgi. Ribosomes are not dependent on a proton pump mechanism and are, therefore, less sensitive to chloroquine. Proinsulin is split into C peptide and insulin in secretory vesicles **(answer b)**. In vivo, C-peptide release can be used to measure production of insulin by a patient's pancreatic β cells. This is particularly useful in patients who are receiving insulin. Glucagon is synthesized by α cells **(answer d)**, and amylase is an exocrine pancreatic product produced by the acinar cells **(answer c)**. Gene and message expression and message stability are also not targets for chloroquine **(answers d and e)**.

48. The answer is b. (*Alberts, pp 815-817, 818, 826-827. Mescher, pp 25-27.*) The structure labeled **B** is the inner membrane of the mitochondrion, which is highly impermeable to small ions because of the presence of cardiolipin. The inner membrane contains the proteins required for the oxidative reactions of the respiratory transport chain; it is the location of the cytochromes, dehydrogenases, and flavoproteins including cytochrome *c* as well as the transmembrane complex (ATP synthase) that is responsible for ATP synthesis. The inner membrane is folded into convolutions called cristae. The number of cristae is directly related to the metabolic activity of the cell. The elementary particles that have been identified on the cristae are composed primarily of ATP synthase complexes. The patient in the vignette is suffering from Leigh disease (subacute necrotizing encephalomyelopathy), a generalized (systemic) form of COX deficiency, characterized by progressive degeneration of the brain and dysfunction of the heart, kidneys, muscles, and liver. Symptoms include loss of acquired motor skills and loss of appetite, vomiting, irritability, and/or seizure activity. As Leigh disease progresses, symptoms include generalized weakness; loss of muscle tone (hypotonia); and/or episodes of lactic acidosis with lactate higher in the CSF than the blood. The region labeled **A** in the electron micrograph of the mitochondrion is the mitochondrial matrix, or intercristal space. The matrix contains the circular DNA of the mitochondrial genome. Most mitochondrial proteins are encoded for by nuclear DNA, but small proportions are encoded within the mitochondrial DNA and are synthesized on mitochondrial ribosomes. The matrix also contains the enzymes responsible for the Krebs (citric acid) cycle. The outer mitochondrial membrane, labeled **C**, is highly permeable to molecules 10,000 Da or less because of the presence of porin, a channel-forming protein. This membrane contains enzymes involved in lipid synthesis and lipid metabolism. Matrix granules represent accumulations of calcium ions **(D)**. The outer membrane also mediates the movement of fatty acids into the mitochondria for use in the formation of acetyl CoA. The intermembrane space **(E)** is the site of cytochrome b and other unique proteins.

49. The answer is c. (*Alberts, pp 917-919, 985. Rubin, pp 1518, 1519. Kumar, p 431. Mescher, pp 418-420, 427.*) The woman in the scenario suffers from retinitis pigmentosa. Vesicles and organelles move unidirectionally along microtubules from the inner segment to the outer segment of the photoreceptor. Opsin, which is needed to sense light, is transported to sites of utilization in the disks of the outer segment. Transport occurs through the connecting, nonmotile cilium, driven by the microtubule motor, kinesin, an ATPase. Microtubules are composed of tubulin and are involved in motility as the principal protein in the composition of the axoneme (the core of the cilium or flagellum). Microfilaments (thin filaments) are composed of actin, the most abundant protein in cells of eukaryotes **(answer a)**. They are involved in cell motility and changes in cell shape. Myosin is the main constituent of the thick filament **(answer b)** that binds to actin and functions as an ATPase activated by actin. Intermediate filaments **(answer d)** that are "intermediate" in diameter (8-10 nm) between thin and thick filaments are of five different types. Type I and type II are the acidic and basic keratins (cytokeratins), respectively, and are found specifically in epithelial cells. Type III intermediate filaments are composed of vimentin, desmin, and GFAP. Vimentin is found in cells of mesenchymal origin, desmin in muscle cells, and GFAP in astrocytes. Type IV intermediate filaments are neurofilament proteins found in neurons. Type V intermediate filaments include the nuclear lamins A, B, and C and are associated with nuclear lamina of all cells. Spectrin heterodimers stabilize the plasma membrane and connect the membrane to actin **(answer e)**.

50. The answer is g. *(Alberts, pp 646-648, 751, 754, 966-970.)* COP-II is the coat protein for vesicles transported in an anterograde direction from the RER → Golgi. Clathrin is an important protein that forms the coating of secretory vesicles transported from the TGN to targets and coated pits and vesicles involved in endocytosis **(answer a)**. It is involved in the retrieval of membrane following exocytosis. Spectrin heterodimers **(answer b)** form tetramers that interact with actin and provide flexibility and support for the membrane. The protein ankyrin **(answer c)** "anchors" the band 3 protein to the spectrin-membrane skeleton indirectly binding band 3 protein to the cytoskeleton (spectrin tetramers) of the red blood cell (RBC). The band 3 protein is known to be an anion transport protein of the RBC. Actin **(answer d)** is the protein found in thin filaments in the RBC cytoplasm. Intermediate filaments are important cytoskeletal elements with specificity that depends on the origin of the cells in question. Vimentin **(answer e)** is the specific intermediate filament protein found in cells derived from mesenchyme, for example, fibroblasts and chondrocytes. COP-I (COat Protein-I) coats vesicles involved in retrograde transport from Golgi → RER **(answer f)**.

51. The answer is c. *(Ross, p 44. Fauci, p 2453. Kumar, pp 150-152. Rubin, pp 254-255.)* The child in the scenario suffers from Tay-Sachs disease, a lysosomal storage disease. Lysosomes contain an array of specific hydrolases. In Tay-Sachs disease, hexosaminidase A is deficient, resulting in the buildup of GM2 ganglioside in lysosomes leading to mental retardation, blindness, and mortality. A pharmacological approach would target reducing GM2 ganglioside levels by increasing hexosaminidase A activity **(answer c)**. Increase in GM2 levels **(answers a and b)** or increased transport **(answer d)** to a lysosome deficient in hexosaminidase would worsen the disease. The table on the next page summarizes the enzyme deficiencies and resulting effects in some of the more prominent lysosomal disorders. Mannose 6-phosphate and its receptor are involved in the trafficking of proteins to the lysosomal compartment. Removal of mannose 6-phosphate **(answer e)**, as occurs in inclusion-cell (I-cell) disease, would result in default of lysosomal enzymes to the secretory pathway, and the hexosaminidase deficiency would worsen.

LYSOSOMAL STORAGE DISEASES

Disease	Enzyme Deficit	Cellular Site	Accumulation	Organ Most Affected
Tay-Sachs	β-N-hexosaminidase-A	Neurons	Glycolipid	CNS
Gaucher	β-D-glycosidase	Macrophages	Glycolipid	Spleen, liver
Hurler	α-L-iduronidase	Fibroblasts, chondroblasts, osteoblasts	Dermatan sulfate	Skeletal system
Niemann-Pick	Sphingomyelinase	Oligodendrocytes, fibroblasts	Sphingomyelin	CNS
Inclusion (I)–cell	N-acetylglucosamine-phosphotransferase	Fibroblasts, macrophages	Glycoproteins and glycolipids	Nervous and skeletal systems (liver unaffected)

52. The answer is a. (*Alberts, pp 742-743, pp 13-35. Rubin, pp 785-787. Kumar, pp 910-911. Fauci, pp 1981-1982.*) The patient in the scenario suffers from Wilson disease in which copper accumulates in the tissues. For example, in the liver the mutation in *ATP7B* prevents translocation of copper from the cytosol to the late endosome blocking biliary copper excretion via lysosomes and resulting in accumulation of copper. The late endosome is part of the endocytic pathway. Cargo proteins from the late endosome reach the lysosome by development into lysosomes, transport to lysosomes via vesicles, or fusion with lysosomes. Clathrin-coated pits and vesicles (**answer b**) endocytose and subsequently deliver proteins to the early endosome in the first stages of the endocytic process. MVBs are the means of transport from early to late endosomes (**answer c**). The CGN (*cis*-Golgi network) receives transitional elements in the form of coatomer-coated vesicles carrying proteins and lipids from the RER and participates in phosphorylation. The remaining Golgi stacks are the *cis*, medial, *trans*, and TGN. The medial compartment is responsible for the removal of mannose and the addition of N-acetylglucosamine. The *trans* face is responsible for the addition of sialic acid and galactose. The TGN serves as a sorting station for proteins destined for various organelles (eg, lysosomes), the plasma membrane, and protein for export from the cell (**answer e**). Golgi-derived transport and secretory vesicles bud off from the TGN. Recycling of receptors occurs from early endosomes to the plasma membrane (**answer d**).

53. The answer is d. (*Mescher, pp 28-30.*) The predominant organelle in the transmission electron micrograph is the RER. Different proteins display different rates of folding in the ER, and those rates determine the time required for transport to the cell surface. Within the ER there are protein chaperones and mechanisms to prevent aberrant protein folding and to catalyze isomerization of correct covalent bonds. Frequently, changes in the extracellular environment result in aberrant protein folding in the ER as occurs in Alzheimer disease from which the patient in the vignette suffers. O-linked glycosylation, sorting of proteins and sulfation (**answers a, b, and c**) occur in the Golgi apparatus and glycogenolysis (**answer e**) occurs in the SER.

Cell Biology: Intracellular Trafficking

Questions

54. A 56-year-old man has been taking atorvastatin because of a poor lipid profile and a family history of cardiovascular disease. The statin family of drugs enhances endocytosis of low density lipoprotein (LDL) from the serum. Endocytosis of LDL differs from phagocytosis of damaged cells in which one of the following ways?

a. Use of membrane-enclosed vesicles in the uptake process
b. Coupling with the lysosomal system
c. Dependence on acidification
d. Use of clathrin-coated pits
e. Use of hydrolases

55. A 21-year-old woman with a history of thin, hyperextensible skin with easy bruising, subcutaneous hematomas, atrophic scarring with large "cigarette paper scars," generalized tissue fragility, and joint hypermobility is referred to the Genetics and Metabolism Division of the Internal Medicine Department. Mutations are found in the *COL5A1* gene in a region specifically encoding the signal peptide domain of preproα1(V)-collagen chain. Which one of the following will directly result from this loss of function mutation?

a. Inability of the peptide to exit the endoplasmic reticulum lumen after translocation
b. Failure of preprotein translocation into the endoplasmic reticulum
c. Directing of preproα1(V)-collagen from the Golgi apparatus to the endoplasmic reticulum (ER)
d. Sorting to the lysosomes
e. Increased release of collagen
f. Inhibition of collagen cross-linking

56. A 65-year-old man presents to the neurology clinic with a several year history in which he has less and less energy and spontaneity, memory loss (especially recent events), and mood swings. He is described by his wife as uncharacteristically slow to learn and react, confused, getting lost easily, exercising poor judgment, and shying away from anything new—preferring the familiar. He scores poorly on the mini-mental status examination. This disease is believed to be caused by protein misfolding. Chaperonins regulate protein folding in which of the following ways?

a. Stimulating aggregation of proteins
b. Contributing folding information to the native protein
c. Controlling the docking of the signal peptide with its receptor on the rough endoplasmic reticulum (RER)
d. Inhibiting proteolytic activity of misfolded proteins
e. Using their ATPase activity to bind and release themselves from hydrophobic regions of the protein

57. A 23-year-old man who is allergic to peanuts has a plain vanilla ice-cream cone at a local ice-cream store. Unfortunately, the server did not sufficiently clean the scoop after serving a cup of peanut brittle ice cream. The young man begins to have an allergic reaction and reaches for his inhalator filled with albuterol, a β-adrenergic drug that binds to β-receptors on the cells of the respiratory airways. The figure below shows the mechanism involved in binding of albuterol to its receptor. Which one of the following statements regarding the molecule labeled "B" in the diagram is true?

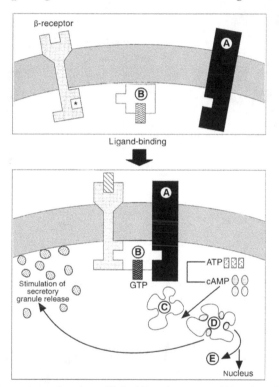

(Modified, with permission, from Avery JK. Oral Development and Histology. 3rd ed. New York, NY: Thieme Medical; 2001.)

a. It is the inactive cyclic AMP (cAMP) kinase.
b. It lacks GTPase activity.
c. It inactivates adenylate cyclase.
d. It is bound to GTP in the inactive state.
e. It is the stimulatory G protein (G_s).

58. A 32-year-old (gravida 2, para 2) woman who gave birth to a baby girl 24 hours before is having difficulty urinating and is retaining urine in her bladder. She is given bethanechol, a muscarinic agonist, which is the ligand shown in the figure below. Which one of the following is the function of molecule A?

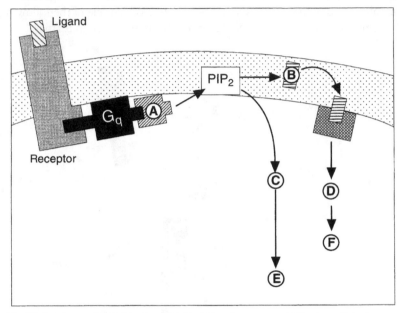

(Modified, with permission, from Avery JK. Oral Development and Histology. 3rd ed. New York, NY: Thieme Medical; 2001.)

a. Directly activates protein kinase C
b. Binds to the ER
c. Hydrolysis of PIP_2 to form diacylglycerol (DAG) and inositol triphosphate (IP_3)
d. Stimulation of inhibitory G protein (G_i) activity through phosphorylation of phosphatidylinositol 4,5-bisphosphate (PIP_2)
e. Stimulation of G_S activity through phosphorylation of PIP_2

59. The two major secretory pathways A → B → C → D (pathway I) and C → E (pathway II) are illustrated in the figure. Albumin secretion by hepatocytes occurs by pathway II. In a patient with cirrhosis, the serum levels of albumin are reduced. Which one of the following is the most likely cause of the reduced secretion of albumin?

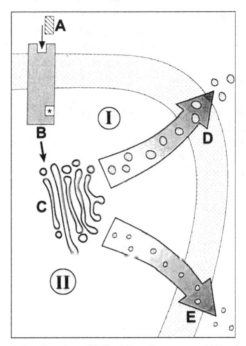

(Modified, with permission, from Avery JK. Oral Development and Histology. 3rd ed. New York, NY: Thieme Medical; 2001.)

a. Reduced binding of "A" to receptors
b. Reduced numbers of functional hepatocytes
c. Down-regulation of "B" on hepatocytes
d. Reduced activity of the cAMP-activated signal transduction system
e. Increased cAMP levels

60. A 6-month-old infant is brought into the pediatric clinic. He weighs 12 lb, 2 oz and is 22 in long. Neither his length nor his weight is on the growth chart for his age; mean weight and height for a 6-month-old are 17 lb, 4 oz and 26.5 in, respectively. Through functional tests, you determine that he is suffering from an inherited condition known as I (inclusion)-cell disease and missing N-acetylglucosamine: undine diphospo (UDP)-N-acetylglucosamine-1-phosphotransferase, which is more conveniently referred to as phosphotransferase. The phosphotransferase enzymes phosphorylate mannose to form mannose 6-phosphate. Electron microscopy is performed on a biopsy, and blood tests are completed. Which one of the following explains the altered cell biological processes in this patient?

a. Lysosomal enzymes missorted back to the Golgi apparatus
b. Peroxisomal proteins missorted to other organelles
c. Abnormal KDEL sequence on vesicles
d. Absence of soluble-N-ethylmaleimide sensitive factor (NSF) attachment protein receptors (SNARE) proteins on vesicles
e. Secretion of lysosomal enzymes into the blood

Cell Biology: Intracellular Trafficking

Answers

54. The answer is d. *(Alberts, pp 789, 791-792.)* Receptor-mediated endocytosis of ligand-receptor complexes is a selective process that requires invagination of the cell membrane to form clathrin-coated pits and vesicles. Clathrin is not involved in phagocytosis. Phagocytosis of damaged cells occurs by evagination to engulf the IgG-coated surface of the target. Both processes use acidification of compartments and hydrolases to uncouple receptor and ligand (receptor-mediated endocytosis) or destroy engulfed material (phagocytosis). Both processes use membrane-enclosed vesicles and are associated with hydrolases and lysosomal activity **(answers a, b, c, and e).**

LDL is the form in which most cholesterol is transported in the blood; cellular uptake of LDL is the classic example of receptor-mediated endocytosis. The receptors are bound to clathrin-coated pits, but the ligand is only directly bound to its cell surface receptor. The LDL-LDL receptor (ligand-receptor) complexes are incorporated into the cell in coated vesicles. The acidic environment of the endosome results in the cleavage of the ligand from its receptor (ie, LDL from its receptor). The LDL receptors are recycled to the membrane for additional exposure to LDL, and the LDL in the endosome is transferred to lysosomes, where it is broken down to cholesterol.

The statins inhibit 3-hydroxy-3-methylglutaryl coenzyme A (HMG-CoA) reductase, thereby blocking hepatic cholesterol synthesis. The decrease in cholesterol synthesis leads to activation of the LDL receptor gene, increased numbers of LDL receptors, enhanced endocytosis of blood LDL, and lower blood LDL levels. Other ligands differ in subtle ways from LDL in their endocytic pathways.

55. The answer is b. *(Alberts, pp 726-730.)* The signal peptide is a key element of the signal hypothesis and is necessary for preprotein translocation into the cisterna of the ER. The signal peptide is present on proteins that are destined either to be secreted or to be membrane components. It is usually at the N-terminus and is normally absent from the mature protein. It interacts with the signal recognition particle (SRP) and directs the ribosome to the ER where co-translational insertion takes place. It is highly hydrophobic, but with some positively charged residues. The signal sequence is normally removed from the growing peptide chain by signal peptidase, a specific protease located on the cisternal face of the RER. Proteins with a KDEL (lys-asp-glu-leu) sequence on the C-terminus are retained in the RER or are routed back to the RER via interaction with the KDEL receptor in the Golgi apparatus (answers a and c). Sorting to lysosomes is regulated by mannose-6-phosphate receptors (answer d). Collagen release and cross-linking (answers e and f) are not directly regulated by the signal peptide.The patient in the vignette has Ehlers-Danlos syndrome (EDS), classic type, a connective tissue disorder characterized by skin hyperextensibility, abnormal wound healing, and joint hypermobility.

56. The answer is e. (Alberts, pp 388-389, 396-397.) The patient in the scenario suffers from Alzheimer disease which is related to protein misfolding leading to neurofibrillary tangles. Three-dimensional folding is required for functional activity of proteins. Native folding of a protein is encoded in its amino acid sequence; however, protein folding inside cells requires molecular chaperones binding and releasing themselves from hydrophobic regions of the newly synthesized protein and ATP to reach their native folded state. Various molecular chaperones protect nonnative protein chains from misfolding and aggregation (answer a), but do not contribute conformational information to the folding process (answer b). Many molecular chaperones are also stress- or heat-shock proteins that stabilize preproteins for membrane translocation, present misfolded proteins for proteolysis (answer d), and regulate the conformation of signaling molecules. The underlying principle in all these functions is the recognition by molecular chaperones of proteins in their nonnative states. Molecular chaperones also inhibit the formation of partially folded intermediates and in conjunction with calreticulin monitor the progress of folding, and ensure that only properly folded proteins are secreted from the cell or shipped to lysosomes. It is hypothesized that this level of ER "quality control" is absent in Alzheimer and other neurodegenerative diseases. Molecular chaperones assist with translocation of proteins across internal membranes (eg, mitochondria) by maintaining precursor proteins in their unfolded state during membrane trafficking. They do not function in the docking of the signal peptide (answer c).

57. The answer is e. *(Alberts, pp 905-907, 919. Mescher, pp 23-25.)* Albuterol binds to the β-receptor initiating a cAMP signal transduction cascade. The structure labeled B is the G_S. The figure illustrates the response of the β-adrenergic receptor to ligand binding. β-Receptors mediate the tissue effects of epinephrine and norepinephrine and respond to pharmacological agents such as albuterol, a β-adrenergic agonist. Signal transduction following ligand binding involves a specific G protein (shorthand for guanosine-triphosphate [GTP]–binding regulatory protein). G proteins associated with increasing cAMP levels in the cell are known as G_S because of their role in enzyme activation. In the inactive state, G_S is bound to GDP. After ligand binding, a G_S binding site is exposed and the G_S protein binds to the β-receptor. The resulting complex is capable of binding GTP in exchange for GDP, activating the G protein. The α-subunit of the activated G_S protein exchanges GDP for GTP and activates adenylate cyclase (**A** in the figure). Intrinsic GTPase activity of the α-subunit is increased resulting in a short activation time for the complex and recycling of the subunits to the inactive state. The inactive cAMP-dependent kinase (PKA) is labeled **C** in the figure. PKA is activated by dissociation of the regulatory subunits leading to activated PKA (**D**). The phosphorylating action of cAMP-dependent protein kinase (kinase A), stimulated by increased intracellular cAMP concentration, affects many aspects of intracellular metabolism and function. Phosphorylation (**E**) stimulates exocytosis and induces nuclear changes, including transcriptional events. The star in the figure delineates the site of ligand-binding-induced conformational change, exposing the G_S-binding site. (See High-Yield Facts Table 6 for a summary of G proteins.)

58. The answer is c. *(Alberts, pp 909-912.)* Bethanechol binds to muscarinic receptors. Molecule A in the figure is phospholipase C that catalyzes the formation of DAG and IP_3 from PIP_2. The phosphoinositide (PI) cycle illustrated in the figure is based on the formation of PIP_2 in the inner leaflet of the plasma membrane. Breakdown of PIP_2 leads to the formation of the key functional agents of the PI cycle. Binding of a ligand to its G protein-linked receptor on the cell surface (Gq) activates a phosphoinositide-specific phospholipase C. PI-specific phospholipase C hydrolyzes PIP_2 to form DAG and IP_3. Those two molecules function differently to regulate intracellular function. IP_3 functions in the mobilization of calcium, while DAG activates protein kinase C (**answer a**), leading to multiple phosphorylations of cytosolic proteins. DAG (**B** in the figure) activates protein kinase C (so called because of its Ca^{2+} dependency), which is labeled **D**. The protein kinase C phosphorylates **(F)** specific serine and threonine residues and may alter gene transcription. In contrast, IP_3 functions to mobilize Ca^{2+} by binding to IP_3-gated channels in the ER membrane **(answer b)**. The two intracellular messenger pathways do interact in that elevated Ca^{2+} translocates protein kinase C from the cytosol to the inner leaflet of the plasma membrane. G_i **(answer d)** is the inhibitory G protein that leads to 5'-AMP production through the action of phosphodiesterase instead of cAMP. G_s is involved in adenylate cyclase signal transduction **(answer e)**.

59. The answer is b. (*Alberts, pp 799-800.*) Cirrhosis damages hepatocytes leading to a reduction in synthesis of serum proteins. Pathway II on the diagram (C → E) is the constitutive (default) pathway, used by fibroblasts for synthesis of proteoglycans, fibronectin, and collagen; serum proteins (albumin, transferrin, and lipoprotein) synthesized by hepatocytes; and plasma-cell-derived immunoglobulins. Pathway I (A → D) is the regulated pathway. It differs from constitutive secretion (C → E) in its requirement for a secretagogue (substance that induces secretion from cells [**answers a and c**]), which binds to a cell-surface receptor. Secretion in the constitutive pathway is not regulated at the level of second messengers **(answers d and e)**. Regulated secretion (pathway I) requires recognition of a receptor **(B)** for its ligand (**A**, resulting in secretagogue-receptor binding). The synthetic processes in the two pathways are similar until the Golgi. The vesicles that bud from the Golgi **(D)** in the regulated pathway are clathrin-coated and contain a receptor involved in the concentration of secretory product. The constitutive pathway shuttles proteins such as integral membrane proteins and lipids in vesicles to the apical and basolateral membranes. The vesicles are nonclathrin-coated in the constitutive pathway. Exocytosis requires vesicle fusion with the membrane in both regulated and constitutive pathways. Ras-superfamily GTPases, members of the protein kinase D family and tethering complexes, like the exocyst that link to microtubules, are involved in constitutive secretion.

60. The answer is e. (*Alberts, pp 721-723, 760, 762-764, 770, 783-786. Mescher, pp 35, 39, 46.*) The child is suffering from inclusion (I)-cell disease (Mucolipidosis type II [ML II]). There is an absence or deficiency of N-acetylglucosamine phosphotransferase and an absence of mannose 6-phosphate

(M6P) on the lysosomal enzymes. The failure to add M6P in the *cis*-Golgi results in inappropriate vesicular segregation by M6P receptors in the *trans*-Golgi network (TGN). The default pathway is transport to the cell membrane and secretion from the cell by exocytosis for proteins lacking M6P. Lysosomal enzymes are secreted into the bloodstream, and undigested substrates build up within the cells. There is no missorting back to the Golgi (**answer a**). Peroxisomal enzymes, which are sorted by the presence of three specific amino acids located at the C-terminus: Ser–Lys–Leu–COO⁻, are not affected (**answer b**). KDEL (**answer c**) is the signal used for retrieval of proteins from the Golgi back to the endoplasmic reticulum. SNAREs are the receptors for SNAPs (soluble-N-ethylmaleimide sensitive factor [NSF] attachment proteins) and bind vesicles to membranes (**answer d**). Trafficking to other structures, such as the nucleus and mitochondria, is regulated by nuclear localization signals (NLSs) or an N-terminal signal peptide, respectively.

Cell Biology: Nucleus

Questions

61. A newborn boy is born with first arch congenital malformations classified as Treacher Collins syndrome, an autosomal dominant inherited disorder. The Treacher Collins-Franceschetti syndrome 1 (*TCOF*) gene encodes the protein treacle. Treacle is localized to the structure labeled with the arrows in the accompanying transmission electron micrograph. Treacle is most likely involved in which one of the following?

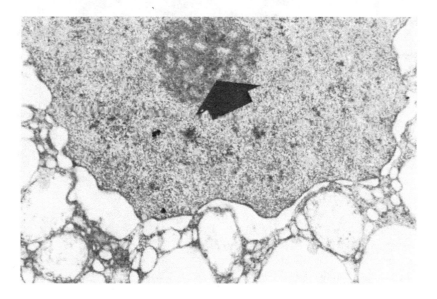

a. Assembly of ribosomal subunits into mature ribosomes
b. Translation of cytosolic proteins
c. Transcription of nuclear proteins
d. Transcription of ribosomal proteins
e. Organelle degradation

62. Dolastatin 11 is a promising chemotherapeutic depsipeptide that arrests mitotic cells in the process shown in the accompanying electron micrograph. Which one of the following would be a possible mechanism for Dolastatin?

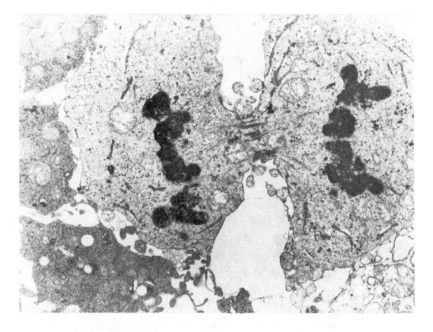

a. Lengthening of kinetochore microtubules
b. Contraction of a ring composed of cytoskeletal elements
c. Shortening of polar microtubules
d. Dysregulation of the M-Cdk complex (MPF)
e. Inhibition of antitubulin antibodies
f. Increased production of tubulin
g. Disruption and rearrangement of cellular actin

63. A 29-year-old woman presents with a 101°F fever, pericardial effusions and Libman-Sacks endocarditis, arthralgias, and facial rash across the malar region ("butterfly rash") that is accentuated by sun exposure. Laboratory tests show creatinine 1.7 mg/dL (normal 0.5–1.1 mg/dL), high titers of antinuclear autoantibodies (ANA), Smith antigen, and antinucleosome antibodies in the serum. Which one of the following is most likely to be directly affected by the disruption of nucleosomes in this patient?

a. Packaging of genetic material in a condensed form
b. Transcribing DNA
c. Forming pores for bilateral nuclear-to-cytoplasmic transport
d. Forming the nuclear matrix
e. Holding together adjacent chromatids

64. A G_1 phase and an M-phase cell are fused together with a Sendai virus. The result is that the chromosomes in the G_1-phase cell condense. Which of the following would be the best possible cell biological explanation?

a. Lamins will be phosphorylated in the G_1 cell.
b. The S-phase activator will be expressed in the M-phase cell.
c. The M-phase cell will reduplicate its DNA.
d. The G_1/S-Cdk complex will be activated in the M-phase cell.
e. A re-replication block will occur in the G_1-phase cell.

65. A middle-aged anatomy professor attends the hottest Indianapolis 500 race in decades and sits with the sun facing him; there is no breeze. He has a history of borderline high uric acid. Dehydration during the race triggers uric acid crystal formation in his foot. The foot becomes sore, red, hot, and swollen. He drinks about 2 L of water and soda at the race and two more liters at home. However, he is anuric for 10 to 12 hours. His physician prescribes colchicine as an anti-inflammatory. A metaphase-blocking dose of colchicine functions through which one of the following mechanisms?

a. Depolymerization of actin
b. Depolymerization of myosin
c. Enhancement of tubulin polymerization
d. Inhibition of tubulin polymerization
e. Binding to and stabilizing microtubules

66. A 29-year-old man is confined to a wheelchair with a diagnosis of Friedreich ataxia. He suffers from cardiomyopathy and cardiac failure. Gate ataxia occurred at age 14 which worsened and spread to his arms and trunk. He developed overall muscle weakness and loss of tendon reflexes in his knees and ankles with gradual loss of sensation in both extremities. About 6 years ago he presented with dysarthria, nystagmus, and scoliosis. Friedreich ataxia is caused by DNA triplet-repeat expansions leading to silencing of the frataxin (*FXN*) gene. The process of gene silencing associated with repetitive DNA sequences is associated with which region (A → E) on the accompanying transmission electron micrograph?

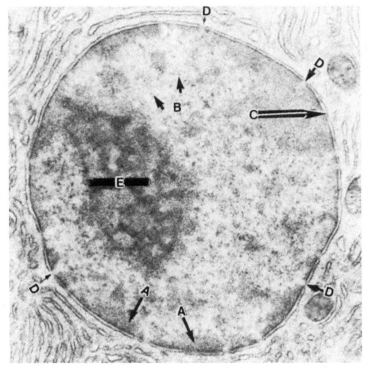

(Reproduced, with permission, from Fawcett DW. A Textbook of Histology. 11th ed. Philadelphia, PA: WB Saunders; 1986.)

a. A
b. B
c. C
d. D
e. E

67. A 55-year-old man with difficulty urinating, blood in the urine, burning during urination, and accelerating prostate-specific antigen (PSA) has a radical prostatectomy. The diagnosis is prostate carcinoma with a Gleason score of 7. Rb, p53, and bcl-2 genes are involved in the development of prostate carcinoma. Which one of the following mechanisms may be involved in the loss of cell cycle control that occurs in prostate carcinoma?

a. Increased CdkI activity
b. Decreased transcription of G_1/S cyclin
c. Decreased expression of bcl-2
d. Increased transcription of gene regulatory proteins such as E2F
e. Dephosphorylation of Rb

68. A 32-year-old man and his 30-year-old wife are referred for a reproductive endocrinology infertility (REI) consult after 2 years of trying to "get pregnant." He is diagnosed with oligozoospermia. Ejaculated mature sperm are collected and analyzed for genetic analysis. Using genetic linkage analysis, his REI specialist determines that he has aberrations in spermatogenic meiotic recombination, including both diminished frequency and suboptimal location, resulting in a high frequency of aneuploid sperm. In the explanation of the problem, she explains meiosis and recombination attributing the problem to a specific phase of meiosis. Which phase of meiosis is most closely associated with recombination?

a. Leptotene
b. Zygotene
c. Pachytene
d. Diplotene
e. Diakinesis

69. A 43-year-old (gravida 2, para 2) pregnant woman requests chorionic villus sampling (CVS) and a karyotype of her fetus because of concerns about Down syndrome. Chorionic villus cells reveal the following karyotype:

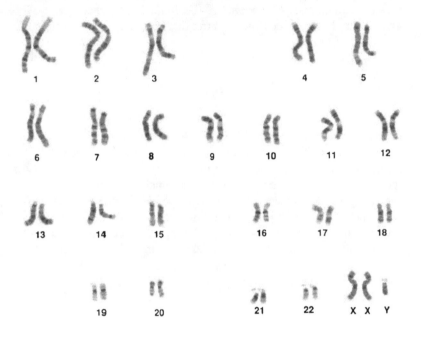

With this karyotype from CVS, discussion of the results with a genetic counselor would include which one of the following?

a. Normal child
b. Male with mild to moderate learning problems and infertility
c. Female with mild to moderate learning problems and delayed puberty
d. Generally normal male, however some degree of short stature and precocious puberty
e. Generally normal female, however some degree of short stature and infertility

70. A 20-month-old boy is diagnosed with Hutchinson-Gilford progerial syndrome (HGPS), a severe form of early-onset premature aging. Fetal and early postnatal development are normal, but there is now severe failure to thrive, some lipoatrophy, bony abnormalities, a small, beaked nose and receding mandible, hair loss, and speckled hypopigmentation with some areas of tight hard skin. His neurological and cognitive tests are normal. Genetic analysis shows a single spontaneous mutation in codon 608 of the *LMNA* gene, which encodes both lamin A and lamin C. Which one of the following would you most likely expect to be a direct effect in cells obtained from this patient?

a. Increased heterochromatin
b. Interference with microtubule treadmilling
c. Increased synthesis of rRNA in the nucleolus
d. Loss of ability to adhere to the basement membrane through integrins
e. Aberrations in nuclear architecture

71. A newborn boy is diagnosed with Apert syndrome. He has craniosynostosis, hypoplasia of the middle part of his face with retrusion of the eyes, and syndactyly that includes fusion of the skin, connective tissue, and muscle of the first, middle, and ring fingers with moderate fusion of the bones of those digits. There is very limited joint mobility past the first joint. Which one of the following is most likely *decreased* in cells in the interdigital region of the developing hand of this newborn child?

a. Random DNA degradation
b. Inflammation
c. Cell swelling
d. bcl-2
e. DNA degradation by endonucleases

72. A 25-year-old man presents with (Allgrove) Triple A syndrome including the clinical triad of adrenal failure, achalasia, and alacrima. The patient shows progressive neurological impairments involving cranial nerves IX, X, XI, and XII, optic atrophy, upper and lower limb muscle weakness, and Horner syndrome. Causative mutations for the disease have been identified in a gene that encodes the protein ALADIN, a component of the structure labeled with the arrows in the transmission electron micrograph. Which one of the following would be directly affected by the mutation?

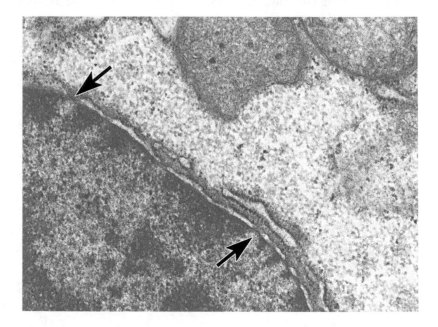

a. Import of macromolecules to the nucleus
b. Reconstitution of the nuclear envelope in telophase
c. Breakdown of the nuclear envelope in prometaphase
d. Condensation of chromatin
e. RNA synthesis

Cell Biology: Nucleus

Answers

61. The answer is d. (*Mescher, pp 52, 56-57. Ross, pp 71, 74-75.*) The *TCOF1* gene encodes treacle. Expression of treacle is critical during early embryonic development in structures that form bones and other facial structures. Treacle is active in the nucleolus, the structure labeled in the transmission electron micrograph. The nucleolus is the site of ribosomal protein transcription and treacle regulates ribosomal DNA transcription and therefore ribosomal RNA (rRNA) synthesis. Ribosomal synthesis occurs in the nucleolus, but the complete assembly and maturation of ribosomes requires transport to the cytoplasm **(answer a)**. Ribosomal proteins as well as all proteins that function in the nucleus are synthesized in the cytosol and transported into the nucleus **(answer b)**. Nuclear proteins are also translated on ribosomes in the cytoplasm and targeted to the nucleus (traveling through the nuclear pores) by specific nuclear localization signals. Cytosolic proteins are synthesized on isolated ribosomes compared with most protein synthesis that occurs on polyribosomes. Nuclear proteins are transcribed on euchromatin **(answer c)**. Lysosomes carry out degradation of organelles **(answer e)**.

62. The answer is g. (*Alberts, pp 1071-1074, 1089-1090, 1092-1094.*) Disruption and rearrangement of cellular actin will interfere with cytokinesis, the stage of mitosis shown in the transmission electron micrograph. Cytokinesis, the cleavage of the cytoplasm to form two cells, occurs after completion of nuclear division (ie, nuclear condensation and separation of the chromosomes that are mediated by microtubules) and requires the action of the contractile ring composed of actin and myosin. The force for cytokinesis is generated by the action of actin and myosin. Dolastatin 11 causes rapid disruption of the actin microfilament network **(answer b)**. Kinetochore microtubules, that attach the kinetochores to the spindle apparatus, shorten and pull the chromatids to opposite poles in anaphase A **(answer a)**. Growth of polar microtubules results in the separation of the spindle poles in anaphase B (**answer c**). M-Cdk complex (MPF) regulates metaphase events through phosphorylation (**answer d**). Antitubulin antibodies block movement of chromosomes (**answer e**). Tubulin is more important in the separation of chromosomes, and nuclear division (**answer f**). The events that occur during each stage of the cell cycle are shown in High Yield Facts, Table 7.

63. The answer is a. (*Alberts, pp 207-211. Mescher, pp 54-55.*) The patient in the scenario suffers from systemic lupus erythematosus (SLE), a chronic autoimmune disease. Autoantibodies against nucleosomes (ANA) are sensitive markers for SLE. Nucleosomes are the basic structural packaging units of chromatin. Chromatin strands that have been treated to unpack the chromatin structure have the appearance of beads on a string in electron micrographs. The beads are formed by a core of histones as an octamer (ie, two of each of the four nucleosomal histones: H2A, H2B, H3, and H4) plus two turns of DNA. The nucleosome beads plus the DNA between beads (ie, linker DNA) constitute the nucleosome. There are additional orders of chromosome packing, including nucleosomal packing. The transcription of DNA is carried out by RNA polymerases I, II, and III, which are responsible for transcription of different types of genes (**answer b**). The nuclear pores are perforations in the nuclear envelope, each composed of a nuclear pore complex (**answer c**). The nuclear matrix is the intranuclear cytoskeleton and forms the scaffolding for nuclear structures (**answer d**). Chromatids are held together at the centromere (**answer e**).

64. The answer is a. (*Alberts, pp 200-201, 1060-1064.*) When a cell in any phase of the cell cycle is fused with a mitotic cell, the mitotic cell dominates. The reason for this is the dominance of M-Cdk complex (formerly called MPF). The G_1-phase cell is quickly pulled or driven into mitosis as the chromosomes condense. The M-Cdk complex will cause the phosphorylation of the lamins. The lamins (nuclear lamina) are a subclass of intermediate filaments including three nuclear proteins: lamins A, B, and C. Phosphorylation of intermediate filaments leads to disassembly, as occurs with the lamins. The disassembly of lamins results in the dissolution of the nuclear envelope in prometaphase of the cell cycle. The S-phase activator cannot be expressed in the M-phase cell, and it also cannot reduplicate its DNA because of the re-replication block (**answers b, c, and d**). A re-replication block cannot occur in the G_1 cell because it has not gone through S-phase (answer e). The lamins differ from other intermediate filament proteins in the presence of a nuclear import signal. The lamins form the core of the nuclear lamina, interact with nuclear envelope proteins, and play a role in the maintenance of the shape of the nucleus. Dephosphorylation of the lamins is associated with the reassembly of the nuclear envelope in telophase.

65. The answer is d. *(Alberts, pp 987-988.)* At a mitosis-inhibiting dose, colchicine binds specifically and irreversibly to tubulin. The colchicine-tubulin complex is added at the positive end of the kinetochore, but it inhibits further addition of tubulin **(answer c)**. The result is a biochemical capping of the tubulin at the growth end, preventing further tubulin addition. Cells are blocked in metaphase and cannot escape because microtubule motors are unable to function in generating the forces required for anaphase. At higher doses of colchicine, cytosolic microtubules depolymerize. Actin and myosin are involved in cytokinesis (the division of cytoplasm [**answers a and b**]), whereas tubulin and the microtubules regulate separation of the daughter nuclei and their contents. Taxol, like colchicine, inhibits mitosis, but it uses a different mechanism. Taxol binds and stabilizes microtubules **(answer e)**, causing a disruption of microtubule dynamics and inhibition of mitosis. Taxol and colchicine are similar in binding only to α,β tubulin dimers and microtubules. The man in the vignette had gout that may be treated with colchicine.

66. The answer is a. *(Mescher, pp 51-52, 56-57. Alberts, pp 200-201, 220-222. Fauci, pp 2570-2571.)* Friedrich ataxia is caused by condensation of chromatin (heterochromatin, A in the image) and gene silencing, associated with large blocks of repetitive DNA sequences. In the light microscope, heterochromatin is visible as condensed basophilic clumps and with electron micrograph as compact, electron-dense material found peripherally along the inner surface of the nuclear envelope. It is transcriptionally inactive during the interphase stage of the cell cycle, when the genetic material is normally duplicated. Heterochromatin is one of two subclassifications of chromatin on a morphologic basis. Euchromatin **(B)** is actively transcribed chromatin and is visible only with the use of electron microscopy. Cells with extensive euchromatin are considered metabolically active. Euchromatic genes repositioned to or near the heterochromatin become silenced which is known as position effect variegation.

The nucleolus (E) is the site of ribosomal RNA synthesis. Tritiated (^{3}H)-uridine may be localized to the nucleolus by use of autoradiography and is often used as a marker of RNA synthesis because uridine is preferentially incorporated into RNA. The RNA is packaged with ribosomal proteins to form ribosomes. The nuclear envelope (C) shields the nucleus from the cytoplasm, which allows the sequestration of the genetic material from mechanical cytoplasmic forces. The separate nuclear compartment also allows for separation of the cellular processes of transcription and translation. The nuclear envelope consists of two concentric unit membranes. The outer membrane is continuous with the rough endoplasmic reticulum. The inner nuclear membrane is associated with fibrous proteins including intermediate filament proteins (lamins) that regulate the assembly and disassembly of the nuclear envelope during mitosis.

Nuclear pores (D) are interruptions in the nuclear envelope that function as aqueous channels for the passage of soluble molecules from the nucleus to the cytoplasm (ribosomal subunits) and from the cytoplasm to the nucleus (nuclear proteins synthesized in the cytoplasm and transported to the nucleus). The nuclear envelope is highly selective, with selection based on pore size, the presence of nuclear import signals, and receptor recognition of RNAs. Translation of mRNA occurs in the cytoplasm.

67. The answer is d. (*Alberts, pp 1103-1105. Kumar pp 287-290. Ross, pp 80-81, 91.*) Increased transcription of the transcription factor, E2F leads to loss of cell cycle control. E2F is regulated through phosphorylation and dephosphorylation of retinoblastoma protein (Rb), a key "negative" regulator of the cell cycle. Cells that enter G_1 have dephosphorylated Rb protein that is subsequently phosphorylated, allowing passage of cells from G_1 to "S." Dephosphorylated Rb is inhibitory because it sequesters E2F. Upon Rb phosphorylation, E2F is released and induces the expression of various genes associated with the initiation of the cell cycle.

The phosphorylation or absence of Rb facilitates E2F binding to DNA (**answer e**). Bcl-2 is an antiapoptotic gene (**answer c**). Accumulation of *bcl-2* has been associated with the increased incidence and severity of prostate carcinoma in African American males. Cell division kinase inhibitors block activation of cyclin-Cdk (cyclin dependent kinase complexes [**answer b**]) and cell cycle progression (**answer a**). *p53* and *Rb* are tumor suppressor genes. In the absence of *Rb* or *p53*, tumor suppression and normal control are lost. *p53* increases in the presence of DNA damage, resulting in the inhibition of cell division. *p53* mutations inhibit cell division kinase (Cdk) inhibitors such as p21, resulting in uncontrolled cell division. The absence of *p53* also permits proliferation of damaged cells. For more details on the regulation of the cell cycle, see High-Yield Facts, Nucleus.

68. The answer is c. (*Alberts, pp 1274-1276. Ross, pp 86-87.*) Pachytene begins as soon as the synapsis is complete and includes the period of crossover. The fully formed synaptonemal complex is present during the pachytene stage. At each point where crossover has occurred between two chromatids of the homologous chromosomes, an attachment point known as a chiasma forms. Meiosis is the mechanism used by the reproductive organs to generate gametes—cells with the haploid number of chromosomes. DNA synthesis occurs before meiotic prophase I begins and is followed by a G_2 phase. Cells then enter meiotic prophase I. During meiotic prophase I, maternal and paternal chromosomes are precisely paired, and recombination occurs in each pair of homologous chromosomes. The first meiotic prophase consists of five substages: leptotene, zygotene, pachytene, diplotene, and diakinesis. During metaphase I, there is random segregation of maternal and paternal chromosomes. Homologous chromosomes are aligned on the metaphase plate of the meiotic spindle in metaphase I. The second meiotic division is responsible for the reduction in the chromosome content of the cell by 50%. In meiotic division II, metaphase consists of daughter chromatids of single homologous chromosomes aligned on a metaphase plate (metaphase II). Condensation of the chromatids occurs in leptotene **(answer a).** In zygotene **(answer b)**, the synaptonemal complex begins to form, which initiates the close association between chromosomes known as synapsis. The bivalent is formed between the two sets of homologous chromosomes (one set maternal and one set paternal equals a pair of maternal chromatids and a pair of paternal chromatids). The four chromatids form a tetrad (bivalent). The formation of chiasmata and desynapsing (separation of the axes of the synaptonemal complex) occurs in the diplotene stage **(answer d).** Diakinesis **(answer e)** is an intermediate phase between diplotene and metaphase of the first meiotic division.

69. The answer is b. (*Fauci, pp 2340-2341. Sadler, pp 20, 21, 258. Moore and Persaud, pp 461, 463, 466.*) The diagnosis is Klinefelter syndrome—a male with mild to moderate learning problems and infertility (**answers a and c → e**). Cells from a patient with the most common form of Klinefelter syndrome (47,XXY genotype) will have one inactive X chromosome. Kline-felter syndrome occurs at a ratio of about 1:500 males and is due to meiotic nondisjunction of the chromosomes. The nondisjunction is more frequent in oogenesis than in spermatogenesis, and increased occurrence is directly proportional to increasing maternal age. Klinefelter symptoms include: abnormal body proportions (long legs, short trunk, shoulder equal to hip size), gynecomastia, less than normal amount of pubic, axillary, and facial hair, small testicles and penis, and height considerably taller than parents or siblings. It may occur as 47,XXY, 48,XXYY, 48,XXXY, and 49,XXXXY. A combination of abnormal and normal genotype occurs in mosaic individuals who generally have less severe symptoms. Females have two X chromosomes, one of maternal and the other of paternal origin. Only one of the X chromosomes is active in the somatic, diploid cells of the female; the other X chromosome remains inactive and is visible in appropriately stained interphase cells as a mass of heterochromatin (Barr body). The genotypic sex of Klinefelter syndrome and XXX individuals would be male and female, respectively, as determined by the presence or absence of the testis-determining Y chromosome. Turner syndrome individuals have an XO genotype and no inactive X chromosome. In comparison, "superfemales" (XXX) would possess two inactive X chromosomes and one active X chromosome. Either amniocentesis or CVS may be used to obtain fetal cells for karyotyping.

70. The answer is e. (*Rubin, p 37. Fauci, p 55.*) In HGPS, an abnormal protein, progerin, is generated and has a "dominant negative" effect on the function of lamins. The lamins are intermediate filament proteins that regulate the nuclear envelope, maintain its stability, and are phosphorylated (prometaphase) and dephosphorylated (telophase) during the cell cycle. In HGPS the results are dramatic abnormalities in the architecture of the nucleus, changes in nuclear shape, loss of heterochromatin (unable to attach to lamins), and an altered distribution of nuclear proteins **(answer a)**. Microtubule treadmilling **(answer b)** and synthesis of ribosomal RNAs in the nucleolus **(answer c)** should not be directly affected. Laminin binds to integrins on the cell surface to facilitate attachment of cells to the basement membrane **(answer d)**.

71. The answer is e. (*Ross, pp 88-91. Kumar, pp 25-32.*) DNA degradation is the hallmark of programmed cell death (apoptosis). Random DNA degradation, inflammation, and cell and nuclear swelling **(answers a → c)**

are involved in necrosis (the response to cell injury or toxins), not apoptosis. Bax and bcl-2 are members of the bcl-2 family of apoptosis regulatory proteins. Bax is a proapoptotic member of that protein family and inhibits the antiapoptotic actions of bcl-2. Bax would be down-regulated and bcl-2 up-regulated in syndactyly where apoptosis has failed (**answer d**). Apoptosis works through several different pathways and ultimately through the action of caspases, which induce DNA degradation by endonucleases.

72. The answer is a. (*Mescher, pp 51-54. Ross, p 78.*) Allgrove syndrome is an autosomal recessive neuroendocrinological disease caused by mutations in a gene that encodes the nucleoporin ALADIN, a component of the nuclear pore complex labeled with the arrows in the electron micrograph. The immediate effect of mutations in the nucleoporins is decreased import of macromolecules from the cytoplasm. Patients with Allgrove syndrome have adrenocorticotrophic (ACTH)-resistant adrenal failure, achalasia (abnormal esophageal motility most often due to inability of the esophageal sphincter to relax), and alacrima (reduced ability to produce tears). The triad of symptoms beginning with the letter "A" has led to the name "triple A" syndrome. Since some consider autonomic neuropathy an integral feature of this condition, others have proposed the name "4 A syndrome." The autonomic disturbance includes Horner syndrome and orthostatic hypotension. Phosphorylation (breakdown) and dephosphorylation (reconstitution) of the lamins regulates nuclear envelope stability during the cell cycle (**answers b and c**). Condensation of chromosomes would not be directly affected (**answer d**) and the nucleolus is the site of RNA synthesis (**answer e**).

Epithelium

Questions

73. A boy is born without the normal structure labeled between the arrows in the accompanying transmission electron micrograph. He presents with refractory diarrhea and is chronically dependent on parenteral nutrition. What is the primary function of the structure labeled between the arrows in the photomicrograph below?

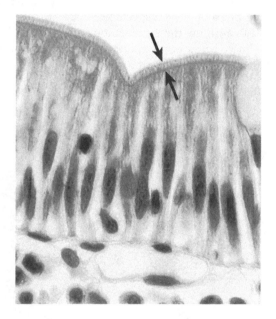

a. Extensive movement of substances over cell surfaces
b. Increase in surface area for absorption
c. Cell motility
d. Transport of intracellular organelles through the cytoplasm
e. Stretch

74. Following a positive α-fetoprotein (AFP) test, a child is born with anencephaly. The development of this open neural tube defect (NTD) is caused by failure of primary neurulation. The mechanism for tube formation as occurs during development of the neural tube could best be explained by which of the following?

a. Contraction of microfilament bundles associated with the zonula adherens
b. Increased condensation of the transmembrane linkers of the desmosomes
c. Expansion of the sealing strands in the zonulae occludentes (tight junctions)
d. Condensation of the gap junctions
e. Contraction of tonofilaments associated with desmosomes

75. In the figure below, A is a transmission electron micrograph, and B is a freeze-fracture preparation of a specific cellular structure. Mutations in the proteins that constitute the intramembranous particles labeled in the freeze-fracture image below occur in humans. Which one of the following would one expect to occur in the presence of loss of function mutations?

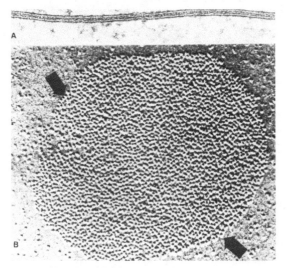

(Micrographs courtesy of Drs. David F. Albertini and Kiyoshi Hama.)

a. Faster conduction of nerve impulses
b. Increased peristalsis in the small intestine
c. Cardiac arrhythmias
d. More rapid mobilization of glycogen to glucose in response to low blood sugar levels
e. Decreased adherence of epithelial cells to the basement membrane

76. Which of the following is a function of the basement membrane?
a. Molecular filtering
b. Contractility
c. Excitability
d. Modification of secreted protein
e. Active ion transport

77. A mother brings her son to the pediatrics clinic. Shortly after birth, the child developed extensive blistering of the skin. He has painful erosions of the oral mucosa and has refused ingestion of milk. He has also had a history of recurrent infections, with sepsis, on one occasion. Antigen mapping of a skin biopsy shows a split within the lamina lucida of the epidermal basement membrane, and junctional epidermolysis bullosa (JEB) is the diagnosis. In which specific layer of the accompanying electron micrograph would one expect to see the disruption?

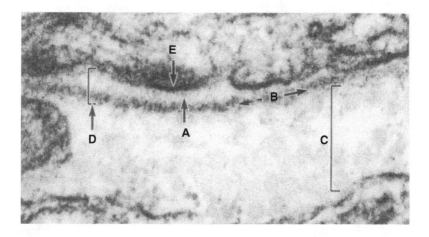

a. A
b. B
c. C
d. D
e. E

78. A 66-year-old man with a 15-year history of heart disease is diagnosed with congestive heart failure. The patient is given digoxin to increase myocardial contractility. Which one of the following is the target for digoxin and definitively characterizes the basolateral membrane of the cardiomyocyte?

a. Sodium-calcium exchanger
b. Proton-potassium ATPase
c. Sodium-potassium ATPase
d. Chloride-bicarbonate exchanger
e. Sodium driven chloride-bicarbonate exchanger
f. Chloride-hydroxyl exchanger

79. A 54-year-old woman presents to the oral surgeon on referral by her general dentist. She complains of pain during eating or even thinking about food. The pain lasts for about 2 to 3 hours after eating. Her dentist observes a firm mass on the anterior right side of the floor of the mouth. A calcified density is identified in the transverse CT film (see arrow in the radiograph below). The calcification blocks the submandibular duct leading to atrophy of the acini and ducts with reduced secretory function. One would expect which of the following functional changes to occur in association with the basal folds of the striated duct cells?

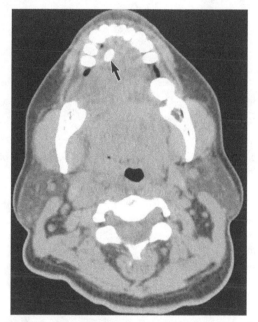

(Radiograph courtesy of Drs. Per-Lennart Westesson and Xiang Liu, University of Rochester, Case #98 http://www.urmc.rochester.edu/smd/Rad/neurocases/Neurocase98.htm.)

a. Increased lipid transport
b. Increased absorption of carbohydrate
c. Decreased active transport
d. Decreased secretion of the primary saliva
e. Decreased lysosomal activity

80. In the electron micrograph below, the structure labeled D primarily does which of the following?

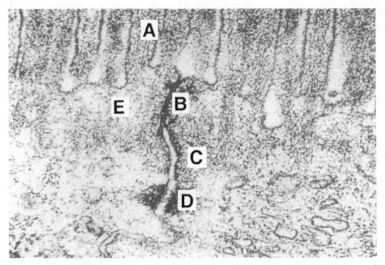

(Reproduced, with permission, from Erlandsen SL, Magney JE. Color Atlas of Histology. St. Louis, MO: CV Mosby; 1992.)

a. Forms a spot weld between cells
b. Interacts with actin in the cytoplasm of the apical cytosol
c. Facilitates communication between adjacent cells
d. Seals membranes between cells
e. Moves microvilli

81. An 11-year-old boy presents with ciliary dyskinesia, sinusitis, and bronchiectasis. He has had persistent infections and otitis media since birth. A PA chest radiograph shows dextrocardia, and he has a negative saccharin test. In the cross-section of the cilium shown below, which one of the following is primarily affected in this disorder?

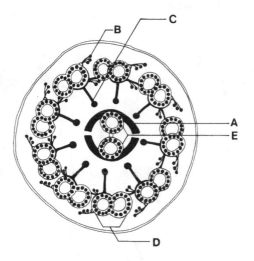

a. Structure A
b. Structure B
c. Structure C
d. Structure D
e. Structure E

82. The conversion of sliding to bending in the cilium is accomplished by which of the following?

a. Restriction of movement by dynein binding of the central microtubules to each other
b. The bending of the basal bodies against the axoneme
c. Sliding of nexin along the adjacent microtubule doublet
d. Sliding of the radial spokes against nexin
e. Restriction of the microtubule doublets by radial spokes, nexin, and basal bodies

83. A 42-year-old woman, of Mediterranean descent, presents with multiple oral blisters (see photograph) and a few cutaneous blisters on her back and buttocks. The bullae are superficial. Vesicles are fragile, some have unroofed to form ulcerated lesions, and there is a positive Nikolsky sign. Sera analysis indicates autoantibodies to a subfamily of cadherins with the distribution shown in the immunofluorescence image (see photomicrograph). Where would one expect to find the lesion?

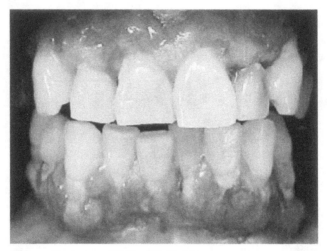

(Micrograph courtesy of Dr. David A. Sirois.)

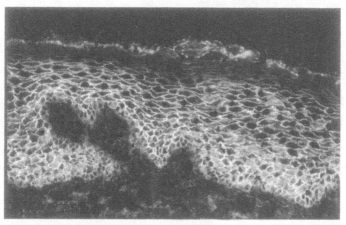

(*Micrograph courtesy of Dr. Erik Dabelsteen.*)

a. Hemidesmosome
b. Zonula occludens
c. Macula adherens
d. Gap junction
e. Lamina densa of the basal lamina

84. The triplet arrangement of microtubules is found in which of the following?

a. Centrioles
b. Cytoplasmic microtubules
c. Flagellae
d. Axonemes
e. Stereocilia

Epithelium

Answers

73. The answer is b. (*Young, pp 5, 88, 93. Mescher, pp 70-72, 266-267, 270.*) The child in the vignette suffers from microvillus inclusion disease (MID) which results in the absence of microvilli in the small intestinal absorptive cell (enterocyte). The brush border is the apical structure labeled between the arrows in the transmission electron micrograph. MID is associated with an inability to absorb even simple nutrients; the disease presents as refractory diarrhea in the early postnatal period with chronic dependency on total parenteral nutrition. In MID, microvilli are found as inclusions in the apical enterocyte. Microvilli increase surface area for specialized uptake of molecules by pinocytosis, receptor-mediated endocytosis, and phagocytosis. The microvilli also contain the brush-border enzymes such as lactase and alkaline phosphatase. Microvilli are supported by a core of microfilaments and are capable of movement; however, cilia (**answer a**) function in the movement of substances, such as mucus and foreign material, over the surface. Cell movement is controlled by interactions between the cytoskeleton and the extracellular matrix (**answer c**), while microtubules facilitate organellar movement within the cytoplasm (**answer d**). Transitional epithelium characteristic of the urinary system facilitates distensibility and stretch (**answer e**).

74. The answer is a. (*Alberts, pp 1370-1372, 1384, 1385.*) Open NTDs, such as anencephaly, are detected by a positive AFP test and are attributed to failure of primary neurulation in which the neural folds (plate) form the neural tube. Tubular structures form from flat sheets by contraction of the microfilament bundles associated with the adhesion belt junctions (zonula adherens). In the apical part of the cells, the actin filament bundles contract, narrowing the cells at their apical ends. The position of the zonula adherens, forming a contractile ring around the circumference of the cell, coupled with the contractile nature of the actin microfilament bundles is ideal for regulating morphogenetic changes. Desmosomes (**answers b and e**) are involved in resisting shear forces and are not directly involved in this process. The zonula occludens (**answer c**) prevent leakage between cells. Gap junctions facilitate communication between cells (**answer d**). See

High-Yield Facts, Table 8, for detailed summary of function of components of the junctional complex.

75. The answer is c. *(Young, pp 88, 91. Kumar, pp 531-532. Mescher, pp 68, 70.)* The transmission and freeze-fracture electron micrographs illustrate the structure of a gap junction. Gap junctions are composed of connexons that traverse the intercellular gap. Gap junctions play an essential role in conduction within cardiac muscle. The action potential is transmitted from cell to cell through the heart, providing the rhythmic contraction of the heartbeat. Abnormalities in the spatial distribution of gap junctions or the proteins (connexins) that compose the connexons will lead to arrhythmias and play a role in obstructive coronary heart disease. Such mutations may also play a role in the racial differences seen in the outcome following myocardial infarction and cardiac disease. For example, alterations in connexin density or distribution may be differentially affected during the development of hypertrophy, thereby increasing the risk of reentrant or nonsustained ventricular tachycardia seen in African American males.

In the freeze-fracture micrograph, the connexons are seen in circular arrangements on the P face of the membrane. When the connexons of adjacent cells are in alignment, a pore of about 1.5 nm is open, and there is continuity between the interior of the two cells. Gap junctions maintain electrical or chemical coupling between cells. Rapid nerve conduction in some systems uses gap junctions to avoid the chemical synapse, which requires the release of neurotransmitter. Mutations in connexins would slow down normal nerve impulse conduction **(answer a)**. Normal peristalsis **(answer b)** requires normal gap junctions between smooth muscle in the small intestine and would be slowed down in the absence of normal gap junctions. Not all hepatocytes are innervated. Innervated and noninnervated hepatocytes are connected by gap junctions, which allow for a more coordinated effect of norepinephrine on hepatocytes to facilitate release of blood glucose from stored glycogen in hepatocytes **(answer d)**. Adherence of epithelial cells to the basement membrane **(answer e)** is dependent on integrins and hemidesmosomes, not gap junctions.

76. The answer is a. *(Alberts, pp 1164-1169. Kumar, pp 94-95. Mescher, pp 66-68.)* Epithelial cells require a basement membrane as a structural support. In most epithelia, the basement membrane prevents penetration from the underlying lamina propria into the epithelium. Basement membranes are a pathway for migrating cells during development and repair processes (eg, healing of skin wounds). In the kidney, the basement membrane of the renal glomerulus forms a selective barrier for the filtration of the plasma. Contractility and excitability (answers b and c) are characteristics that are associated with muscle and nerve, respectively, not with the basement membrane. Modification of secretory proteins and active ion transport (answers d and e) are characteristics of the epithelia that are positioned on the basement membrane, not of the basement membrane itself.

77. The answer is a. (Alberts, pp 1164-1169. Mescher, pp 66-68.) The regions labeled in the electron micrograph are A (lamina rara, also known as the lamina lucida), B (lamina densa), C (reticular lamina), D (basal lamina), and E (basal cell membrane). JEB represents a disruption between laminin, specifically the beta and gamma chains, and integrins. The split occurs through the lamina lucida of the basal lamina, which contains primarily laminin and its connections with the integrins. At the light microscopic level, a uniform basement membrane is visible under epithelia. Ultrastructurally, basement membranes are composed of one or two electron-lucent areas (laminae rarae) that contain laminin, proteoglycans, and adhesive proteins. Deep to the lamina rara is the lamina densa with its electron-dense type IV collagen. The third layer is the reticular layer that is formed by the underlying connective tissue. This reticular lamina is composed of collagen fibrils formed by the connective tissue below the epithelium (basement membrane = basal lamina + reticular lamina). See High-Yield Facts, Table 9, which summarizes the components of the basal lamina/basement membrane.

78. The answer is c. (Mescher, p 81.) The sodium-potassium ATPase (Na^+-K^+ ATPase) characterizes the basolateral membrane of all eukaryotic cells and is responsible for generating the Na^+, K^+ gradient of the cell. Na^+, is pumped out of the cell, and K^+ is pumped into the cell by this ATP-dependent pump (answers a, b, d, e, and f). Digoxin inhibits the cardiomyocyte Na^+-K^+ ATPase, reducing the transport of Na^+ from the cell and leading to increased intracellular Na^+. Higher intracellular Na^+ levels cause a decrease in Ca^{2+} efflux and an increase in Ca^{2+} influx. In response to the rise in intracellular calcium, the sarcoplasmic reticulum of the digoxin-exposed cardiomyocyte sequesters more Ca^{2+}. When cardiomyocytes exposed to digoxin depolarize in response to an action potential, there are more Ca^{2+} available to bind troponin C, and stronger contraction is facilitated.

79. The answer is c. (*Mescher, pp 82, 283, 284. Ross, pp 121, 131-132.*) Distal tubule cells of the kidney and striated duct cells of the submandibular glands possess prominent basal infoldings that are observed at the light microscopic level as basal striations. Basal folds are modifications of the basal region of the cell. These deep infoldings of the basal plasma membrane increase surface area and compartmentalize numerous mitochondria that provide energy for ionic and water transport. The primary (isotonic) saliva (**answer d**) is formed by acinar cells and modified by the striated duct cells which resorb Na^+ and excrete K^+. Other activities listed (**answers a, b, and e**) are not directly associated with the basal folds.

80. The answer is a. (*Young, pp 70-74, 88. Mescher, pp 67-70.*) The structure labeled **D** in the transmission electron micrograph is the macula adherens (desmosome). It forms a spot weld or rivet between the adjacent cells and resists shearing forces on the epithelium. The transmission electron micrograph illustrates a junctional complex between two enterocytes in the small intestine. Label **A** represents the microvilli, which constitute the brush border. The brush border is covered by the glycocalyx and in the small intestine contains enzymes involved in the degradation of food in the lumen. The structure labeled **B** is the zonula occludens, which provides a tight seal between the epithelial cells. Label **C** marks the zonula adherens, which interacts with actin that comprises the terminal web (label **E**).

81. The answer is b. (*Alberts, pp 1014-1015, 1033. Young, p 92. Mescher, pp 42, 46, 298, 302, 379. Kierszenbaum, pp 27, 55.*) The patient in the scenario presents with Kartagener syndrome, also known as immotile cilia syndrome, and has cilia that do not function normally. This leads to chronic infections (otitis media) and infertility (immotile sperm or suboptimal oviductal ciliary function in females). In this disorder, abnormalities occur in the organization of axonemal (ciliary) dynein arms (**answer b**) that bridge the nine outer doublet microtubules (**answer d**) to each other. Dynein is a high-molecular weight ATPase. When dynein is activated, it produces the sliding motion of the microtubules as it walks along the adjacent doublet. The protein nexin links the outer microtubular doublets, creating a strap-like arrangement of paired microtubules around the central microtubule doublet. The radial spokes (**answer c**) restrain the sliding movement of the outer doublets, so those doublets are held in place and sliding is limited lengthwise. The inner sheath (**answer a**) surrounds the central microtubule doublet (answer e). The basal body that anchors the microtubules also plays an essential role in converting the sliding of the outer microtubules into the bending of the cilium.

Bronchiectasis is the irreversible, abnormal dilation of one or more bronchi associated with various lung conditions, commonly accompanied by chronic infection. In Kartagener syndrome it has been found that uncoordinated dyskinesia is more prevalent than immotile cilia. There is therefore a movement in the literature to call this syndrome primary ciliary dyskinesia, and Kartagener syndrome would be a subclassification of that group of disorders. Dextrocardia (cardiac apex to the right) occurs in mild cases and situs inversus in more severe cases. In situs inversus, the morphologic right atrium is on the left, and the morphologic left atrium is on the right. Pulmonary structures (ie, right and left lungs) as well as abdominal organs may also be reversed in a mirror image of normal. The development of right-left asymmetry is at least partially regulated by ciliary beat at Hensen node.

The saccharin test is a test of nasal mucociliary clearance. It is carried out by placing a small amount of saccharin behind the anterior end of the inferior turbinate. In the presence of normal mucociliary action, the saccharin will be swept backward to the nasopharynx and a sweet taste perceived. Failure of sweetness to be detected within about 20 minutes indicates delayed mucociliary clearance.

82. The answer is e. (*Kierszenbaum, pp 26-27. Alberts, pp 1031-1034, Mescher, pp 43, 46. Ross, pp 104-106.*) Nexin, the radial spokes, and the basal body all play a role in restricting the sliding motion and converting it to the bending of the axoneme in relation to the basal body. When dynein is activated, it produces the sliding motion of the microtubules as it walks along the adjacent doublet (answer a). The basal body (answer b) anchors the microtubules and also plays an essential role in converting the sliding of the outer microtubules into the bending of the cilium. The basal bodies resist the sliding movement generated by dynein activation. Nexin (answer c) links the outer microtubular doublets, creating a strap-like arrangement of paired microtubules around the central microtubule doublet. The radial spokes hold the microtubule doublets in place, and sliding is limited lengthwise. The radial spokes (answer d) are rigid and do not slide against nexin.

83. The answer is c. (*Fauci, pp 336-337. Mescher, p 321. Kierszenbaum, pp 15, 35. Alberts, p 1144.*) In pemphigus vulgaris, autoantibodies to desmogleins (a member of the cadherin protein family) result in disruption of the macula adherens (desmosomes). The desmogleins are the transmembrane linker proteins of the desmosome. Specific desmogleins are the target of the autoantibodies in different forms of the disease. Cadherins are Ca^{2+}-dependent transmembrane linker molecules essential for cell-cell contact, so their disruption in pemphigus leads to severe blistering of the skin because of disrupted cell-cell interactions early in the differentiation of the keratinocytes (epidermal cells) and excessive fluid loss. The other parts of the junctional complex: zonula occludens (**answer b**) and gap junctions (**answer d**) are not affected in pemphigus. The connections to the basal lamina, hemidesmosomes (**answer a**), as well as the basal lamina itself, are not part of the etiology of pemphigus. This is in contrast to the subepidermal disease, bullous pemphigoid (BP), where the BP antigens (BPAG1 and BPAG2) cause the separation of the epithelium from the basal lamina. Cadherins are also critical molecules in the maintenance of the zonula adherens, but the autoantibodies in pemphigus are specific to the desmogleins. Pemphigus vulgaris, which is described in the clinical scenario, often begins as oral lesions and subsequently appears cutaneously. The Nikolsky sign is positive (pressure at the edge of a blister causes extension of the bulla into adjacent normal skin) in pemphigus, while in bullous pemphigoid the Nikolsky sign is negative. Epidermolysis bullosa acquisita (EBA) is a distinct blistering disease. The EBA antigen is localized within and subjacent to the lamina densa. It is a constituent molecule of anchoring fibrils attaching the basal lamina to the underlying dermis (**answer e**). For more details on junctional complexes, see High-Yield Facts, Table 8. (Also, see Questions and Answers to 196 and 198.)

84. The answer is a. (*Mescher, pp 39-43, 46, 71, 381-382, 437.*) The centriole consists of nine microtubule triplets arranged together by linking proteins to form a cartwheel arrangement. Microtubules are found in different structural patterns within the cell. The basal body is a centriole-like structure associated with the ciliary axoneme. It too has a nine-triplet arrangement of microtubules. Cytoplasmic microtubules (**answer b**) are found in the singlet form and undergo constant association and dissociation of tubulin at their plus ends and minus ends, respectively. Flagella (**answer c**) have the same "9 + 2" arrangement as cilia, but are limited to one per cell and in adult humans are found only in sperm. The axoneme (**answer d**) has the classic "9 + 2" arrangement of microtubules. Stereocilia (**answer e**) are large, modified microvilli, found in the epididymis and on hair cells in the organ of Corti, therefore, they are not composed of microtubules.

Connective Tissue

Questions

85. A 27-year-old, 5 ft 10 in tall woman presents in the emergency room with a pneumothorax but is afebrile. On physical examination it is noted that she has scoliosis, pectus excavatum, ectopia lentis, and myopia. Her musculoskeletal examination reveals long upper and lower extremities, including the fingers and toes, and an overall gangly, lanky appearance. Her arm span (6 ft 3 in) noticeably exceeds her height. She has very flexible fingers and a narrow face as well as a narrow mouth with overcrowded teeth. There are stretch marks across her buttocks. Which part of the cardiovascular system would often be adversely affected in this syndrome?

a. Middle cerebral artery
b. Basilar artery
c. Aorta
d. Lymphatic vessels
e. Superior vena cava

86. The extracellular matrix and the cytoskeleton communicate across the cell membrane through which one of the following?

a. Proteoglycans
b. Integrins
c. Cadherins
d. Intermediate filaments
e. Microtubules

87. A pregnant 29-year-old woman diagnosed with type I diabetes two decades ago, taking humulin three times per day, is referred to the ophthalmology clinic. She is complaining of "floaters" and difficulty with nighttime driving. Dilated indirect ophthalmoscopy coupled with biomicroscopy and fundus photography detect the presence of proliferative diabetic retinopathy with leaky retinal vessels indicative of increased vascular permeability, growth of new, fragile vessels on the retina and posterior surface of the vitreous, and macular edema. Overexpression of fibronectin is a histological marker of diabetic microangiopathy. Which of the following is the primary function of fibronectin in the basement membrane?

a. Elasticity
b. Cell attachment and adhesion
c. Binding to selectins
d. Binding to cadherins
e. Binding to actin filaments

88. A 36-year-old man is referred by his family medicine physician to the pulmonary clinic. He complains of shortness of breath following physical activity and a decreased capacity for exercise. He says that strenuous exercise including yard work is impossible without sitting down and resting every few minutes. After he takes several deep breaths during the physical examination, he begins to wheeze. He is not a smoker and as an office worker he is not exposed to dust, fumes, or other irritants at work. He appears slightly jaundiced. Serum alpha-1-antitrypsin (AAT) concentration is below normal and is followed up with AAT phenotype and DNA testing indicating one copy of S and one of Z (SZ) mutations and 40% abnormal AAT protein production. Desmosine and isodesmosine are elevated in the urine. Desmosine and isodesmosine contribute to the elasticity of the lung by which one of the following mechanisms?

a. Cross-linking fibrillin
b. Cross-linking tropoelastin
c. Activating elastase
d. Inactivating AAT
e. Binding type IV collagen to elastin

89. A 63-year-old homeless woman who has lived on the streets for more than 3 years presents at the free clinic. She has smoked cigarettes since age 10. It is estimated that alcohol accounts for half of her dietary caloric intake. She has vitamin E, B_1, and C intakes below the recommendations for adults in the United States. She has only six teeth, brittle bones with fractures, and bleeding tendencies with bruising and bleeding periodontium. Which one of the following is the most likely explanation for her symptoms?

a. Ascorbic acid deficiency results in insufficient hydroxylation of collagen.
b. α-Tocopherol deficiency results in decreased collagen synthesis in connective tissues.
c. α-Tocopherol deficiency results in increased collagenolytic activity in connective tissues.
d. Thiamine deficiency results in increased collagenolytic activity in connective tissues.
e. Thiamine deficiency results in decreased collagen synthesis in connective tissues.

90. Tropocollagen is not assembled in the cell because of which one of the following?

a. Action of lysyl oxidase in the Golgi apparatus
b. Cross-linking of tropocollagen in the rough endoplasmic reticulum (RER)
c. Presence of nonhelical registration peptides at the ends of the triple helix
d. Presence of specific collagenases in the RER and Golgi apparatus
e. Presence of procollagen peptidases in the Golgi apparatus

91. A 31-year-old woman presents to her primary care physician. She complains of fatigue, generalized joint pain with swelling of her wrists and knees, and a "butterfly" skin rash that occurs after being in the sun. She has frequent mouth sores and excessive, recent hair loss. Her white blood cell count is 3.2 (normal >4), hematocrit 25% (normal for age >38%) and erythrocyte sedimentation rate 120 mm/h (normal <20), and her blood pressure is 132/86 mm Hg. Her serum creatinine is 1.6 mg/dL (normal = 0.8-1.4 mg/dL); her urine protein-to-creatinine ratio is 2.1 (normal <0.1); and 24-hour urine creatinine is 2500 mg/day (normal range from 500-2000 mg/day). In addition to a positive antinuclear antibody (ANA) test and DNA antibodies, autoantibodies are detected to entactin (nidogen). The autoantibodies to entactin are significant because its primary function is to crosslink which of the following molecules?

a. Laminin to collagen
b. Cells to the basal lamina
c. Cells to the extracellular matrix
d. Collagen
e. Actin

92. A 14-year-old boy presents with thin, translucent skin, and a history of easy bruising. Biochemical studies of the patient's dermal fibroblasts cultured from a skin biopsy show abnormal electrophoretic mobility and abnormal secretion of type III procollagen. A mutation in the *COL3A1* gene is identified by molecular testing. Which one of the following symptoms would be most expected in this patient?

a. Rupture of the intestinal or aortic walls
b. Hyperextensibility of the integument
c. Hypermobility of synovial joints
d. Increased degradation of proteoglycans in articular cartilages
e. Imperfections in dentin formation (dentinogenesis imperfecta)

93. A full-term newborn boy develops firm, erythematous nodules and plaques over his trunk, arms, buttocks, thighs, and cheeks 10 days after birth. His mother's pregnancy was complicated by placenta previa and his airway was cleared of meconium aspiration immediately after birth. A biopsy of subcutaneous tissue shows necrosis of the tissue in the accompanying photomicrograph. The tissue shown in the photomicrograph differs from white adipose tissue in which one of the following ways?

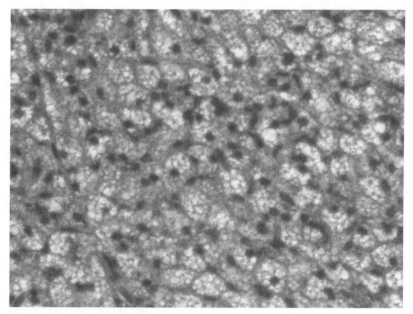

(*Micrograph courtesy of Dr. WenFang Wang.*)

a. Export of fatty acids
b. Role as a thermal insulator
c. Use of fatty acids to produce heat
d. Activation of the adenylate cyclase system
e. Initiation of shivering

94. A newborn boy presents with delayed umbilical cord separation (normal separation is 3-45 days, mean = 10 days) is observed with an elevated WBC count (>20 X 10^9/L) in the absence of infection. He is diagnosed with primary immunodeficiency, leukocyte adhesion deficiency. A loss of function mutation in integrin expression on lymphocytes (beta 2 integrin, CD18) is identified. Which one of the following would be the most likely consequence?

a. Leukopenia
b. Leukocytosis
c. Lymphadenopathy
d. Lymphocyte apoptosis
e. Increased numbers of plasma cells in the blood

95. A 33-year-old homeless woman has been living in an abandoned building eating dried meat and bread from the trash cans outside a bakery. She smokes cigarettes she "bums" from others. She presents at the free clinic with bleeding under the skin particularly around hair follicles with bruises on her arms and legs. She is irritable, clinically depressed, and fatigued with general muscle weakness. Her gums are bleeding, swollen, purple, and spongy. Her incisors and second molars are loose. She has an infected toe, which may be broken. She is afebrile, a glucose finger stick is normal, and urine dipstick shows no sugar, protein, or ketones. You suspect a vitamin deficiency. What might be the underlying mechanism for the symptoms in this patient?

a. Decreased degradation of collagen
b. Stimulation of prolyl hydroxylase
c. Formation of unstable collagen helices
d. Excessive callus formation in healing fractures
e. Organ fibrosis

96. A 53-year-old man who has been a type I diabetic since childhood is referred to an orthopedic surgeon with Charcot foot neuroarthropathy and weakness in his calf muscles. Patients with neuroarthropathy have significantly altered tensile strength in their Achilles tendons compared to tendons from nondiabetic patients. Which one of the following is a major contributor to the tensile strength of collagen?

a. Interactions with the FACIT collagens
b. The double helical arrangement of collagen
c. Electrostatic interactions
d. Intramolecular and intermolecular cross-links
e. Low concentrations of lysine

97. An 11-year-old boy presents with extreme fragility of the skin and mucous membranes. Genetic analysis shows a mutational defect in laminin 5. Laminin functions in which one of following ways?

a. As an integrin
b. In cell-cell adhesion
c. As the insoluble scaffolding of the basal lamina
d. As the filtration molecule in the basement membrane
e. In adherence of epithelia to the basement membrane

98. A 40-year-old woman is referred to a dermatologist with more than 100 oval or round red-brown macules on her back. There is a positive Darier sign. The dermatologist takes a skin biopsy, which is stained with toluidine blue. There are an excessive number of the metachromatically-stained cells labeled with the arrows and shown in the inset to the lower left in the photomicrograph below. Which one of the following would be the most likely expected symptom in the patient?

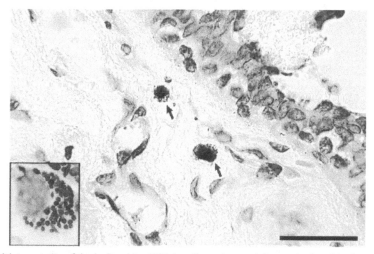

(With permission of the JayDoc Histo Web:http://www.kumc.edu/instruction/medicine/ anatomy/histoweb/.)

a. Inhibition of HCl production by parietal cells
b. Darkening of the skin
c. Osteoporosis
d. Anemia
e. Edema

99. A 46-year-old woman who has been a type I diabetic for 35 years visits her family physician's clinic. She has foot ulcers on both her right and left feet. You prescribe Becaplermin gel, a prescription drug for the treatment of diabetic foot ulcers. It contains platelet-derived growth factor (PDGF). Which one of the following is the most likely mechanism for the action of PDGF in the improvement of wound healing?

a. Acceleration of chemotaxis of monocytes-macrophages
b. Inhibition of vascular smooth-muscle cell proliferation
c. Inhibition of fibroblast proliferation
d. Inhibition of granulation tissue formation
e. Secretion of type II collagen from fibroblasts

100. A 55-year-old Caucasian man presented with generalized back pain. His physical examination reveals slight right-sided muscular weakness and a pulse of 78/min, regular; blood pressure 140/82 mm Hg. X-ray examination of the spine showed two wedged thoracic vertebrae, T7 and T8; no osteolytic lesions are observed. Peripheral blood: Hb 11 g/dL, WBC 6.0 × 10^9/L (polymorphs 81%, lymphocytes 16%, monocytes 2%, eosinophils 1%), platelets 300 × 10^9/L (300,000/mm^3). The blood film was normal. The bone marrow shows an increase in the cells shown in the accompanying light micrograph. Other tests were all normal. The cells in the light micrograph synthesize which of the following?

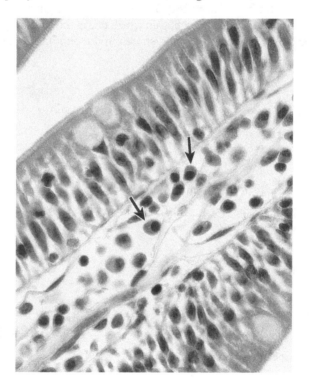

a. Collagen
b. Heparin and histamine
c. Histaminase
d. IgA
e. Myeloperoxidase

101. A 44-year-old African American woman visits her family physician for a physical examination at the urging of her husband. She has no current complaints and is taking no medications. She is allergic to erythromycin. She works as a software developer and lives with her 52-year-old husband and 12-year-old daughter. She is a nonsmoker, and drinks an occasional glass of wine when she and her husband go out to dinner. She is involved in no regular exercise. Her mother is 66 and suffers from type II diabetes, hyperlipidemia, and hypertension and had a myocardial infarction last year. The patient's father died of a stroke last year at the age of 72. On examination, the patient's blood pressure is 155/100 mm Hg, pulse 84, weight 215 lb (increased from 180, 3 years ago), and height 5 ft 7 in. In this patient, during the period of weight gain which one of the following responses would be most expected in the cells shown in the photomicrograph?

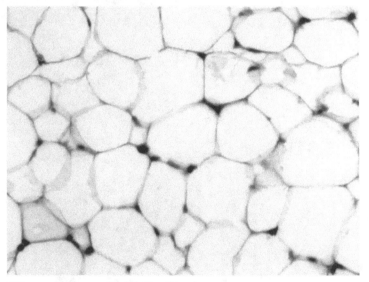

(Micrograph courtesy of Dr. WenFang Wang.)

a. Up-regulation of leptin receptors
b. Decreased synthesis of leptin
c. Decreased release of leptin into the serum
d. Increased secretion of neuropeptide Y
e. Increased release of norepinephrine from nerve terminals in adipose tissue

102. A 65-year-old African American man who has a history of both urinary tract infections and urinary stones presents at the urology clinic with hematuria. He has a dietary history high in saturated fats and has been exposed to second-hand smoke both at home (his wife smokes) and at work where many of his coworkers smoke. His work as a machinist exposed him to metal parts. Before working as a machinist he worked as a commercial painter. Cystoscopy identified several bladder tumors and was followed by transurethral resection and biopsy (TURB). The biopsy shows a transitional cell carcinoma 4.5 cm in diameter staged as "T3aN1M2." Which one of the following would facilitate the processes involved in the "M2" classification?

a. Lysyl oxidase
b. Metalloproteinases
c. Plasminogen
d. Serpins
e. Tissue inhibitors of metalloproteases (TIMPs)

Connective Tissue

Answers

85. The answer is c. (*Alberts, p 1190-1191. Fauci, p 2468.*) The patient in the scenario suffers from Marfan syndrome, an autosomal dominant disease in which persons develop abnormal elastic tissue. Decreased elasticity of lung tissue causes an increased tendency toward spontaneous pneumothorax, also known as a collapsed lung. The aorta is the most affected organ because of the extensive elastin in the wall, and dissecting aortic aneurysms are common in these patients **(answers a, b, d, and e)**. Marfan malformations include cardiovascular (valve problems as well as aortic aneurysm), skeletal (abnormal height and severe chest deformities), and ocular systems. The molecular basis of the disease is a mutation in the fibrillin gene. The lens is also often affected in patients with Marfan syndrome. The result is the dislocation of the lens because of loss of elasticity in the suspensory ligament.

86. The answer is b. (*Alberts, pp 1169-1178.*) The integrins are transmembrane heterodimers (integral membrane proteins) that act as membrane receptors for extracellular matrix components. Examples are the fibronectin receptor and the laminin receptor. The receptor structure includes an intracytosolic portion that binds to the actin cytoskeleton through the attachment proteins talin or α-actinin. The extracellular portion has specificity for extracellular matrix molecules. Proteoglycans **(answer a)** are located on the extracellular surface of the plasma membrane and throughout the extracellular matrix. The cadherins **(answer c)** function as transmembrane glycoproteins involved in the formation of parts of the intercellular junctional complexes. Cadherins are components of the desmosome and zonula adherens. Intermediate filaments and microtubules **(answers d and e)** are found intracellularly and constitute the cytoskeleton.

87. The answer is b. (*Alberts, pp 1133-1136, 1191-1193. Mescher, pp 101-102, 104.*) Fibronectin is an adhesive glycoprotein that is important for cell attachment and adhesion. It is important for modulation of cell migration in the adult and during development. Neural crest and other cells appear to be guided along fibronectin-coated pathways in the embryo. Fibronectin is found in three forms: a plasma form that is involved in blood clotting; a cell-surface form, which binds to the cell surface transiently; and a matrix form, which is fibrillar in arrangement. Fibronectin contains a cell-binding domain (RGD sequence), a collagen-binding domain, and a heparin-binding domain. Elastin and type III collagen are responsible for elasticity seen in large arteries and the pinna of the ear **(answer a)**. Cell-cell interactions involve both transient and more long-term, stable processes. Cell adhesion is mediated by transmembrane proteins (cell adhesion molecules) which include the calcium or magnesium-dependent selectins, integrins, and cadherins **(answers c and d)** and the non-calcium-dependent immunoglobulin (Ig) superfamily. The stable adhesion junction, known as the zonula adherens, links the cytoskeleton of adjacent cells through cadherins (transmembrane linker proteins) to actin filaments inside the cell, **answer e** (also, see answer for Questions 196 and 198).

88. The answer is b. (*Mescher, p 314. Fauci, pp 1636-1637. Kumar, pp 864-866.*) The patient is diagnosed with AAT emphysema. AAT protects the lung from neutrophil-derived elastase, which breaks down elastic fibers **(answer d)**, that are composed of a core of elastin with a surrounding network of fibrillin. Desmosine and isodesmosine are amino acids unique to elastin and responsible for the covalent binding of elastin fibers to each other. Lysyl oxidase catalyzes the cross-linking of tropoelastin **(answer a)**. Microfibrils, composed of fibrillin, facilitate formation of the elastin molecules, but are not directly involved in cross-linking. Elastase **(answer c)** is a serine protease that specifically degrades elastin. Interactions occur between type III collagen and elastic fibers **(answer e)**. The collagen may serve to limit the stretch of the elastic components. Elasticity is conferred through the highly hydrophobic nature of elastin. One-third of elastin is composed of the hydrophobic amino acid glycine, which is randomly distributed throughout the elastin molecule. This is in contrast to the even distribution of glycine in collagen. The random distribution of glycine makes elastin hydrophobic. The overall hydrophobicity of elastin molecules allows for their distensibility and facilitates their capacity to slide over one another.

89. The answer is a. (*Alberts, pp 1186-1187. Kierszenbaum, pp 110-112. Mescher, pp 98, 99, 259.*) Although Vitamin E ([α-tocopherol], **answers b**

and c) and B₁ ([thiamine] **answers d and e**) affect collagen synthesis, the symptoms described in the woman in the vignette are characteristic of scurvy, vitamin C (ascorbic acid) deficiency. Vitamin C is required as a cofactor and reducing agent in the hydroxylation of proline and lysine by prolyl and lysyl hydroxylase, respectively. In scurvy, there is a deficiency in ascorbic acid resulting in insufficient hydroxylation of collagen and abnormal collagen fibrils. Prolyl and lysyl hydroxylase are the two enzymes that carry out hydroxylation of proline and lysine, two amino acids characteristic of collagen. Hydroxyproline, which constitutes 10% of collagen, is often used to determine the collagen content of various tissues. Hydroxylation of proline stabilizes the triple helix through interchain hydrogen bonds, and hydroxylation of lysine is critical for the cross-linking stage of collagen assembly.

90. The answer is c. *(Alberts, pp 1186-1189. Mescher, pp 95-97.)* Nonhelical registration peptides at the ends of the triple helix prevent tropocollagen assembly in the RER, Golgi apparatus, and secretory vesicles. Collagen is synthesized as pro-α–chains, which are assembled into procollagen molecules (triple helix) in the RER. Procollagen is subsequently transported in transfer vesicles to the Golgi for packaging into secretory vesicles. Transport of secretory vesicles is an energy- and microtubule-dependent process. Outside of the cell, N-terminal and C-terminal specific procollagen peptidases (**answer e**) cleave the nonhelical registration peptides, which results in the formation of tropocollagen. Tropocollagen spontaneously assembles in a staggered array to form collagen fibrils. Lysyl oxidase (**answer a**) is an extracellular enzyme responsible for the formation of covalent cross-links between tropocollagen molecules (**answer b**). Fibrils form collagen fibers under the influence of other extracellular matrix constituents, such as proteoglycans and glycoproteins. Collagenases (**answer d**) specifically cleave tropocollagen in the extracellular matrix.

91. The answer is a. *(Alberts, pp 1006-1008, 1165-1169, 1186.)* The primary function of entactin (nidogen) is to cross-link laminin to type IV collagen. The basal lamina is formed by interactions between type IV collagen, laminin, entactin, and the proteoglycan perlecan. Integrins like laminin receptors (**answer b**) bind cells to the basal lamina; fibronectin receptors bind cells to the extracellular matrix (**answer c**). Laminin receptors in the cell membrane also organize the assembly of the basal lamina.

Collagen (answer d) is cross-linked by covalent intramolecular and intermolecular cross-links that form primarily between the nonhelical segments at the ends of the collagen molecules. Lysyl oxidase is a key enzyme in the cross-linking process; it deaminates lysine and hydroxylysine to form aldehyde groups that react with each other to form the covalent bonds. Actin is cross-linked (answer e) into bundles by actin-binding proteins such as the bundling protein α-actinin and the gel-forming protein (fimbrin). The diagnosis of the patient in this vignette is lupus erythematosus (SLE) with the major criteria of leukopenia, positive ANA, positive anti-dsDNA, arthritis, and nephritis.

92. The answer is a. (*Mescher, pp 98, 99, 322. Alberts, p 1187. Kierszenbaum, pp 110, 112.*) The patient in the vignette is suffering from Ehlers-Danlos Syndrome (EDS) type IV (also known as EDS of the vascular type). In that disorder there is improperly formed type III collagen, which is responsible for the elasticity of the intestinal and aortic walls. There are errors in the transcription of type III collagen mRNA or in translation of this mRNA. Hyperextensible skin (answer b) occurs in Ehlers-Danlos type VI disorder, in which problems with the hydroxylation of the amino acid lysine and subsequent cross-linking result in enhanced elasticity. Type VII EDS involves a specific deficiency in an amino terminal procollagen peptidase. This results from a genetic mutation that alters the propeptide sequence in such a way that the molecular orientation and cross-linking are adversely affected. The result is hypermobility (answer c) of synovial joints. Increased degradation of proteoglycans occurs in osteoarthritis (answer d). Type I collagen is found in dentin (answer e). Also, see High Yield Facts, Table 12.

93. The answer is c. (*Mescher, pp 109, 112-113.*) The photomicrograph illustrates the microscopic structure of brown adipose tissue. The patient in the vignette has subcutaneous fat necrosis of the newborn (SCFN), characterized by firm, erythematous nodules and plaques that appear on full-term newborns in the first few weeks of life. SCFN may be induced by cold or stress-induced injury to immature fat resulting in solidification and necrosis.

Both types of fat tissues (brown and white) are highly vascularized and function in protection from the cold. Brown fat specifically is involved in heat production, whereas white fat is a true thermal insulator. Brown adipose tissue is multilocular and is found in the human fetus and neonate.

Brown fat is involved in nonshivering thermogenesis and generates heat (answer c), probably as a protective device for developing organs in the fetus and neonate. White adipose tissue is specialized for lipid storage and functions as a thermal insulator (answer b) and shock absorber. White adipose tissue is unilocular, and the cells have a single, large lipid droplet in the cytoplasm that provides the "signet-ring" appearance often described for fat cells. Brown adipose tissue has a multilocular appearance and is brown because of numerous mitochondria.

In fat, norepinephrine activates the cyclic AMP (answer d) cascade through adenylate cyclase. Cyclic AMP activates hormone-sensitive lipase, which removes triglycerides from the stored lipid and hydrolyzes free fatty acids. In white adipocytes, the released fatty acids and glycerol are exported from the cells. In brown adipose tissue, the fatty acids are used within the cell (answer a). However, the electron transport system is uncoupled from oxidative phosphorylation, which results in the production of heat (answer c) instead of ATP. Heat is transferred to the blood by the extensive capillary networks found in brown adipose tissue. Shivering (answer e), as caused by hypothermia, initiates the mobilization of lipid in white adipose tissue because shivering requires energy.

94. The answer is b. (*Alberts, pp 1145-1146. Kierszenbaum, p 8.*) A mutation resulting in loss of integrin function would prevent leukocytes from extravasating from the blood to the lymphoid compartment (see High-Yield Facts, Figure 5) and sites of inflammation resulting in increased lymphocytes in the blood (leukocytosis), not leukopenia (answer a) or lymphadenopathy (answer c). In a rare congenital immunodeficiency disease, known as lymphocyte adhesion disease (LAD), patients suffer from recurrent bacterial infections in which the leukocytes from affected children fail to adhere to endothelial cells and migrate to the site of infection (answer c) due to defects in the leukocyte integrin CD18 subunit. Initial diagnosis is by blood test following failure of separation of the umbilical cord. In different forms of LAD there may be structural defects in the integrin molecule or a deficiency or absence of CD18. Lymphocyte apoptosis (answer d) is not regulated directly by integrins and plasma cells do not normally enter the blood (answer e). The leukocyte adhesion cascade involves several precise ordered steps: rolling, integrin activation, and firm adhesion of the leukocytes, all necessary prerequisites to transendothelial migration. Therefore, in LAD, extravasation of leukocytes is not possible leading to an increased white cell count. Alterations of lymphocyte integrins have been identified in the inflammatory bowel diseases: Crohn disease and ulcerative colitis.

95. The answer is c. (*Alberts, pp 1186-1187. Mescher, pp 98, 99, 259.*) Vitamin C deficiency causes scurvy. The woman in the scenario smokes and has a diet deficient in fresh fruits and vegetables. Scurvy, or vitamin C deficiency, results in an inability to form normal collagen triple helices. In scurvy, the resulting collagen is less stable and is subject to denaturation and proteolytic breakdown **(answer a)**. That instability results partially from slower secretion of collagen from fibroblasts. The collagen formed is not normally hydroxylated at proline and lysine residues because of the absence of vitamin C, which is a specific cofactor for hydroxylation of proline and lysine **(answer b)**. Bone structure and dentition may be abnormal and wound and fracture healing delayed **(answer d)**. General tissue instability may occur because collagen synthesis is necessary for maintenance of structural support **(answer e)**. Periodontal bleeding and ulceration are also common symptoms in scurvy.

96. The answer is d. (*Alberts, pp 1184-1189.*) The fibrillar collagens establish tensile strength at a number of levels including intra- and intermolecular cross-links. Covalent binding occurs through the OH⁻ groups of hydroxylysine and hydroxyproline and serves to stabilize the triple helix. The triple helix **(answer b)** itself functions to resist tensile forces. The degree of cross-linking varies from tissue to tissue. For example, it is highly extensive in tendons. The organization of collagen in tissues also varies, depending on function, from the layered appearance in bone to the axial parallel bundles in tendons and the wickered pattern in skin. The interactions with fibril-associated collagens (with interrupted triple helices) regulate orientation and are also important in establishing tissue organization and flexibility **(answer a)**. Electrostatic interactions **(answer c)** do not play a significant role in maintenance of collagen tensile strength. Lysine, along with hydroxylysine, is the substrate for lysyl oxidase that catalyzes the formation of cross-links **(answer e)**.

97. The answer is e. (*Alberts, pp 1165-1167. Kierszenbaum, pp 17-19. Mescher, pp 66, 101-102, 104.*) Laminin is a glycoprotein and a major component of all basement membranes that is involved in cell adherence to the basal lamina. The patient in the vignette has junctional epidermolysis bullosa in which blisters form at the level of the lamina lucida within the basal lamina. Laminin in the lamina rara (lucida) of the basal lamina binds to the laminin receptor (integrin) on the epithelial cell **(answer a).** Cell-cell interactions **(answer b)** are modulated by the cell adhesion molecules (eg, the Ca^{2+}-dependent cadherins and selectins and the Ca^{2+}-independent CAMs, such as the neural cell adhesion molecule [N-CAM]). Laminin contains cell-binding sites as well as binding sites for collagen, entactin (nidogen), and heparan sulfate proteoglycan. Type IV collagen forms the insoluble scaffolding of the basal lamina **(answer c).** The highly charged glycosaminoglycans are responsible for the filtration characteristics **(answer d)** of the basement membrane (eg, renal glomerular basement membrane).

98. The answer is e. *(Fauci, pp 300, 324, 2067-2068. Mescher, pp 90-93, 126, 133, 268.)* Mastocytosis is a disease in which there is excessive production of mast cells by the bone marrow. The cells in the biopsy are mast cells that stain metachromatically (change color of the stain from blue to purple). Like basophils, they synthesize and secrete heparin and histamine. The result of mastocytosis is an excessive release of the bioactive products contained in mast cell granules: histamine, heparin, eosinophil chemotactic factor of anaphylaxis (ECF-A), slow-reacting substance of anaphylaxis (SRS-A), and leukotrienes. Mastocytosis induces urticaria pigmentosa (the skin condition from which the patient in the scenario suffers), including edema (caused by the increased vascular permeability induced by histamine and SRS-A). In mastocytosis, there is infiltration of eosinophils (attracted by ECF-A), which causes itching. Excessive production of acid by the parietal cells of the stomach **(answer a)** occurs because of overstimulation of histamine receptors on those cells and can result in peptic ulcers and gastritis. Lower GI tract symptoms include increased motility and diarrhea due to the stimulation by mast cell contents. Periportal fibrosis of the liver often occurs in systemic mastocytosis due to the extensive infiltration of mast cells into the liver. Melanocytes **(answer b)** are not affected. Osteoporosis and anemia **(answers c and d)** would occur in either multiple myeloma or plasmacytosis, where there are excessive numbers of plasma cells. The excessive production of plasma cells in the bone marrow disrupts normal hematopoiesis including the production of RBCs, causing anemia. Plasma cells release interleukins (IL-1 and IL-6) and tumor necrosis factor-alpha (TNF-α) that stimulate osteoclastic activity and induce osteoporosis (see clinical case questions in the chapter on the specialized connective tissues, bone, and cartilage). The positive Darier sign is a red wheal and surrounding erythema around the lesions after rubbing due to the release of histamine.

99. The answer is a. (*Alberts, pp 923, 925, 1102, 1441, 1450. Kumar, pp 87, 88, 1138. Rubin, pp 86-88, 103.*) PDGF stimulates chemotaxis of monocytes and macrophages as well as fibroblasts to the site of a wound. PDGF also induces proliferation of vascular smooth muscle cells **(answer b)** to facilitate blood vessel repair and fibroblasts **(answer c)** to synthesize type I collagen. PDGF stimulates the formation of granulation tissue **(answer d)** consisting of new connective tissue and small blood vessels that form in the wound site. Type II collagen **(answer e)** is synthesized by chondrocytes in hyaline and elastic cartilage. Wound healing is a complex process initiated by damage to capillaries in the dermis. The clot forms through the interaction of integrins on the surface of blood platelets with fibrinogen and fibronectin. Fibrin is the primary protein that constructs the three-dimensional structure of the clot. A scar is formed as a very dense region of type I collagen fibers. Macrophages remove debris at the wound site and are also involved in the remodeling of the scar. All wound healing processes are slower in diabetics, and the presence of advanced-glycation end products (AGE) and their interaction with the receptor for AGE (RAGE) as well as the endogenous ligand for RAGE (ENRAGE) appear to contribute to inhibited healing in diabetes. AGE are produced by the nonenzymatic glycation and oxidation of proteins/lipids and alter those molecules and therefore the function and structure of tissues and organs such as the kidney (diabetic nephropathy), peripheral nerves (neuropathy), and the retina (diabetic retinopathy).

100. The answer is d. (*Fauci, pp 701-703. Young, pp 207, 209, 218. Kindt, pp 9, 33, 36-37, 76-78, 88-94.*) The patient in the scenario suffers from multiple myeloma with an increase in the number of plasma cells responsible for producing immunoglobulins (antibodies). The cells delineated by the arrows in the photomicrograph are plasma cells characterized by eccentric nuclei with coarse granules of heterochromatin arranged in a radial pattern about the nuclear envelope. Membrane-bound ribosomes are extremely plentiful, providing the cytoplasm with a characteristic intense basophilia. The ribosomes are involved in antibody production, principally immunoglobulin G (IgG).

The juxtanuclear region, which does not stain, represents the Golgi complex, in which the antibodies are processed for secretion. Plasma cells produce all the immunoglobulins—IgG, IgA, IgM, IgD, and IgE—and are derived from B lymphocytes. The differentiation of plasma cells requires antigen-presenting cells (macrophages, dendritic cells, or B cells that phagocytose and present antigen-MHC II complex) and T helper (T_H) cells. Fibroblasts synthesize collagen (**answer a**), mast cells synthesize heparin and histamine (**answer b**), eosinophils synthesize histaminase (**answer c**), and neutrophils synthesize myeloperoxidase (**answer e**).

101. The answer is e. (*Mescher, p 111. Ross, pp 239-241.*) Leptin is a protein hormone produced by adipocytes (shown in the photomicrograph). Leptin binds to receptors in the hypothalamus and has multiple effects including increased release of norepinephrine (NE) from sympathetic nerve terminals that innervate adipose tissue. Adipocyte adrenergic receptors bind NE leading to increased metabolism of fatty acids with dissipation of the energy as heat. As weight increases and adipocytes accumulate triglycerides, the "obese" (*ob*) gene is up-regulated in adipocytes and leptin synthesis and serum levels of leptin are increased (**answers b and c**). Leptin-receptors in the hypothalamus are up-regulated as leptin levels increase (**answer a**). Leptin inhibits hypothalamic synthesis and secretion of neuropeptide Y, an appetite (orexigenic) peptide (**answer d**).

102. The answer is b. (*Kumar, pp 298-301.*) The patient is diagnosed with transitional cell carcinoma (TCC) that is highly aggressive having penetrated the muscle of the bladder (T3a), with lymph node involvement and metastases (M2). TCC metastasizes primarily to the lymph nodes, lung, bone, liver, and brain. The tumor cells normally adhere to the basement membrane. To undergo metastasis they must dissolve the basement membrane and extracellular matrix in order to reach the bloodstream and subsequently migrate to a new site, where they reaggregate and reestablish cell-cell and cell-basal lamina interactions. Metalloproteinases such as the serine, cysteine, and metalloproteinases (MMPs), including type IV collagenase (MMP-2), play a key role in freeing tumor cells to migrate to metastatic sites. Lysyl oxidase (**answer a**) is an extracellular enzyme that is responsible for cross-linking of collagen by deamination of lysine and hydroxylysine residues to form aldehydes. Those aldehydes then interact with each other or with other lysyl side chains to form collagen cross-links.

A similar process occurs in the synthesis of elastin. Plasminogen (**answer c**) is an inactive form of plasmin that occurs in plasma and is converted to plasmin by organic solvents. Serpins (**answer d**) are serine protease inhibitors. Members of that gene family regulate cell division and migration, neurite extension, tumor cell metastasis, and blood coagulation. The serpins act as specific inhibitors of cell-surface and extracellular matrix serine proteases that participate in cascade mechanisms in those biological processes. TIMPs (**answer e**), are the tissue inhibitors of the metalloproteases and, like serpins, inhibit the degradation of the extracellular matrix.

Specialized Connective Tissues: Bone and Cartilage

Questions

103. Intramembranous ossification differs from endochondral ossification in which one of the following ways?

a. Action of osteoblasts
b. Light microscopic appearance of the adult bone
c. Ultrastructural appearance of the adult bone
d. Presence of woven bone early in the ossification process
e. Microenvironment in which ossification occurs

104. A 7-year-old boy is referred to the endocrine clinic with short stature, rhizomelic shortening of the arms and legs, a disproportionately long trunk, trident hands, midfacial hypoplasia, prominent forehead (frontal bossing), thoracolumbar gibbus, and megalencephaly. Radiological examination by MRI reveals caudal narrowing of the interpedicular spaces of T1 and T2 vertebrae and spinal stenosis at L2 to L4. Genetic analysis reveals a gain of function mutation, G1138A, in the fibroblast growth factor receptor-3 (FGFR3), band 4p16.3. His parents are requesting the initiation of treatment with growth hormone. The endocrinologist is concerned about harmful growth hormone effects: deposition of abnormally formed bone and worsening of the patient's kyphoscoliosis. During this child's postnatal development, which one of the following is the most likely effect of the FGFR3 gene mutation?

a. Decreased bone deposition under the periosteum
b. Decreased proliferation of osteoblasts in the primary ossification center
c. Decreased proliferation of osteoblasts in the secondary ossification center
d. Decreased appositional growth of chondroblasts in the primary ossification center
e. Decreased interstitial growth of chondroblasts in the epiphyses

105. The molecular basis for shock absorption within articular cartilage is which one of the following?

a. Electrostatic interaction of proteoglycans with type IV collagen
b. Ability of glycosaminoglycans to bind anions
c. Noncovalent binding of glycosaminoglycans to protein cores
d. Sialic acid residues in the glycoproteins
e. Hydration of glycosaminoglycans

106. A 16-year-old adolescent presents to the pediatric genetic and endocrine clinic with short stature, Tanner stage 2 of pubertal development, and lack of menstruation. She is 49 in tall (normal range for age is 59-68 in, mean 64 in) and weighs 65 lb (normal range for age is 92-158 lb, mean is 126 lb). She has a short, broad, webbed neck, short fingers and toes, and *cubitus valgus*. Hormonal profile reveals high levels of the gonadotrophins LH and FSH, and very low levels of estrogen. Ultrasound studies show uterine hypoplasia and poorly-defined gonadal streaks. Genetic analysis shows a 45, X0 pattern. The short stature has been linked to reduced protein expression of the short stature homeobox gene (*SHOX*). This gene working through specific transcription factors would influence the production of which one of the following by the cells delineated by the box in the accompanying photomicrograph?

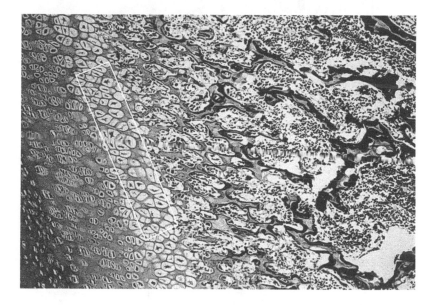

a. Cyclins
b. Acid phosphatase
c. Alkaline phosphatase
d. Type I collagen
e. Osteocalcin

107. A 22-year-old man presents with persistent joint pain and a history of recurrent fractures of the humerus and femur, numerous dental caries, and associated abscesses. Serum acid phosphatase is 4 units (normal 0.5-2) and hematocrit is 35 (normal 41%-50%, mean 47%). Other blood tests are normal. He complains of joint pain. "Sandwich" vertebrae with thickening of the vertebral end-plates, abnormal thickening of the long bones and basilar sclerosis are seen on x-rays. The cell type primarily affected in this patient is shown in the accompanying transmission electron micrograph (A) and labeled as "C" in the light micrograph (B). The activation and stimulation of those cells is involved in which one of the following?

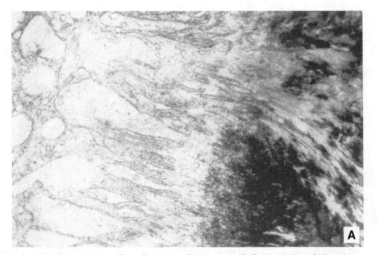

(Reproduced, with permission, from Erlandsen SL, Magney JE. Color Atlas of Histology. St. Louis, MO: CV Mosby; 1992.)

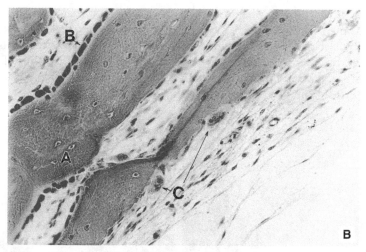

(Micrograph courtesy of Dr. John K. Young.)

a. Mechanical grinding of the bone matrix
b. Synthesis of alkaline phosphatase
c. Response to vitamin D through receptors on its cell membrane
d. Regulation by parathyroid hormone (PTH) receptors on its cell membrane
e. Proton pump activity similar to a parietal cell

108. A 64-year-old woman presents with symmetric polyarticular joint pain, swelling, joint stiffness lasting an hour or more (particularly in the morning), malaise, fatigue, tenderness and pain, and is seropositive for anti-cyclic citrullinated peptide (anti-CCP) antibodies. Analysis of synovial fluid reveals synovitis with a white blood cell count of 2500 (normal less than 2000/mm^3). Physical examination shows decreased abduction and external rotation of the right and left shoulders. She has swelling in her right and left metacarpal-phalangeal joints with full range of motion. Which joint changes will most likely be associated with this patient's disease?

a. Loss of the proteoglycan matrix and fibrillation in the articular cartilage during the early stages
b. Decreased levels of fibrinogen in the synovial fluid
c. Formation of osteophytes at the articular margins and eburnation of large weight-bearing joints in the later stages
d. Decreased number of leukocytes including PMNs in the synovial fluid
e. Heterologous autoantibodies directed against the synovium

109. A 42-year-old woman, who has been a type I diabetic for 30 years, falls when she trips over her vacuum cleaner hose. She tried to break her fall by placing her hand out to save herself and in the process her wrist is forced backward. She arrives in the emergency room and an x-ray of her wrist is shown in the accompanying x-ray. Which one of the following is the first step in the healing of this injury?

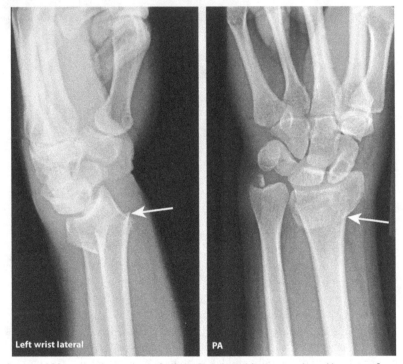

Left wrist lateral   PA

(Image 6120, used with permission from the Radiological Anatomy website, University of Kansas, School of Medicine, http://classes. Kumc.edu/SOM/radanatomy/.)

a. Internal callus
b. External callus
c. Clot
d. Pannus
e. Granulation tissue

110. A 55-year-old woman presents with pain in her right hip and thigh. The pain started approximately 6 months ago and is a deep ache that worsens when she stands or walks. Your examination reveals increased warmth over the right thigh. The only laboratory abnormalities are alkaline phosphatase 656 IU/L (normal 23-110 IU/L), elevated 24-hour urine hydroxyproline, and osteocalcin 13 ng/mL (normal 6 ng/mL). X-ray of hips and pelvis shows osteolytic lesions and regions with excessive osteoblastic activity. Bone scan shows significant uptake in the right proximal femur. Which one of the following should be included in the differential diagnosis?

a. Paget disease
b. Multiple myeloma
c. Osteomalacia
d. Osteoporosis
e. Hypoparathyroidism

111. A 66-year-old man with no previous significant illness presents with back pain. The patient had felt well except for an increase in fatigue over the past few months. He suddenly felt severe low back pain while raising his garage door. Physical examination reveals a well-developed white male in acute pain. His pulse is 88 beats per minute and blood pressure is 150/90 mm Hg. The conjunctivae are pale. There is marked tenderness to percussion over the lumbar spine. The following laboratory data are obtained: hemoglobin 11.0 g/dL (normal 13-16 g/dL), serum calcium 12.3 mg/dL (normal 8.5-11 mg/dL), abnormal serum protein electrophoresis with a monoclonal IgG spike, urine positive for Bence Jones protein, and abnormal bone marrow smear. X-rays reveal lytic lesions of the skull and pelvis and a compression fracture of lumbar vertebrae. A potential underlying mechanism for the symptoms observed in this case is which one of the following?

a. Increased IL-1, IL-6, and TNF-α by plasma cells
b. Increased release of histamine from mast cells
c. Decreased RANK expression on osteoclasts
d. Decreased RANK-L levels
e. Decreased production of M-CSF
f. Increased osteoprotegerin

112. A 46-year-old woman presents with pain in the left leg that worsens on weight bearing. An x-ray shows demineralization, and a decalcified (EDTA-treated) biopsy shows reduction in bone quantity. The patient had undergone menopause at age 45 without estrogen replacement. She reports long-standing diarrhea. In addition, laboratory tests show low levels of 1,25-hydroxyvitamin D, calcium and phosphorus, and elevated alkaline phosphatase. A second bone biopsy, which was not decalcified, shows uncalcified osteoid on all the bone surfaces. On the basis of those data, the best diagnosis would be which one of the following?

a. Osteoporosis
b. Osteomalacia
c. Scurvy
d. Paget disease
e. Hypoparathyroidism

113. Patients with Cushing syndrome often show osteoporotic changes. Which one of the following is involved in the etiology of osteoporosis induced by Cushing syndrome?

a. Decreased glucocorticoid levels that result in decreased quality of the bone deposited
b. Excess deposition of osteoid
c. Stimulation of intestinal calcium absorption
d. Decreased PTH levels
e. Bone fragility resulting from excess bone resorption

114. A newborn girl is born with a small mouth, rather widely spaced eyes, and low-set ears. Genetic analysis shows a microdeletion on chromosome 22q11.2 leading to a diagnosis of an anomaly which results from failure of the normal development of the third and fourth branchial pouches during embryonic development. Which one of the following would be expected to occur in a child with this anomaly?

a. Absence of the parafollicular (C) cells
b. Increased numbers of cells in the deep cortex of the lymph nodes
c. Tetany
d. Excess activity of osteoclasts
e. Increased Ca^{2+} levels in the blood

115. A 56-year-old man with a history of hypertension, type II diabetes, and a 2-year history of end-stage renal disease requiring hemodialysis returns to the internal medicine clinic. The patient has hyperparathyroidism (parathyroid hormone, 234 pg/mL; normal 10-55 pg/mL) and is hypercalcemic (calcium, 12.2 mg/dL). He also has elevated levels of serum urea nitrogen (52 mg/dL), creatinine (5.2 mg/dL), and hyperphosphatemia (phosphorus, 9.1 mg/dL). Serum levels of 1,25-dihydroxyvitamin D are decreased (10 pg/mL; reference range, 24-65 pg/mL). He has been receiving large doses of calcium supplemented with vitamin D to bind the phosphate. He complains of bone and chest pain, increasing fatigue, and extreme dyspnea. His coronary arteries are examined by electron-beam computed tomography and are found to be calcified. The production of calcified soft tissues is mediated by the matrix vesicles shown in the accompanying transmission electron micrograph. Which one of the following is a possible mechanism of action for matrix vesicles?

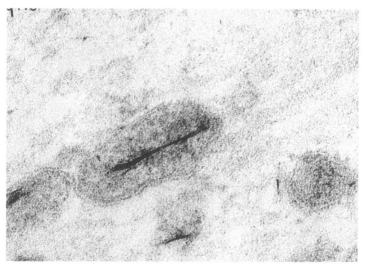

(Micrograph courtesy of Dr. H. Clarke Anderson.)

a. Increased secretion of acid phosphatase
b. Inhibition of alkaline phosphatase
c. Accumulation of calcium and phosphate
d. Increased secretion of osteoprotegerin
e. Increased synthesis of type I collagen

116. The collagenous protein in bone subserves which of the following functions?

a. Growth factor
b. Binding of ionic calcium and physiologic hydroxyapatite
c. Formation of the three-dimensional lattice of the matrix
d. Cell attachment
e. Binding of mineral components to the matrix

117. In the diagram of a joint below, the structure labeled C is which one of the following?

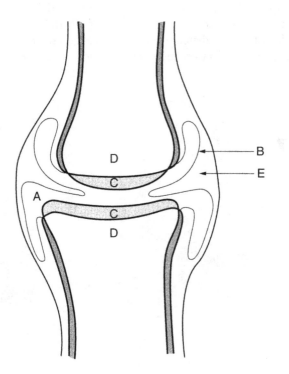

a. Site of macrophage-like cells that phagocytose particles from the synovial fluid
b. Site of cells that synthesize the synovial fluid
c. Initial site of damage in osteoarthritis
d. Initial site of inflammation in rheumatoid arthritis
e. Perichondrium

118. A 58-year-old Caucasian woman is seen in the endocrine clinic. She has been followed for type I diabetes for the past decade. She sustained a Colles' fracture last year when she fell over the hose while watering the garden. She took hormone replacement therapy (HRT) for 3 years at the start of menopause, but was taken off HRT 5 years ago because of her concerns about ovarian cancer. She drinks three glasses of milk a day and eats other dairy products frequently. She drinks socially, a drink, a glass of wine, or a beer twice/week. She does not smoke. She once was a "runner," but now walks 2 miles twice/week when weather permits. She is 5 ft 4 in and she weighs 122 lb. Her height has decreased by an inch over the past 5 years and her weight has increased by 12 lb. Blood chemistries and CBC are normal. Her "T" score on dual-energy absorptiometry (DXA) is −2 for spine and −2.5 for hip. Bisphosphonates are prescribed. Which one of the following is the most likely mechanism of action for the bisphosphonates?

a. Inhibition of osteoblastic activity
b. Increased RANK-L secretion by osteoblasts
c. Increased M-CSF secretion by osteoblasts
d. Apoptosis of osteoclasts
e. Increased RANK expression by osteoclasts

119. A 12-year-old boy who has grown 3 in. in the past 2 months presents with pain and swelling in his femur just above the knee. Any exercise results in intense pain, and the boy now walks with a limp. X ray shows a fracture at the distal end of the right femur. Overall, the bone appears immature in the distal femur and there is increased density extending into the metaphysis. There appears to be a soft tissue mass expanding outside the bone. There is also some cortical bone destruction above the lateral condyle. A CT scan shows bone-forming cells in the lung. Once the osteosarcoma cells reach the lungs, enter the lung parenchyma, and clonally expand, they produce bone. In that process, the tumor cells synthesize which one of the following?

a. Type III collagen
b. Type II collagen
c. Acid phosphatase
d. Alkaline phosphatase
e. Elastin

120. If a laboratory were designing an effective therapy to prevent the spread of metastatic osteosarcoma, which one of the following approaches would most likely be successful?

a. Enhancement of fibronectin-integrin interactions
b. Enhancement of laminin-integrin interactions
c. Up-regulation of selectins on endothelial cells
d. Up-regulation of tissue inhibitors of matrix metalloproteinases (TIMPs) at the primary tumor site
e. Down-regulation of angiostatin or endostatin at the primary tumor site

121. A 28-year-old woman visits the family medicine clinic complaining of loss of sense of smell, nosebleeds, problems with swallowing, and hoarseness. She admits to "casual, social use" of cocaine on a regular basis since her sophomore year of college when her "boyfriend turned her on to cocaine at a party." A complete examination of her nose with a speculum and otoscope determines that she has rhinitis (inflammation). There is also perforation and collapse of the nasal cartilage resulting in a "saddle nose" deformity. Erosions in the enamel of her front teeth are noted. The breakdown of the nasal cartilage releases collagen fibers primarily of which type?

a. Type I
b. Type II
c. Type III
d. Type IV
e. Type VII

Specialized Connective Tissues: Bone and Cartilage

Answers

103. The answer is e. (*Mescher, pp 129-131. Ross, pp 232-235.*) The difference between endochondral and intramembranous ossification is the microenvironment in which bone formation occurs. In both cases, bone development occurs by essentially the same process, the synthesis of collagen and other matrix components by osteoblasts **(answer a)** and the calcification of the matrix through the action of alkaline phosphatase from osteoblasts. Bone development occurs in two different locations, which differ in the presence or absence of cartilage models of the bones. For example, in the flat bones of the skull, bone formation occurs through the differentiation of osteoprogenitor cells from mesoderm and is accompanied by vascularization. This is known as intramembranous ossification. In the other form of ossification (endochondral), chondrocytes establish a cartilage model of the long bone that is subsequently replaced by bone. This method occurs in bones such as the humerus and femur. The cartilage model of each bone is used as a scaffolding for bone formation. Bone formed by the two methods cannot be distinguished with the light or electron microscope **(answers b and c)**. In both endochondral and intramembranous ossification, the first bone formed is woven bone **(answer d)**, also known as primary bone. This bone is replaced by adult, lamellar bone through a remodeling process.

104. The answer is e. (*Sadler, pp 132-134.*) In achondroplasia, the common mutations cause a gain of function of the *FGFR3* gene, resulting in decreased endochondral ossification, inhibited proliferation of chondroblasts in growth plate cartilage, decreased cellular hypertrophy, and decreased cartilage matrix production. Growth in the length of long bones after birth (postnatally) occurs through cell proliferation of chondroblasts (immature chondrocytes) in the secondary ossification centers of the epiphyses. The primary ossification centers "close" soon after birth (answer d). Fetal development of long bones occurs by the process of endochondral ossification in which a cartilage model is replaced by bone. Before birth, growth in length of the long bone occurs primarily through the proliferation of chondroblasts within the diaphysis of the cartilage model (primary ossification center). Growth in the width of the long bone occurs by the addition of osteoblasts from the periosteum and deposition of a periosteal collar (answer a). This is appositional growth without a cartilage intermediate (intramembranous ossification). It is one of the best examples of intramembranous ossification, even though it occurs in the development of a long bone. The action of osteoblasts is to deposit bone matrix and secrete alkaline phosphatase; they do not proliferate in either the primary or the secondary ossification centers (answers b and c).

105. The answer is e. (*Alberts, pp 1182-1184. Mescher, pp 114-115.*) Hydration of the glycosaminoglycans plays an important role in shock absorption and enhances the resiliency of the cartilage. This role is particularly important in the articular cartilages, which receive pressure during joint movement and are required to resist strong compressive forces. Proteoglycans are the major component of the ground substance of cartilage. They possess a large anionic charge because of the presence of sulfate, hydroxyl, and carboxyl groups within the glycosaminoglycans, which join to form proteoglycan subunits by linking with a core protein (answer c). The proteoglycan subunits (monomers) subsequently form an aggregate by linking noncovalently to hyaluronic acid (answer c). Those aggregates establish the rigidity of hyaline cartilage by reacting electrostatically with type II collagen (answer a), probably through the sulfate groups of the glycosaminoglycans. The negative charge of the glycosaminoglycans facilitates the binding of cations (answer b) and the transport of electrolytes and water within the matrix. This is an important aspect of cartilage metabolism because the chondrocytes depend on diffusion to obtain nutrients or to dispose of waste products. Glycoproteins (answer d) are not a major constituent of the cartilage matrix.

106. The answer is c. (*Kumar, pp 165-167. Fauci, pp 2341-2342.*) The child in the vignette is diagnosed with Turner syndrome, gonadal dysgenesis, in which the 45, X karyotype results in multiple medical problems. The short stature has been attributed to the *SHOX* (short stature homeobox) gene which affects various stages of endochondral development. The light micrograph illustrates a developing long bone. The region in the box is the zone of chondrocyte hypertrophy, where chondrocytes synthesize alkaline phosphatase which calcifies the cartilage matrix, eventually leading to chondrocyte death because of dependence on diffusion to obtain oxygen and nutrients from the matrix. During long bone development, specific zones are established, as a cartilage model of a long bone is converted to mature bone. The zones from the epiphysis toward the center of the shaft (diaphysis) are: resting zone, proliferative zone, hypertrophy zone, and zone of calcified cartilage that is used as the scaffolding for the deposition of bone. The periosteal bud represents the ingrowth of blood vessels (angiogenesis) bringing bone marrow precursors and osteoprogenitor cells into the diaphysis. Angiogenesis is required for bone formation. Bone is formed by the action of osteoblasts forming type I collagen, noncollagenous proteins (eg, osteocalcin, osteopontin, and osteonectin), and alkaline phosphatase, which plays an essential role in mineralization of the osteoid. Cyclins are synthesized by cells passing through the cell cycle, ie, cells in the proliferative zone **(answer a)**; acid phosphatase **(answer b)** is synthesized by osteoclasts; and type I collagen and osteocalcin **(answers d and e)** are synthesized by osteoblasts.

107. The answer is e. (*Alberts, pp 1470-1472, 1474. Costanzo, p 432. Fauci, pp 671, 2411. Mescher, pp 125-126. Kumar, pp 1126, 1208, 1212-1215.*) The patient in the vignette is diagnosed with type II autosomal dominant osteopetrosis (type II ADO), also known as Albers-Schönberg disease with a characteristic radiological image of "sandwich vertebrae." The targets in this disease are the osteoclasts which are indicated in the micrographs. Osteoclast function is altered in osteopetrosis. Osteoclasts function by release of lytic enzymes and protons (derived from carbonic acid) into the calcified matrix beneath the ruffled border and not through a grinding action **(answer a)**. The bone compartment around the ruffled border of the osteoclast is, therefore, analogous to a secondary lysosome in function, albeit extracellular. Osteoclasts use protons derived from carbonic acid, catalyzed by carbonic anhydrase, in similar fashion to parietal cells of the stomach. Alkaline phosphatase is synthesized by osteoblasts **(answer b)**; PTH and vitamin D receptors are found on osteoblasts **(answers c and d)**, not osteoclasts.

The electron micrograph illustrates the typical ultrastructure of an osteoclast with its distinctive ruffled border. The light micrograph illustrates the position of the osteoclasts (multinucleate cells) in small depressions in the bone (Howship lacunae). The cell membrane of the osteoclast adjacent to the resorbing bone surface is thrown into folds and villous-like processes with tips that reach and even enter the bone surface (ruffled border). The osteoclast is attached to the bone surface, and the resorption area is sealed off by the presence of contractile proteins in the cytoplasm lateral to the site of the ruffled border. The basolateral membrane of the osteoclast posseses a Na^+-K^+-ATPase pump as do all human cells.

Osteoclasts are of hematopoietic origin and arise from the monocytic lineage. Osteoclasts are responsive to a number of hormones including PTH, calcitonin, and 1,25(OH) 2-vitamin D_3. PTH is the major regulator of osteoclastic activity, increasing the number of osteoclasts as well as ruffled-border activity. The osteoclasts respond to low serum Ca^{2+} by removing calcium from bone. PTH receptors are located on osteoblasts, not osteoclasts **(answer d)**, and so PTH affects osteoblasts to release soluble factors (RANK-L and M-CSF) that stimulate osteoclasts. Vitamin D receptors are also present on osteoblasts but absent from the plasma membrane of osteoclasts **(answer c)**. This indirect receptor effect links the osteoblast and osteoclast in the so-called "ARF cycle" (Activation of osteoclasts → Resorption → Formation of new bone). Calcitonin is responsible for transient changes in bone resorption. In the presence of high Ca^{2+}, calcitonin is synthesized and released from C (interfollicular, parafollicular) cells of the thyroid, which decreases ruffled-border activity. Calcitonin receptors are located on osteoclasts. Long-term responses to elevated Ca^{2+} are mediated by lowering of PTH levels rather than increased calcitonin production. This is exemplified in patients with an absence of calcitonin secretion (eg, after thyroidectomy), or with stimulated levels of calcitonin (eg, in medullary thyroid carcinoma) who exhibit relatively normal bone metabolism. However, calcitonin measurements are an important tool in the diagnosis of medullary thyroid carcinoma, a malignancy of thyroid cells. Calcitonin may be used as a nasal spray for osteoporosis when patients cannot tolerate bisphosphonates. Bisphosphonates are analogues of pyrophosphate and the primary means of treating osteoporosis and Paget disease. They function by inhibiting osteoclastic activity through apoptosis of osteoclasts.

108. The answer is e. *(Kumar, pp 1235-1240.)* Arthritis involves inflammatory changes in a joint. The patient in the vignette suffers from rheumatoid arthritis; an autoimmune disease in which rheumatoid factor (RF) composed of heterologous autoantibodies directed against serum gamma globulin (IgG) appears. Anti-CCP antibodies are used to diagnose rheumatoid arthritis and appear to be superior over IgM RF in predicting an erosive disease course. RF is present in the serum of 85% to 90% of patients with rheumatoid arthritis. Deposition of RF can be pathogenic and leads to inflammatory destruction of the joint surface. Cell-mediated immunity is also involved in rheumatoid arthritis. Alteration of the synovial membrane results in the formation of a pannus, or inflammatory, hypertrophic synovial villus. The presence of the pannus and release of lysosomal enzymes from the pannus result in degradation of the cartilage. This is followed by hypertrophy and hyperplasia of the articular cartilages, which often leads to bone formation across the joint with welding of the bones together (ankylosis). Because of the inflammation in rheumatoid arthritis, there are elevated numbers of leukocytes (**answer d**), in particular PMNs, in the synovial fluid. During rheumatoid arthritis, fibrinogen (**answer b**), another indicator of inflammatory responses, is elevated. Osteoarthritis begins with loss of hydrated glycosaminoglycans, followed by death of chondrocytes, fibrillation, and development of fissures in the articular cartilage matrix (**answer a**). The severe wear and tear of osteoarthritis increases with age. During the breakdown of the articular cartilages, the width of the underlying bone increases. Osteoarthritis typically includes the formation of reactive bone spurs called osteophytes (**answer c**), which may break off to form foreign bodies in the joint space (ie, "joint mice"). In the fingers, osteoarthritis primarily affects distal interphalangeal joints, where it produces painful nodular enlargements called Heberden nodes. Large weight-bearing joints are also usually involved in osteoarthritis and often exhibit eburnation in the late stages, when the articular cartilages have been worn down, and result in an osseous articular surface.

109. The answer is c. (*Mescher, pp 131-132. Kumar, pp 1219-1220.*) The most common type of wrist fracture is a Colles' fracture. The location of the break is approximately 2 cm from the wrist joint at the point where the radius narrows from cancellous bone forming the joint to the cortical bone of the shaft. In the healing of fractures, the first step is clotting of extravasated blood. The clot is organized into a callus by granulation tissue (**answer e**) that consists of fibroblasts, osteogenic cells, and budding capillaries. An internal, bony callus (**answer a**) forms where local bone factors are most active (ie, in close proximity to the periosteum and endosteum that retain osteogenic potential). An external, cartilaginous (answer b) callus forms bone by endochondral ossification following initial chondrogenesis. These steps involve repetition of the cellular events involved in the histogenesis of bone. A bone graft is more important as a method of forming a temporary bridge in a severe defect than a source of osteoprogenitor cells. Other methods useful in stimulating bone repair include electrical forces and bone morphogenetic protein (BMP), a bone growth factor obtained from decalcified bone matrix. BMP stimulates bone formation when implanted at the fracture site. Pannus formation is an inflammatory event within the synovial membrane in patients with rheumatoid arthritis (answer d).

110. The answer is a. (*Favus, pp 321-323. Kumar, pp 1216-1218. Greenspan, pp 338-341. Fauci, pp 2408-2409.*) The correct diagnosis is Paget disease, also known as osteitis deformans because of its deforming capabilities (eg, skull or femoral head enlargement). In this disease the serum calcium is normal, but there is an increase in osteoclastic activity (osteolytic lesions and elevated 24-hour urine hydroxyproline) and an increase in osteoblastic activity (elevated osteocalcin and alkaline phosphatase). Patients with Paget disease exhibit a marked increase in osteoid, and the bone actually enlarges. The osteoid is never normally mineralized in this disease. In this patient, the bone scan shows significant uptake of labeled bisphosphonates, which are incorporated into newly formed osteoid during bone formation. Her proximal femur is enlarged and no longer fits properly into the acetabulum, which results in the hip pain. The test results are characteristic of Paget, not multiple myeloma, osteomalacia, osteoporosis, or hypoparathyroidism (answers b → e).

There are a number of useful biochemical markers of bone metabolism. Osteoclasts synthesize tartrate-resistant acid phosphatase so that increased osteoclastic activity is reflected in increased serum levels of tartrate-resistant acid phosphatase. Bone resorption fragments of type I collagen and noncollagenous proteins increase as bone matrix is resorbed. Hydroxyproline is a good urinary marker of bone metabolism because hydroxyproline is released and excreted in the urine as collagen is broken down. The presence of pyridinoline cross-links, which are involved in the bundling of type I collagen, is used for measurement of bone resorption. Those cross-links are released only during degradation of mineralized collagen fibrils as occurs in bone resorption. Usually, pyridinoline cross-links are measured by immunoassay over a 24-hour period to detect excess bone resorption and collagen breakdown in disorders such as Paget disease.

Markers of bone formation include osteocalcin, alkaline phosphatase, and the extension peptides of type I collagen. Osteocalcin is a vitamin K–dependent γ-carboxyglutamic acid protein, that is, synthesized by osteoblasts and secreted into the serum in an unchanged state. Serum concentrations of osteocalcin are, therefore, directly related to osteoblastic activity. It is a more specific marker than alkaline phosphatase, because other organs, such as the liver and kidney, produce that enzyme.

Radiologic methods such as conventional x-ray can be used to detect osteoporosis, but only after patients have lost 30% to 50% of their bone mass. Dual-beam photon absorptiometry allows a much more accurate diagnosis of loss of bone mass.

111. The answer is a. *(Favus, pp 378-379. Kumar, pp 609-611. Fauci, pp 701-704.)* The patient is diagnosed with multiple myeloma, which causes increased plasma cell activity and anemia (hemoglobin data and increasing fatigue). Those plasma cells produce elevated levels of interleukin 1 (IL-1), which functions as an osteoclast activation factor, resulting in elevated serum calcium (12.3 mg/dL). Depletion of bone calcium results in lytic lesions of the skull and pelvis as well as compression fractures of the spine. The Bence Jones protein represents free-immunoglobulin light chains, a diagnostic feature (Bence Jones proteinuria) in the urine of patients with multiple myeloma. RANK is found on osteoclasts, binds to RANK-L produced by osteoblasts, and stimulates osteoclastic activity (see High-Yield Facts, Figure 7). Mast cells (**answer b**) are not directly involved, and RANK, RANK-L, and M-CSF are up-regulated (**answers c → e**), while osteoprotegerin (**answer f**) levels are decreased in multiple myeloma.

112. The answer is b. *(Favus, pp 330-335. Kumar, pp 433, 435-436. Greenspan, pp 331-334. Mescher, pp 125, 133. Fauci, pp 2375, 2694.)* The patient suffers from osteomalacia, a disease related to malnutrition, specifically vitamin D deficiency. On the basis of the first bone biopsy in which the tissue was decalcified, one could make a diagnosis of osteoporosis (**answer a**). The second, nondecalcified bone biopsy indicates that osteoid is being formed, but is not undergoing mineralization (**rules out diagnoses answers a, c → e**). This correlates with the low 25-hydroxyvitamin D levels. Vitamin D replacement and calcium supplementation would be prescribed for this patient.

113. The answer is e. (*Favus, pp 398-401. Kumar, pp 1214-1216. Greenspan, pp 302, 322, 324-325. Fauci, pp 2397, 2401-2402.*) Excess glucocorticoid induces osteoporosis. For example, in Cushing syndrome, patients produce high levels of corticosteroids that interfere with bone metabolism (**rules out answers a → d**). A similar pattern may be seen during prolonged steroid therapy. The result is increased bone resorption compared with bone deposition. Intestinal calcium absorption is inhibited and PTH levels may be increased.

Osteoporosis is a major problem of normal aging in both sexes, sixth decade in women and seventh decade in men. In that disease, the balance between bone deposition and bone resorption is lost. The disease is prevalent in postmenopausal women because the protective effect of estrogens is no longer present. Osteoporosis may also be induced by other diseases (eg, diabetes mellitus, hyperthyroidism) or drugs (eg, alcohol and caffeine).

114. The answer is c. (*Sadler, pp 177, 185, 276-277. Moore and Persaud, pp 173, 468.*) The child in the vignette is suffering from DiGeorge anomaly, which results in the absence of the thymus and parathyroid glands, which arise from the third and fourth pairs of branchial (pharyngeal) pouches. The absence of the thymus results in a deficiency in T lymphocyte–dependent areas of the immune system. These areas include the deep cortex of the lymph nodes (**answer b**), periarterial lymphatic sheath of the spleen, and interfollicular areas of the Peyer patches. PTH stimulates the development of osteoclasts and the formation of ruffled borders in osteoclasts. The absence of PTH results in: (1) a drastic reduction in numbers and activity of osteoclasts (**answer d**), (2) reduced Ca^{2+} levels in the blood (**answer e**), (3) denser bone, (4) spastic contractions of muscle called tetany, and (5) excessive excitability of the nervous system. The parafollicular (C) cells arise from the ultimobranchial body that migrates into the thyroid gland and should form normally (**answer a**).

115. The answer is c. (*Ross, p 209. Mescher, p 124.*) The transmission electron micrograph is a high magnification view of matrix vesicles, which are derived from the cell membrane of osteoblasts, hypertrophied chondrocytes, ameloblasts, and odontoblasts depending on the location. After budding off from the cell membrane, matrix vesicles accumulate calcium and phosphate in the form of hydroxyapatite crystals and serve as seed crystals for calcification. Exposure of those crystals to the extracellular fluid leads to seeding of the osteoid between the spaces in the collagen fibrils located in the matrix. Matrix vesicular alkaline phosphatase (**answers a and b**) results in local increases in the Ca^{2+}/PO_4^{2-} ratio. Adult lamellar bone contains very few matrix vesicles, suggesting that mineralization in remodeling of adult bone occurs by other mechanisms. The three-dimensional arrangement of collagen with the presence of holes or pores where hydroxyapatite crystals form is involved in the mineralization of adult bone. Osteoprotegerin inhibits osteoclastic activity (**answer d**) and osteoblasts synthesize type I collagen (**answer e**).

116. The answer is c. (*Kumar, pp 1207-1209. Ross, pp 202-203.*) Type I collagen is responsible for the three-dimensional fiber structure of the matrix. It is synthesized by osteoblasts and accounts for 85% to 90% of total bone protein. The noncollagenous bone proteins are primarily synthesized by osteoblasts and constitute 10% to 15% of bone protein. Some plasma proteins are preferentially absorbed by the bone matrix. The noncollagenous proteins include cytokines and growth factors (**answer a**), which are synthesized endogenously and become trapped in the matrix. Also included in the category of noncollagenous proteins are the cell attachment proteins (fibronectin and osteopontin [**answer d**]); proteoglycans (eg, chondroitin 4-sulfate and chondroitin 6-sulfate), which appear to play a role in collagen fibrillogenesis; and the GLA (containing γ-carboxyglutamic acid) proteins, such as osteocalcin, which binds Ca^{2+} and mineral components to the matrix (**answers b and e**).

117. The answer is c. (*Young, pp 202-203. Kumar, pp 1235-1240. Ross, pp 189, 205.*) The structure labeled **C** is the articular cartilage that is the site of wear-and-tear damage, which is the hallmark of osteoarthritis. The disease begins with the production of metalloproteinases, such as collagenases, that proteolytically destroy the cartilage matrix. Erosion of the articular cartilage leads to release of proteoglycan and collagen fragments into the synovial fluid. Joint architecture is altered and induces bone overgrowth in a response to stabilize the joint.

The joint shown in the diagram is a freely movable joint known as a diarthrosis. Other joints allow limited or no movement (synarthroses) and may be classified by the uniting connective tissue: hyaline cartilage (synchondroses), bone (synostoses), or dense connective tissue (syndesmoses).

The joint cavity (**A**) is lined by an epithelium (**B**), which is surrounded by an external fibrous layer (**E**). The synovial fluid is formed from the synovial capillary ultrafiltrate as well as mucins, hyaluronic acid, and glycoproteins produced by fibroblast-like cells in the synovial epithelium (B) that lines the fluid-filled joint cavity (A). Macrophage-like cells in the epithelium perform a phagocytic function. The ends of the bone (D) are covered by hyaline cartilage that lacks a perichondrium. Synovial fluid, which differs from blood serum in its reduced protein content, acts as a lubricant and becomes more viscous with age. It may be used to diagnose joint disorders such as arthritis. Rheumatoid arthritis is an autoimmune disease in which infiltration of cells from the immune system leads to the destruction of the synovial capsule and the articular cartilages. Inflammation of the synovium leads to the formation of a pannus and eventually to changes in the articular cartilage converting it into a fibrocollagenous structure.

118. The answer is d. (*Favus, pp 58-59, 150-152, 277-282. Kierszenbaum, pp 140-142, 145, 545-546. Kumar, pp 1126, 1208. Reszka, pp 45-52.*) The woman in the vignette is diagnosed with osteoporosis. The DXA "T" score of −2 indicates that she is four times more likely to have a spine fracture than a person with a normal bone mineral density (BMD). The −2.5 "T" score indicates she is five times more likely to have a hip fracture than a person with a normal BMD. Bisphosphonate treatment is the most effective current treatment for osteoporosis. Bisphosphonates are analogues of the pyrophosphates and suppress bone resorption by osteoclasts. Inhibition of osteoblastic activity **(answer a)** would block new bone deposition but also inhibit the production of RANK-L (receptor for activation of nuclear factor kappa beta-ligand) and M-CSF (macrophage colony-stimulating factor) by osteoblasts. RANK-L binds to RANK on the osteoclast and stimulates osteoclastic activity. M-CSF stimulates the differentiation of monocytes into osteoclasts. Increased RANK-L **(answer b)** and M-CSF **(answer c)** secretion by osteoblasts and up-regulation of RANK **(answer e)** on the surface of osteoclasts will all increase osteoclastic activity. Some of the bisphosphonates are metabolized to a toxic analogue that targets mitochondria and apoptosis of the osteoclasts. Others interfere with cholesterol-dependent pathways in the osteoclast. The interactions of RANK, RANK-L, and osteoprotegerin are shown in High-Yield Facts, Figure 7.

119. The answer is d. (*Kumar, pp 1225-1227.*) The patient in the scenario has an osteosarcoma that has metastasized to the lungs. The osteosarcoma cells synthesize bone and function similarly to osteoblasts, from which they are derived. Osteoblasts and osteosarcoma cells synthesize alkaline phosphatase, which is critical in increasing the local calcium: phosphate ratio, thereby inducing the calcification of osteoid (prebone) to form bone. Osteoblasts synthesize type I collagen. Fibroblasts in highly cellular organs such as the spleen synthesize type III collagen (**answer a**), the primary component of reticular fibers. Chondrocytes in hyaline and elastic cartilage synthesize type II collagen (**answer b**). Acid phosphatase (**answer c**) is synthesized by osteoclasts and is essential for the dissolution of bone and its subsequent resorption. Elastin (**answer e**) is synthesized by smooth-muscle cells, endothelial and microvascular cells, chondrocytes, and fibroblasts.

120. The answer is d. *(Kierszenbaum, pp 10-12. Kumar, pp 269-271, 298-300. Favus, pp 372-373.)* One possible target for therapy of metastatic tumors, such as osteosarcoma, is to reduce metastases by up-regulation of TIMPs at the primary tumor site. TIMPs inhibit the proteolytic activity of the matrix metalloproteinases (MMPs) by inhibiting tumor invasion of the basement membrane or by restraining tumor angiogenesis. TIMPs also appear to modulate tumor growth and apoptosis of tumor cells. Downregulation of the anti-angiogenic peptides, angiostatin and endostatin, would enhance tumor growth (**answer e**). Angiostatin is a cleavage product of plasminogen; endostatin is a cleavage product of type XVIII collagen (see High-Yield Facts, Vasculature: Vasculogenesis versus Angiogenesis, for more information on angiogenesis). Antibodies to fibronectin, integrins, and laminin interfere with metastasis. Enhancement of integrin-integrin receptor interactions would facilitate metastasis (**answers a and b**). Overexpression of selectins (**answer c**) on endothelial cells could enhance sticking of tumor cells to the endothelium and eventual extravasation.

121. The answer is b. *(Mescher, pp 114-115.)* Type II collagen is found in the nasal septum. Type I collagen (**answer a**) is ubiquitous, type III collagen forms a reticular network in highly cellular organs (**answer c**), type IV collagen is found in the basement membrane (**answer d**) and type VII collagen (**answer e**) is found in the basement membrane of skin and forms anchoring fibrils (see High-Yield Facts, Table 12).

Muscle and Cell Motility

Questions

122. A 5-year-old boy sustains a tear in his gastrocnemius muscle when he is involved in a bicycle accident. Regeneration of the muscle will occur through which one of the following mechanisms?

a. Differentiation of satellite cells
b. Dedifferentiation of myocytes into myoblasts
c. Fusion of damaged myofibers to form new myotubes
d. Hyperplasia of existing myofibers
e. Differentiation of fibroblasts to form myocytes

123. A healthy, 32-year-old man lifts weights regularly as part of his workout. In one of his biceps muscle fibers at rest, the length of the I band is 1.0 μm and the A band is 1.5 μm. Contraction of that muscle fiber results in a 10% shortening of the length of the sarcomere. What is the length of the A band after the shortening produced by muscle contraction?

a. 1.50 μm
b. 1.35 μm
c. 1.00 μm
d. 0.90 μm
e. 0.45 μm

124. A 66-year-old man who lives alone has a severe myocardial infarction and dies during the night. The medical examiner's office is called the following morning and describes the man's body as being in *rigor mortis*. The state of *rigor mortis* is due to which one of the following?

a. Inhibition of Ca^{++} leakage from the extracellular fluid and sarcoplasmic reticulum (SR)
b. Enhanced retrieval of calcium by the sarcoplasmic reticulum
c. Failure to disengage tropomyosin and troponin from the myosin active sites
d. Absence of ATP preventing detachment of the myosin heads from actin
e. Increased lactic acid production

125. The sarcoplasmic reticulum of skeletal muscle functions in which one of the following ways?

a. Cellular Ca^{2+} storage
b. Cellular glycogen storage
c. Glycogen degradation
d. Transport of Ca^{2+} into the terminal cisternae during muscle contraction
e. Ca^{2+} release from the transverse tubules during muscle relaxation

126. Observation of a histologic preparation of muscle reveals cross-striations and peripherally located nuclei. The use of histochemistry shows a strong staining reaction for succinic dehydrogenase. The same tissue prepared for electron microscopy shows many mitochondria in rows between myofibrils and underneath the sarcolemma. Which one of the following is the best description of this tissue?

a. White muscle fibers
b. Fibers that contract rapidly, but are incapable of sustaining continuous heavy work
c. Red muscle fibers
d. Cardiac muscle
e. Smooth muscle

127. In skeletal muscle contraction, the "powerstroke" is initiated by which one of the following?

a. The initial binding of ATP to the myosin heads
b. Release of Pi from the myosin heads
c. Release of ADP and subsequent addition of an ATP molecule
d. Detachment of the myosin head from the actin
e. Phosphorylation of the myosin light chains

128. In muscular dystrophy, the actin-binding protein dystrophin is absent or defective. Dystrophin has similar actin-binding domains and structure to the spectrins (I and II) and α-actinin. Which of the following is most likely to occur as a result of this deficiency?

a. Enhanced smooth-muscle contractility
b. Deficiency in skeletal muscle actin synthesis
c. Loss of binding of the I and M bands to the cell membrane
d. Loss of organelle and vesicle transport throughout the muscle cell
e. Loss of integrity of the desmosomal components of the intercalated discs of cardiac muscle

129. A 32-year-old homosexual man is seropositive for HIV. He has HIV-associated periodontitis and intraoral candidiasis. Peripheral neutrophils (PMNs) from this patient have increased activity as measured by oxidative burst and F-actin assays compared to control patients. Which one of the following cellular events would most likely be increased in the peripheral blood PMNs from this patient?

a. Phagocytosis
b. Bidirectional transport of vesicles
c. Fast axoplasmic transport
d. Chromosomal movements
e. Ciliary movement

130. Which one of the following is absent in smooth-muscle cells compared to skeletal muscle cells?

a. Troponin
b. Calmodulin
c. Calcium
d. Myosin light-chain kinase
e. Actin and tropomyosin interactions

131. In the transmission electron micrograph of skeletal muscle shown below, which one of the following is true of the zone labeled C?

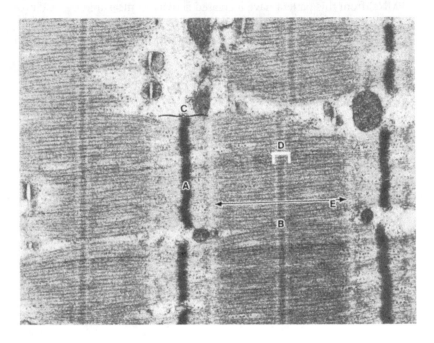

a. It defines the sarcomere.
b. Thin filaments are anchored to this structure.
c. This structure bisects the H band and is formed predominantly of creatine kinase.
d. No overlap of thick and thin filaments occurs in this zone.
e. This portion of the A band consists solely of the rodlike portions of myosin.

132. The mechanochemical enzyme that can be found on the surfaces of cellular organelles where it mediates movement toward the plus end of microtubules is which one of the following?

a. Myosin (myosin II)
b. Minimyosin (myosin I)
c. Dynein
d. Kinesin
e. Filamin

Muscle and Cell Motility

Answers

122. The answer is a. (*Kierszenbaum, pp 209-210. Kumar, pp 82, 85-86. Alberts, p 1466.*) Satellite cells in skeletal muscle proliferate and reconstitute the damaged part of the myofibers. They are supportive cells for maintenance of muscle and a source of new myofibers after injury or after increased load. There is no dedifferentiation of myocytes into myoblasts (**answer b**), or fusion of damaged myofibers to form new myotubes (**answer c**). Hypertrophy, not hyperplasia (**answer d**), occurs in existing myofibers in response to increased load. Proliferation of fibroblasts may occur in the damaged area but leads to fibrosis, not repair of skeletal muscle. Fibroblasts do not differentiate into myocytes (**answer e**). The multinucleate organization of skeletal muscle is derived developmentally by fusion and not by amitosis (failure of cytokinesis after DNA synthesis). Mitotic activity is terminated after fusion occurs. In the development of skeletal muscle, myoblasts of mesodermal origin undergo cell proliferation. Myocyte cell division ceases soon after birth. Myoblasts, which are mononucleate cells, fuse with each other end to end to form myotubes. This process requires cell recognition between myoblasts, alignment, and subsequent fusion.

123. The answer is a. (*Alberts, pp 1026, 1028. Mescher, p 177.*) During contraction, the sarcomere, the distance between adjacent Z lines, decreases in length, and the length of the A band is almost constant (**answers b → e**). However, as the degree of overlap of thick and thin filaments is altered, the thin filaments, which form the I band and are anchored to the Z line, are pulled toward the center of the sarcomere. As this occurs, the I band decreases in length and the H band is no longer visible. The filaments themselves do not decrease in length; they slide past one another in the sliding-filament model of muscle contraction. The average length of a sarcomere is 2.5 μm, measured from Z line to Z line. If the resting length of the A band is 1.5 μm and the length of the I band is 1.0 μm and there is a 10% contraction of the muscle (contraction to

90% of its length), the sarcomere is reduced in length from 2.5 to 2.25 µm. The size of the A band remains unchanged, therefore the length of the I band is reduced from 1.0 to 0.775 µm and "compensates" for the 0.25 µm reduction in length during the muscle contraction. The processes of skeletal muscle contraction and relaxation are shown in High-Yield Facts, Figure 9.

124. The answer is d. (*Alberts, p 1019. Mescher, p 171.*) There is some small amount of production of ATP after death through anaerobic and phosphagen pathways. However, there is insufficient ATP to induce the detachment of the myosin heads from actin. Ca^{2+} ions continue to leak from the extracellular fluid and the sarcoplasmic reticulum (**answer a**), however, the sarcoplasmic reticulum is no longer able to retrieve the Ca^{2+} ions (**answer b**). Tropomyosin and troponin are disengaged from the myosin active sites (**answer c**). Lactic acid is produced during *rigor mortis* through anaerobic pathways. The high levels of lactic acid cause deterioration of the skeletal muscle and end the state of *rigor mortis* (**answer e**).

125. The answer is a. (*Alberts, pp 1026-1030. Mescher, pp 169-175.*) Ca^{2+} is responsible for the coupling of excitation and contraction in skeletal muscle. The SR is a modified smooth endoplasmic reticulum. Ca^{2+} is concentrated in the lumen of the SR. Depolarization of the muscle cell membrane during an action potential triggers the opening of ryanodine receptor channels in the membrane of the SR. Ca^{2+} passes through the open ryanodine receptor channels, traveling from the lumen of the SR into the muscle cell cytoplasm. When Ca^{2+} in the muscle cell cytoplasm is high, the Ca^{2+} binds to the troponin complex. The binding of Ca^{2+} to the troponin complex results in a conformational change in the complex, thereby allowing myosin to interact with actin. The interaction of myosin and actin produces force. Ca^{2+} is constantly pumped back into the lumen of the SR by Ca^{2+}-ATPases (**answer d**). As the Ca^{2+} in the cytoplasm is pumped back into the SR, the concentration of Ca^{2+} in the cytoplasm drops, and Ca^{2+} dissociates from the troponin complex. The troponin complex subsequently reverts to the conformational state in which the troponin complex blocks the interaction of myosin with actin. Glycogen is stored as particles or droplets in the cytoplasm, which contains the enzymes required for the synthesis and breakdown of glycogen (**answers b and c**). The transverse tubule system, or T system, is an extension of the plasma membrane of the myofiber (sarcolemma). The T system allows for simultaneous contraction of all myofibrils since it encircles the A-I bands in each sarcomere of every myofibril. In combination with the paired terminal cisternae, the transverse tubules form a triad. Two triads are found in each sarcomere of skeletal muscle—one at each junction of dark (A) and light (I) bands. Depolarization of the T system during contraction is transmitted to the sarcoplasmic reticulum at the triad (**answer e**). Cardiac muscle also has a T system, although it is not as elaborate and well organized as that found in skeletal muscle (eg, diads are present rather than the triads of skeletal muscle and there are fewer T tubules in atrial compared to ventricular muscle).

126. The answer is c. (*Kumar, pp 1260-1261. Mescher, p 175, 178-179.*) The histologic sample contains red (oxidative) fibers (type I, slow). The deductive process is based on the fact that the sample must be skeletal or cardiac muscle due to the presence of cross-striations (**answer e**). The presence of peripherally placed nuclei eliminates cardiac muscle as a possibility (**answer d**). Skeletal muscle may be subclassified into three muscle fiber types: red, white, and intermediate fibers. Red muscle fibers have a high content of cytochrome and myoglobin and, beneath the sarcolemma, contain many mitochondria required for the high metabolism of these cells. Mitochondria are also found in a longitudinal array surrounding the myofibrils. The presence of numerous mitochondria provides a strong staining reaction with the use of cytochemical stains such as that for succinic dehydrogenase. Physiologically, red fibers are capable of continuous contraction (high concentrations of myosin ATPase), but are incapable of rapid contraction (**answer b**). The term "red (type I) fibers" is due to the presence of large concentrations of myoglobin, the colored oxygen-binding protein. White (type IIb, fast, white glycolytic) muscle fibers (**answer a**) are fast-twitch in function, stain very lightly for succinic dehydrogenase and myosin ATPase, and few mitochondria would be visible at the ultrastructural level. White fibers are capable of rapid contraction, but are unable to sustain continuous heavy work. They are larger than red fibers and have more prominent innervation. The white fibers contain relatively little myoglobin. The intermediate (oxidative-glycolytic, type IIa, fast) fibers possess characteristics including a size and innervation pattern intermediate between red and white muscle fibers. The intermediate fibers contain a concentration of myoglobin between white and red muscle fibers.

127. The answer is b. (*Alberts, p 1016. Mescher, pp 171-177.*) The "powerstroke" is initiated by the release of Pi from the myosin heads, leading to the tight binding of actin and myosin. The tight binding induces a conformational change in the myosin head. The myosin head subsequently pulls against the actin filament to cause the "powerstroke" of the myosin head walking along the actin filament. This walking process is unidirectional and is based on the polarity of the actin filament (ie, walking occurs from the minus to the plus end of the actin filament). The cycle of ATP-actin-myosin interactions during contraction begins with the resting state. In the quiescent period, ATP binds to myosin heads (**answer a**); however, hydrolysis occurs slowly and only allows the weak binding of myosin heads to the actin filaments. Tight binding occurs only when Pi is released from myosin heads, leading to the "powerstroke." Recycling occurs through the release of ADP and the subsequent addition of an ATP molecule (**answer c**) and detachment of the myosin head from actin (**answer d**). Rigor results from the lack of ATP because one ATP molecule is required for each myosin molecule present in the muscle. *Rigor mortis* occurs from the absence of ATP. In skeletal muscle, phosphorylation of the light chain is not required for binding to actin (**answer e**).

128. The answer is c. (*Alberts, p 1466. Fauci, pp 2682-2684. Kumar, pp 1268-1269.*) Dystrophin, like α-actinin and spectrin, is an actin-binding protein. It binds actin to the skeletal muscle membrane and therefore binds the I and M bands to the cell membrane. The inability to bind actin to the plasma membrane of skeletal muscle leads to disruption of the contraction process, weakness of muscle, and abnormal running, hopping, and jumping. The Gower maneuver is the method used by persons suffering from muscular dystrophy to stand from a sitting position. Respiratory failure occurs in those persons because of disruption of diaphragmatic function. Dystrophin is found in all muscle types and is part of a complex that regulates interactions of the sarcolemma with the extracellular matrix through associated glycoproteins (dystrophin-glycoprotein complex). Therefore, loss of dystrophin causes destabilization and decreased contractility (**answer a**). Muscular dystrophy refers to a group of progressive hereditary disorders (1/3500 male births) that involve mutations in the dystrophin gene. Dystrophin is similar in structure to spectrins I and II and α-actinin. Dystrophin is absent in Duchenne muscular dystrophy. Becker muscular dystrophy is a less severe dystrophy in which dystrophin is defective.

Synthesis of actin **(answer b)** is not reduced in skeletal muscle from these patients; in fact, hypertrophy and pseudohypertrophy (replacement of muscle with connective tissue and fat) occurs. Microtubules perform vesicular and organelle transport functions **(answer d)**, and intermediate filaments, not actin, form the intracellular connection in desmosomes **(answer e)**.

129. The answer is a. *(Alberts, pp 965-969.)* The patient's peripheral blood PMNs have increased activity as measured by oxidative burst and F-actin assays. Actin maintains the mechanical strength of the cytoplasm of the cell and is essential for cellular functions that require surface motility. Those functions include phagocytosis, cytokinesis, and cell locomotion. Movement of vesicles along filaments is regulated by minimyosins (myosin I), movement of vesicles and organelles is predominantly a function of microtubules **(answers b and c)** under the influence of the unidirectional motors kinesin and dynein. The movements of chromosomes **(answer d)** as well as the cilia and flagella **(answer e)** are driven by dynein, and chromosomal movements occur through microtubular kinetics.

130. The answer is a. *(Alberts, p 1030. Mescher, pp 180-183.)* Smooth muscle is the least specialized type of muscle and contains no troponin. The contractile process is similar to the actin-myosin interactions that occur in motility of nonmuscle cells. In the smooth-muscle cell, actin and myosin are attached to intermediate filaments at dense bodies in the sarcolemma and cytoplasm. Dense bodies contain α-actinin and, therefore, resemble the Z-lines of skeletal muscle. Contraction causes cell shortening and a change in shape from elongate to globular. Contraction occurs by a sliding filament action analogous to the mechanism used by thick and thin filaments in striated muscle. The connections to the plasma membrane allow all the smooth-muscle cells in the same region to act as a functional unit. The sarcoplasmic reticulum is not as well developed as that in the striated muscles. There are no T tubules present; however, endocytic vesicles called caveolae are believed to function in a fashion similar to the T tubule system of skeletal muscle.

When intracellular calcium levels increase, the calcium is bound to the Ca^{2+}-binding protein, calmodulin. Ca^{2+}-calmodulin **(answers b and c)** is required and is bound to myosin light-chain kinase **(answer d)** to form a Ca^{2+}-calmodulin-kinase complex. This complex catalyzes the phosphorylation of one of the two myosin light chains on the myosin heads. That phosphorylation allows the binding of actin to myosin. A specific phosphatase dephosphorylates the myosin light chain, which returns the actin and myosin to the inactive, resting state. The actin-tropomyosin interactions (answer e) are similar in smooth and skeletal muscle.

Smooth-muscle cells (eg, vascular smooth-muscle cells) also differ from skeletal muscle cells in that like fibroblasts, they are capable of collagen, elastin, and proteoglycan synthesis.

131. The answer is d. (Mescher, pp 174, 177.) Myofibrils are composed of sarcomeres, which are repeating units that extend from Z disc (A on the transmission electron micrograph [TEM]) to Z disc in the TEM. With the use of polarizing microscopy, the A (anisotropic) bands (E on the TEM) are visible as dark, birefringent structures, and the I (isotropic) bands are visible as light-staining bands (C on the TEM). The I band consists of thin filaments without overlap of thick filaments. At the center of the myofibril and consisting of thick filaments is the A band, which interdigitates with the I band. Each I band is bisected by the Z disc. The Z disc is composed mostly of the intermediate filament protein desmin and other proteins such as α-actinin, filamin, and amorphin, as well as Z protein. In the center of the A band is a lighter-staining area that consists only of thick (rodlike portions of myosin) filaments and is known as the H band (D on the TEM). Lateral connections occur between adjacent thick filaments in the region of the M line (B on the TEM), which bisects the H zone and is composed primarily of creatine kinase, an enzyme that catalyzes the formation of ATP.

132. The answer is d. (Alberts, pp 1006-1008, 1014-1015. Mescher, pp 40, 145, 298, 379.) Kinesin moves vesicles unidirectionally from the minus end to the plus end of the microtubule—for example, from the cell body to the axon terminus in fast axonal transport. Myosin, minimyosin, dynein, dynamin, and kinesin (answers a, b, c, and e) are all mechanochemical enzymes or molecular "motors" that hydrolyze ATP and undergo conformational changes that are converted into movement. Cytoplasmic dynein is responsible for movement toward the minus end of the microtubules. Remember kinesin kicks out and dynein drags them in (see answer to Question 41). Ciliary and flagellar bending is the classic model for microtubule-based motility. The motor is dynein, which causes the relative sliding between microtubules in the axoneme. Structural constraints within the axoneme as a whole convert sliding into ciliary bending.

Dynamin is another ATPase motor that mediates sliding between adjacent cytoplasmic microtubules.

Filamin or other actin cross-linking proteins form a gel network in the cell cortex (the area just beneath the cell membrane). The presence of the actin gel in the cell cortex contributes to the rigidity of the cell and is also involved in changes in cell shape and chromosome movements during mitosis. The sarcomere extends from Z disc (line) to Z disc. The H band is located between the ends of the thin (actin) filaments. The A band is defined by the width of the thick (myosin) filaments. The I bands are not shown completely on the figure because they are found between adjacent A bands.

The sarcomere extends from Z disc (line) to Z disc. The H band is located between the ends of the thin (actin) filaments. The A band is defined by the width of the thick (myosin) filaments. The I bands are not shown completely on the figure (see High-Yield Facts, Figure 9), because they are found between adjacent A bands.

Nervous System

Questions

133. A 4-year-old boy is referred to the pediatric neurology clinic. He has difficulty in expressing needs, uses gestures instead of words, and repeats words in place of normal responsive language. In the examination room he wanders around repeatedly singing "Baa Baa Black Sheep," then cries and laughs for no apparent reason. His parents say he is nervous, excitable, "will not cuddle or be cuddled," and is hyperactive. He has no apparent fear of danger and a constant need to spin objects and jumps while twiddling his fingers. MRI showed a significant reduction in total gray matter volume with localized gray matter reductions within fronto-striatal, parietal, and ventral and superior temporal gray matter. FMRI showed an abnormal activation pattern in cortical as well as limbic/striatal areas. The neurons in the frontal, parietal, and temporal cortex originate from which region embryologically?

a. Subventricular zone
b. Marginal zone
c. Intermediate zone
d. Mantle zone
e. Sulcus limitans

134. The action potential in the neuron is initiated by which one of the following mechanisms?

a. Hyperpolarization
b. The opening of K^+ channels
c. The opening of Na^+ channels
d. Inward flux of K^+
e. Pumping of Na^+ from the neuron

135. An 18-month-old girl flexes the great toe toward the top of her foot and the other toes fan out after the sole of her foot has been firmly stroked by the pediatrician. A year later, the response cannot be evoked by the same stimulus. The change in response is due to which postnatal event?

a. Apoptosis of exuberant neurons in the cortex by microglia
b. Maturation of the cerebellar cortex
c. Myelination of the lumbar spinal nerves by Schwann cells
d. Myelination of the corticospinal tract by oligodendrocytes
e. Formation of new neurons in the cerebral cortex

136. A 2-year-old boy has an acute inflammatory reaction in the region shown in this photomicrograph, several weeks after suffering from chicken-pox. Which one of the following is the most likely symptom?

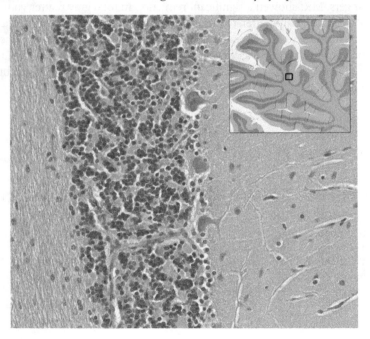

a. Amnesia
b. Ataxia
c. Loss of spinal cord reflex responses
d. Loss of pain sensation
e. Aphasia

137. A febrile 52-year-old male patient receiving glucocorticoid treatment presents with vesicular lesions with intense itching, burning, and sharp pain along the back in a specific dermatomal pattern covering his nipple and extending onto the right side of his back. The vesicular lesions do not cross the midline. A Tzanck test is positive. The cause of this illness is the movement of virus from the structures shown in the photomicrograph toward the surface of the skin. This movement occurs in which direction and by which molecular motor?

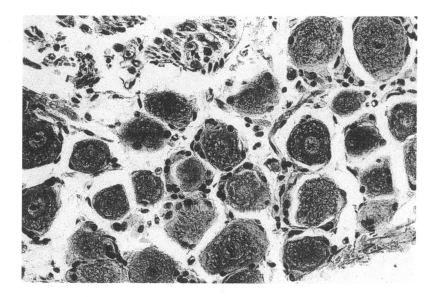

a. Minus end to plus end, dynein
b. Minus end to plus end, kinesin
c. Plus end to minus end, dynein
d. Plus end to minus end, kinesin
e. Minus end to plus end, myosin II

138. A 22-year-old man receives a severe, traumatic compression injury to his radial nerve during a motorcycle crash. He shows an advancing Tinel sign. Which one of the following is true about regeneration of axons after his nerve injury?

a. It occurs in the absence of motor unit potentials.
b. It occurs at a rate of 100 mm/day.
c. It occurs by a mechanism that is dependent on the proliferation of Schwann cells.
d. It occurs in conjunction with degeneration and phagocytosis of endoneurial tubes.
e. It occurs in the segment distal to the damage.

139. A 14-year-old adolescent presents with slowly progressive degeneration of his fibularis muscles, foot-drop walking gait, foot bone abnormalities, high arches and hammertoes, problems with balance, problems with hand function, occasional lower leg and forearm muscle cramping, scoliosis, and some occasional breathing difficulties. He is diagnosed with Charcot Marie Tooth syndrome. In this syndrome, gene mutations result in a thick myelin sheath and reduced nerve conduction velocity. Recent studies have shown alterations in the characteristics of the nodes of Ranvier in those patients. The nodes of Ranvier increase the efficiency of neural transmission by means of which one of the following mechanisms?

a. Decelerating the closing of Na^+-gated channels
b. Enhancing myelination of the internodal segment
c. Sequestration of Na^+ entry into the axon
d. Multiple firings due to local ionic currents around the node
e. Decreasing threshold for the action potential

140. A 47-year-old man is diagnosed with AIDS-dementia complex including aseptic meningitis, encephalitis, leukoencephalopathy, myelopathy, neuropathy, and myopathy. He has shown progressive memory loss, intellectual deterioration, behavioral changes, ataxia, and motor deficits over the past 2 years. The original entry of the HIV virus into the brain in this patient is most likely through which one of the following mechanisms?

a. HIV-infected monocytes entering through fenestrations between capillary endothelial cells
b. HIV transport in vesicles by a transcytotic mechanism
c. HIV-infected monocytes passing through occluding junctions between endothelial cells
d. B lymphocytes passing through occluding junctions between endothelial cells
e. T lymphocytes entering through fenestrations between capillary endothelial cells
f. Paracellular transport of viral particles by passive transport
g. Active transport of viral particles
h. Passage of viral particles through gap junctions between the endothelial cells

141. A 48-year-old man initially presents with progressive dysphonia of 20-months duration and subsequent dysarthria for the past 4 months. More recently he has experienced progressive muscle weakness in his hands and feet. He reports muscle twitches in his lower limb muscles and aches in his upper limb muscles. Physical examination reveals a Hoffmann sign, Babinski sign, and clonus. MRI rules out other possible causes and the diagnosis is amyotrophic lateral sclerosis (ALS). Which one of the following would be involved in the disrupted and defective neuromuscular transmission that occurs in ALS?

a. Ca^{2+}-gated channels
b. Na^+-gated channels
c. K^+-gated channels
d. Cl^--gated channels
e. Gap junctions

142. Following a vehicular accident, a 45-year-old man is transported to the emergency room by ambulance. He presents with motor deficits on his right side, is unable to move his right arm and leg, and has slurred speech. The injury has most likely occurred on which side and affects which of the following cells, which predominate in the accompanying photomicrograph?

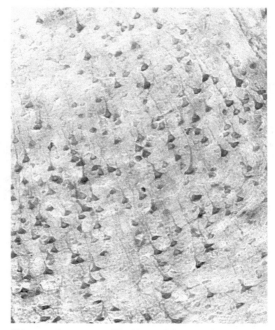

(Micrograph courtesy of Dr. Nancy E. J. Berman.)

a. Right, Purkinje cells
b. Left, Purkinje cells
c. Right, pyramidal cells
d. Left, pyramidal cells
e. Left, basket cells

143. A 36-year-old woman internist completes a 4 week medical mission to rural Bahia, Brazil. Eighteen months after her return she complains of loss of sensation in her hands and feet. Neurologic examination reveals loss of temperature, light touch, pain, and deep pressure on her hands and feet. A hypopigmented macula is present on the dorsum of her hand. A lepromin test is positive and a biopsy reveals inflammation of the structure labeled C in the accompanying photomicrograph. The structure labeled C is which one of the following?

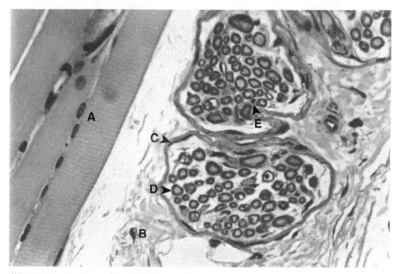

(*Micrograph courtesy of Dr. John K. Young.*)

a. Perineurium
b. Epineurium
c. Endomysium
d. Perimysium
e. Tunica media

144. A 2-year-old boy presents with hearing impairment, poliosis (a white shock of hair), complete heterochromia and sectoral heterochromia, hypertelorism, a low hairline with eyebrows that touch in the middle, white pigmentation on the skin, and suspected neurologic deficits. He is diagnosed with Waardenburg syndrome with a mutation in the *PAX-3* gene that affects neural crest differentiation. Which one of the following structures would most likely be affected in this patient?

a. Zona glomerulosa of the adrenal gland
b. Pyramidal cells
c. Ventral horn cells
d. Astrocytes
e. Sensory neurons of the cranial ganglia

145. During labor an infant girl went into fetal distress. The child was delivered by a mid-forceps delivery, had seizures soon after birth, and developed an intracranial hemorrhage with left-sided hemiplegia. She is 6 years old, has an IQ of about 80, walks with a very severe limp, and has a contracted hand on the left side. She barely speaks despite therapy. She is treated with atropine for her sialorrhea. Which one of the following best describes the effects of atropine on the structure labeled with the arrow?

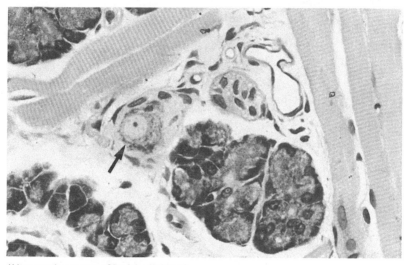

(Micrograph courtesy of Dr. John K. Young.)

a. Block parasympathetic pathways
b. Stimulate parasympathetic pathways
c. Block sympathetic pathways
d. Stimulate sympathetic pathways
e. Bind to acinar cells

146. A 45-year-old man presents at the neurology clinic with memory loss, mood swings, and clinical depression. Laboratory results reveal a CD4 level of 170/mm³ (normal range is 500-1200) and a CD4 percentage of 12% (normal approximately 40%). His viral load is 12,000 copies/mL. He has previously been treated for pneumocystis pneumonia. The cells in the accompanying photomicrograph, labeled with anti-glial fibrillary acidic protein (GFAP), are involved in the progress of this disease. These cells function to do which one of the following?

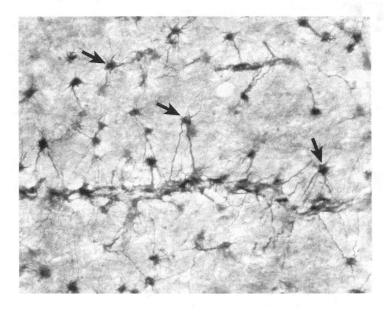

a. Form synaptic contacts with neurons
b. Present antigen
c. Phagocytose dying neurons
d. Form a glial scar following damage
e. Form myelin in the CNS

147. A 47-year-old man is treated with fluoxetine hydrochloride (Prozac) for clinical depression. This pharmaceutical agent functions through a mechanism that involves the structure labeled "C" in the transmission electron micrograph below. The structure labeled "C" in the accompanying transmission electron micrograph is the site of which one of the following?

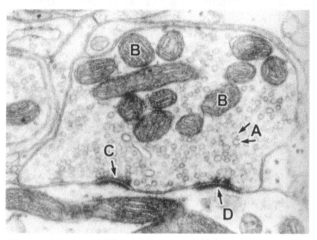

(Micrograph courtesy of Drs. J. F. Heuser and T. S. Reese.)

a. Neurotransmitter reuptake in synaptic vesicles
b. Binding of neurotransmitter to postsynaptic receptors
c. Neurotransmitter-induced alteration of membrane permeability
d. Membrane continuity between adjacent neurons
e. Degradation of neurotransmitter

148. A 35-year-old woman presents with weakness and spasticity in the left lower extremity, visual impairment and throbbing in her left eye, difficulties with balance, fatigue, and malaise. There is an increase in cerebrospinal fluid (CSF) protein, elevated gamma globulin, and moderate pleocytosis. MRI confirms areas of demyelination in the anterior corpus callosum. Imaging identifies plaques which are hyperintense on T2-weighted and fluid attenuated inversion recovery (FLAIR) images, and hypointense on T1-weighted scans. Which one of the following cells are specifically targeted in her condition?

a. Microglia
b. Oligodendrocytes
c. Astrocytes
d. Schwann cells
e. Axons of multipolar neurons

149. A 33-year-old woman is referred to the neurology clinic complaining of weakness of her eye muscles which began 2 months ago. Subsequently she has had diplopia and increasing difficulty in swallowing. Her speech is slurred and she has difficulty clearly enunciating and pronouncing many words. Physical examination reveals bilateral ptosis and an unstable, waddling gait, and some shortness of breath. Laboratory and diagnostic tests reveal a positive edrophonium chloride (Tensilon) test and autoantibodies to the acetylcholine receptor. On the accompanying transmission electron micrograph, which region is most affected in this disease?

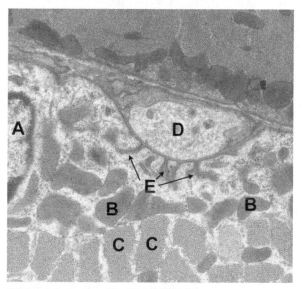

(Micrograph courtesy of Dr. Michael J. Werle.)

a. A
b. B
c. C
d. D
e. E

Nervous System

Answers

133. The answer is a. (*Sadler, pp 296-298, 306-307, 310-312. Moore and Persaud, pp 381, 386-387, 404.*) Abnormalities in the anatomy and connectivity of cortical regions and the so-called social brain regions (limbic–striatal systems) contribute to the behavioral and brain metabolic differences in autism. In the cerebral cortex, neurons originate from the ventricular and subventricular zones. Layers I to VI form by waves of proliferation and migration from deep to superficial layers, with new cells arising from the subventricular zone. Before neural tube closure, cell proliferation is the predominant process. After neural tube closure, neurons differentiate. Three layers differentiate from the wall of the neural tube. Mitotic activity occurs in the ventricular zone, closest to the lumen. The mantle (intermediate) zone **(answers c and d)**, is where cell bodies of differentiating motoneurons are located. The most peripheral zone is the marginal zone **(answer b)**, which contains the myelinated axons of the developing motoneurons (adult white matter). In the spinal cord, the layers differentiate into peripheral white matter with a central H-shaped region of gray matter from the marginal and mantle zones, respectively. The sulcus limitans separates the alar (sensory) and basal (motor) plates in the developing brainstem **(answer e)**. The macroglia (astrocytes and oligodendrocytes), arise from the neural epithelium. Microglia (the macrophages of the brain) are bone marrow–derived, arising from monocytes. Cerebral and cerebellar cortices are areas of peripheral gray matter formed through a second wave of cell proliferation. In cerebellar development, the second wave comes from the external granular layer.

134. The answer is c. (*Alberts, pp 677-679. Mescher, pp 140, 146. Kandel, pp 29-39, 147-148. Waxman, pp 20-22.*) In the resting state, the presence of Na^+/K^+ ATPase builds up high ionic gradients across the axolemma. There are many more Na^+ on the outside of the axon; the inside of the axon is negative relative to the outside (-70 mV resting potential). An action potential is initiated by an exchange of ions across the axonal membrane that will displace the membrane potential toward zero. The first step is the presence of a stimulus that causes Na⁺-gated channels to open, Na⁺ ions flow through the channels into the neuron. The positive charge of Na⁺ makes the axon more positive and depolarized. There is a delay in the opening of K⁺ channels. The opening of K⁺ channels causes the flow of K⁺ out of the cell, reversing the depolarization. Na⁺ channels start to close at about this time, causing the action potential to return toward −70 mV and repolarizing the membrane. The membrane actually hyperpolarizes (**answer a**) as the potential passes −70 mV. This is due to the fact that the K⁺ channels remain open longer than required to return to −70 mV. Gradually, the ion concentrations return to resting levels and the membrane returns to −70 mV. K⁺ channels (**answer b**) serve to bring the membrane potential to the hyperpolarized state. Inward flux of K⁺ (**answer d**) combined with the closing of Na⁺ channels (**answer e**), is important in return to the resting membrane potential. The action potential is an all-or-none phenomenon and occurs with constant amplitude and duration for a given axon. Myelination increases conduction of the action potential.

135. The answer is d. (*Young, pp 127-131. Mescher, pp 159-161. Kandel, pp 20, 147-148. Waxman, p 61.*) The Babinski sign or extensor plantar reflex is an infantile reflex present in children until the age of 2 years, but abnormal in older children or adults. The Babinski sign is an indication of immaturity of the corticospinal tract which is myelinated after birth (**answers a and e**); the process of myelination is completed by oligodendrocytes in the CNS (**answer c**). Cerebellar cortical development (**answer b**) begins in the second trimester and continues until several years after birth, but is not involved in the Babinski reflex. Also, please see the brief review of myelination in High-Yield Facts.

136. The answer is b. (*Fauci, pp 152-153. Young, p 396. Mescher, pp 152, 155. Waxman, pp 2, 189, 193, 288.*) The region shown in the photomicrograph is the cerebellum. An acute childhood infection in the cerebellum (cerebellitis) would result in ataxia: inability to coordinate voluntary muscle movements, unsteady movements, and staggering gait. Ataxia may be classified as axial (trunk) or limb ataxia. In the sitting position, the child's trunk may move side to side and/or back to front and then resume a vertical position in a jerky motion. Nystagmus (jerky eye movements) may also occur. Limb ataxia manifests itself with loss of fine motor control of the hands or legs and appears as though the person is able to coordinate his or her movements. For example, a hand may sway back and forth when reaching for an object. Most often, the cerebellar ataxia that follows a viral infection subsides without treatment over a period of weeks to months. Occasionally, a child will be left with a persistent movement disorder or behavioral problem. Amnesia (**answer a**) would result from a cortical injury; reflexive actions (**answer c**) would occur at the level of the ventral horn cells in the spinal cord; loss of pain sensation (**answer d**) is complex and could involve the dorsal root or trigeminal ganglion, the sensory and frontal cortex, limbic system, and thalamus, but not the cerebellar cortex; and total or partial loss of ability to use or understand language, aphasia (**answer e**), would be the result of a cortical injury. Damage to the perirhinal–entorhinal–hippocampal–mammillary body–thalamus circuit, the fornix, or the temporal lobe can cause amnesia. There are different types of memory. For example, working memory can be affected by prefrontal lesions or by lesions to specific temperoparietal regions subserving the modality being used. Aphasia can involve several different areas of the cortex including the frontal, parietal, and/or temporal lobes.

Note the three layers forming the cerebellar cortex (molecular layer at left/top, the large Purkinje cell layer, and the granular layer). The mnemonic MPG: **M**olecular, **P**urkinje, and **G**ranular may help you remember the layers. White matter is inside of the three layers of gray matter. Basket cells, Purkinje cells, and granule cells compose the cerebellar cortex. Basket cells make profuse inhibitory dendritic contacts with the flask-shaped Purkinje cells. Each Purkinje cell receives about 2×10^5 synapses, mostly onto its dendritic spines which splay out across the molecular layer. Granule cells are small neurons located in the vicinity of the Purkinje cells. Granule cell axons form the parallel fibers that make excitatory synapses onto Purkinje cell dendrites. Each parallel fiber synapses on about 200 Purkinje cells creating an excitation strip across the cerebellum.

137. The answer is b. (*Alberts, pp1047-1050. Young, p 26. Mescher, p 145. Kierszenbaum, pp 27-29. Fauci, pp 1102-1104. Moore, pp 96-97. Waxman, p 8.*) Kinesin is a motor protein that uses energy from ATP hydrolysis to move vesicles (– → +) from the cell body in the dorsal root ganglion (shown in the photomicrograph) in an anterograde direction toward the axon terminal (**answer d**). The patient in question has shingles caused by the herpes virus known as the varicella-zoster virus (VZV). Shingles begins as erythematous maculopapular eruptions and rapidly evolves to vesicles;

it often presents with fever. The patient had chickenpox as a child. Chickenpox is also caused by VZV. The virus is stored in the dorsal root ganglion, primarily in the satellite cells surrounding the perikarya (cell bodies). Kinesin walks along the microtubule toward the plus end of the microtubule. The dyneins (answers a and c) are minus-end directed microtubule motors that move organelles, including vesicles, in a retrograde direction toward the cell body (in this case toward the cell bodies of the dorsal root ganglia). The dyneins involved in axonal transport are the cytoplasmic dyneins as compared to the axonemal dyneins seen in cilia and flagella. Myosin II (answer e) is an actin-based motor protein that generates the force of muscle contraction. The Tzanck test is a method of testing for the virus; it can detect the presence of the herpes virus in the cells scraped from a lesion. It cannot detect the difference between herpes simplex virus (HSV) and VZV. PCR of the DNA is required for absolute detection.

The patient's shingles involve dermatomal segment T4, which surrounds the nipple. The nipples are normally found in the middle of T4, although T5 may also innervate this region. A dermatome is the area of skin supplied by nerves originating from a single spinal nerve root.

138. The answer is c. *(Mescher, pp 163-166. Ross, p 351. Kierszenbaum, pp 244-245. Kandel, pp 99-103, 1108-1109. Waxman, pp 15, 16-17.)* Regeneration depends on the proliferation of Schwann cells, which guide sprouting axons from the proximal segment toward the target organ. The injury causes Wallerian (orthograde) degeneration distal to the level of injury and proximal axonal degeneration to at least the next node of Ranvier. In more severe traumatic injuries, the proximal degeneration may extend beyond the next node of Ranvier. Electrodiagnostic studies demonstrate denervation changes in the affected muscles, and in cases of reinnervation, motor unit potentials (MUPs) are present (answer a). Axonal regeneration occurs at the rate of 1 mm/day (answer b) or 1 in/month and can be monitored with an advancing Tinel sign. The Tinel sign is observed when tapping over nerve trunk that has been damaged or is regenerating following trauma causes a sensation of tingling and pins in its distribution up to the site of regeneration. If this sign is absent, there is a poor prognosis. The endoneurial tubes remain intact (answer d), and, therefore, recovery is complete, with axons reinnervating their original motor and sensory targets.

Axonal regeneration occurs in neurons if the perikarya survive following damage. The segment distal (answer e) to the wound, including the myelin, is phagocytosed and removed by macrophages. Macrophages also produce cytokines that activate nerve growth factor and other neurotrophins in Schwann cells. The proximal segment is capable of regeneration because it remains in continuity with the perikaryon. Chromatolysis (literally disintegration of color) is the first step in the regeneration process, in which there is breakdown of the Nissl substance (RER, ribosomes), swelling of the perikaryon, and migration of the nucleus peripherally. Degeneration of perikarya and neuronal processes occurs when there is extensive neuronal damage. Axonal regeneration in the peripheral nervous system is much more successful than in the central nervous system.

139. The answer is c. (*Kierszenbaum, pp 229-231. Mescher, pp 154, 171, 174. Kandel, pp 21-22, 148, 160.*) The nodes of Ranvier increase the efficiency of nodal conduction because of restriction (sequestration) of energy-dependent Na^+ influx to the node (**answers a, b, d, and e**). The nodes of Ranvier represent the space between adjacent units of myelination. That area is bare in the CNS, whereas in the PNS the axons in the nodes are partially covered by the cytoplasmic tongues of adjacent Schwann cells. Most of the Na^+-gated channels are located in the bare areas. Therefore, spread of depolarization from the nodal region along the axon occurs until it reaches the next node. This is often described as a series of jumps from node to node, or saltatory conduction.

140. The answer is c. (*Fauci, pp 1162, 1181. Kierszenbaum, pp 240-242. Mescher, p 154. Kandel, pp 1288-1295. Waxman, pp 9, 22.*) HIV entry into the brain occurs when infected CD4$^+$ lymphocytes and monocytes (**answer d**) enter through occluding junctions (**answers f and g**) of the blood-brain barrier. The barrier function of the blood-brain barrier is formed by occluding (tight) junctions (zonulae occludentes) between endothelial cells that comprise the lining of brain capillaries. Adding to the impermeability are the non-fenestrated nature of the capillary endothelium (**answers a and e**) and the paucity or absence of pinocytotic vesicles (**answer b**) that represent the physiological pores seen in other endothelia. Astrocytes form foot processes around the brain capillaries that induce and maintain the blood-brain barrier. Surrounding the CNS is a basal lamina with a lining of astrocyte foot processes that form the glia limitans. Microglia, the macrophages of the brain, phagocytose dying infected CD4$^+$ lymphocytes or endocytose free viral particles. Pathologically, HIV encephalitis is characterized by diffuse myelin damage (spongy myelinopathy), gliosis, neuronal loss, vascular damage, microglial nodules, and lymphocytic infiltrates. HIV envelope gly-coproteins cause the membranes of HIV-infected macrophages to fuse, forming multinucleate giant cells, the hallmark of HIV encephalitis. Gap junctions facilitate communication between cells **(answer h)**.

141. The answer is a. (*Alberts, pp 682-684, 1149. Fauci, pp 2572-2574. Mescher, pp 146, 147-148. Kierszenbaum, pp 225-226, 235-236. Kandel, pp 43, 175-177, 183, 210-211. Waxman, p 29.*) Ca^{2+} entry through specific channels results in fusion of acetylcholine-containing synaptic vesicles with the presynaptic membrane and ultimately the release of neurotransmitter. Neuromuscular (myoneural) junctions represent the site at which end feet (boutons terminaux) approximate the surface of skeletal muscle cells. The arrangement is similar to the synapse; a neuromuscular junction can be considered the best-studied synapse. Na^+, K^+, and Cl^- voltage-gated channels **(answers b, c, and d)** are involved in transmission of nerve impulses, but do not couple action potentials (an electrical signal) to neurotransmitter release (a chemical alteration). Ca^{2+} influx into the end feet may have a direct effect on phosphorylation of synapsin I, a vesicular membrane protein, which in its nonphosphorylated state blocks vesicle fusion with the presynaptic membrane. Gap junctions are not involved **(answer e)**. In ALS, continuous denervation and reinnervation does not allow sufficient time for maturation of newly formed neuromuscular junctions. Antibodies against voltage-gated Ca^{2+} channels are found in patients with sporadic ALS.

142. The answer is d. (*Mescher, pp 142-144, 152-154. Waxman, pp 136-141.*) The left hemisphere regulates language and speech and the right hemisphere controls nonverbal, spatial skills such as the ability to draw or play music. If the right side of the cerebrum is damaged, movement in the left arm and leg, vision to the left, or hearing in the left ear, may be affected. An injury to the left side of the cerebrum affects speech and movement on the right side of the body **(answers a → c and e)**. Pyramidal neurons are present throughout the photomicrograph. Axons are evident in the histologic section arising from the axon hillock. Neither the axon nor the axon hillock contains Nissl substance, RER, which is dispersed throughout the soma and dendrites. Dendrites generally are wider than axons, are of nonuniform diameter, and taper to a point. Motor neurons, such as those illustrated in the photomicrograph, usually display large amounts of euchromatin, distinct nucleoli, and Nissl (if stained appropriately) characteristic of high synthetic activity.

143. The answer is a. (*Mescher, pp 161-162. Fauci, pp 1021-1024.*) The woman in the scenario has contracted leprosy with infection of the peripheral nerves by *Mycobacterium leprae*. Perineurial inflammation of cutaneous nerves leads to distal anesthesia and paralysis, which are major clinical features of the early stages of leprosy. These neuropathic changes are eventually responsible for the deformities that elicit most of the social stigma associated with leprosy. The neuropathy of leprosy primarily affects the facial, ulnar radial, and fibular nerves with ascending degeneration of the nerves. In the later stages, endoneurial inflammation, infection of Schwann cells, demyelination, and reduced conduction velocity occurs. In the high-magnification light micrograph, several cross-sections through small peripheral nerves are visible. **C** indicates the perineurium, a layer of two to three fibroblast-like cells with contractile properties that surround individual fascicles. Cells of the perineurium are joined by tight junctions and form a barrier to macromolecules. **B** indicates the dense, irregular connective tissue part of the epineurium surrounding the entire nerve. There are numerous nerve fibers surrounded by myelin sheaths (**D**) produced by Schwann cells (nucleus visible at **E**). Other nuclei visible within the fascicle include those of fibroblasts, which secrete the reticular connective tissue elements forming the endoneurium surrounding the individual neuronal fibers, and nuclei of capillary endothelial cells. Neuronal perikarya are not present in peripheral nerves. Label **A** indicates skeletal muscle, identifiable by its striations and peripherally located nuclei.

144. The answer is e. (*Sadler, pp 73, 294, 299. Mescher, pp 140-141, 143. Kandel, pp 880, 883, 1027, 1046-1048. Moore and Persaud, pp 62-64, 75, 77, 179, 383.*) The neural crest forms most of the peripheral nervous system, in contrast to the neural tube, which is the embryonic source of the central nervous system. The sensory neurons of the cranial and spinal sensory ganglia (eg, dorsal root ganglia), sympathetic chain ganglia, and postganglionic sympathetic and parasympathetic fibers of the autonomic nervous system, cells of the pia and arachnoid, Schwann cells, and satellite cells of the dorsal root ganglia are neural elements derived from the neural crest. Nonneuronal structures formed from the neural crest include melanocytes of the skin, odontoblasts in teeth, derivatives of the branchial arch cartilages (eg, pinnae of ear), and the adrenal medulla, but not the adrenal cortex, for example, zona glomerulosa (**answer a**). The adrenal medulla represents postganglionic sympathetic fibers that respond to inputs from preganglionic sympathetic fibers in splanchnic nerves. Ventral horn and pyramidal cells (**answers b and c**) as well as astrocytes (**answer d**) are derived from the neuroepithelium of the neural tube.

145. The answer is a. (*Mescher, pp 164-165. Ross, p 336. Fauci, pp 151, 238. Kumar, p 1286.*) The structure in the photomicrograph delineated by the arrow is a single intramural parasympathetic ganglion cell distinctly characterized by its large, euchromatic nucleus and prominent nucleolus. Several small satellite cells surround the ganglion cell. Parasympathetic stimulation of the salivary glands produces a profuse, watery secretion. Atropine blocks parasympathetic responses (**answers b → e**). The child in the scenario is suffering from cerebral palsy (CP). Sialorrhea is excessive drooling and is a common symptom in children with CP. Children with CP are at increased risk of aspiration, skin maceration, and infection. Sialorrhea also impedes social integration. Parasympathetic ganglia are located in close proximity to or in the wall of the organs they innervate. Other structures within the field include serous acini from an exocrine gland, a small peripheral nerve, a venule, and several skeletal muscle fibers.

146. The answer is d. (*Mescher, pp 147-152, 158-159. Waxman, pp 13-14.*) The cells labeled with GFAP are activated astrocytes. Astrocytes are the most abundant cell type in the human brain. Astrocytes are activated following CNS damage and form the glial scar. These glial cells interact with neurons, blood vessels, and the pia mater by their stellate processes. Regulation of the microenvironment including the concentrations of ions, metabolites, and neurotransmitters (eg, glutamate) is an important function of astrocytes. Astrocytes are also the source of the most common glioma, astrocytoma. The barrier function of the blood-brain barrier is established by tight junctions (*zonula occludentes*) between endothelial cells in the blood vessels of the brain. However, astrocytes establish and maintain the blood-brain barrier and thus control the entry of compounds into the brain parenchyma. During development, the astrocytes are critical to normal migration of developing neurons. The patient in the vignette suffers from NeuroAIDS. In that disease, astrocytes are believed to be infected with the AIDS virus. Astrocytes can be infected with HIV-1, however, there appears to be only limited replication. Infection can lead to changes in gene expression (of the cell) and some of the released products can have deleterious effects on neurons. Astrocytes integrate neuronal inputs, exhibit calcium excitability, and communicate bidirectionally with neighboring neurons and synapses, but do not synapse with neurons (answer a). Microglia present antigen and phagocytose dying neurons (answers b and c). Oligodendrocytes myelinate axons in the CNS (answer e).

147. The answer is a. (*Fauci, pp 2717-2718. Mescher, pp 146-148, 166-169. Kandel, pp 265-269.*) Clinical depression is associated with reduced levels of the monoamines, such as 5-hydroxytryptamine (serotonin, 5-HT) in the CNS. The selective serotonin reuptake inhibitors (SSRIs), such as fluoxetine hydrochloride (Prozac), bind to the 5-HT reuptake transporter in the presynaptic membrane, blocking reuptake, and subsequent degradation of serotonin in the synaptic cleft (answer e). Therefore, serotonin levels increase in the synaptic cleft as a result of SSRI treatment. The structure labeled "D" in the transmission electron micrograph is the postsynaptic membrane. Other regions of the synapse are the presynaptic membrane (C), mitochondria (B), and synaptic vesicles (A). Recycling of synaptic vesicle membrane occurs at the presynaptic membrane in conjunction with neurotransmitter release by exocytosis. Neurotransmitter release is induced by membrane depolarization, leading to transient opening of calcium channels followed by calcium influx. There is no cytoplasmic continuity between adjacent neurons (answer d). Transmission from neuron to neuron occurs by chemical transmission in the form of neurotransmitter release. The neurotransmitter (from the synaptic vesicles) crosses the synaptic cleft (between the pre- and postsynaptic membranes) and interacts with receptors on the postsynaptic membrane (answer b), which results in changes in the permeability of this membrane (answer c). Numerous mitochondria and synaptic vesicles are typically found on the presynaptic side of the synapse. The postsynaptic surface typically is denser than the presynaptic membrane.

148. The answer is b. (*Fauci, pp 2611-2614. Kumar, pp 1310-1312. Kierszenbaum, pp 233-235. Mescher, p 151. Waxman, pp 24, 35, 292.*) The patient is suffering from multiple sclerosis (MS), a demyelinating disease in which both CD4+ and CD8+-T cells as well as autoantibodies are targeted against oligodendrocytes. MS is twice as prevalent in women as in men and demyelination is most commonly found in the anterior corpus callosum. Alterations in the CSF shows pleocytosis (increase in the number of mononuclear cells above normal levels), increase in protein, elevated gamma globulin (antibodies to oligodendrocytes as represented by oligo-clonal bands on gel electrophoresis). Microglia **(answer a)** are the phago-cytes of the CNS, astrocytes **(answer c)** induce and maintain the blood-brain barrier and form the glial scar following injury, and Schwann cells **(answer d)** are responsible for myelination in the PNS. On autopsy, plaques are found that contain lymphocytes and monocytes in infiltrates around small veins in what is known as perivascular cuffing. Axons **(answer e)** are generally preserved. The main identifying feature on histopathological examination is the paucity of oligodendrocytes. Astro-cytic proliferation and gliosis may increase with the duration of MS.

149. The answer is e. *(Mescher, pp 171-172, 175. Ross, pp 291-292, 311-313. Fauci, pp 2672-2674. Kumar, pp 1275-1276. Waxman, pp 30, 61, 283, 287.)* The junctional folds are the site of acetylcholine (ACh) receptors which are reduced in number in myasthenia gravis. The normal neuromuscular junc-tion releases ACh from the motor nerve terminal in discrete packages (quanta). The ACh quanta diffuse across the synaptic cleft and bind to recep-tors on the folded muscle end-plate membrane. Stimulation of the motor nerve releases many ACh quanta that depolarize the muscle end-plate region and then the muscle membrane causing muscle contraction. In myasthenia gravis, the postsynaptic muscle membrane is smooth and lacks the normal folded shape. The concentration of ACh receptors on the muscle end-plate membrane is reduced, and antibodies are attached to the membrane. ACh is released normally, but its effect on the postsynaptic membrane is reduced. The postjunctional membrane is less sensitive to applied ACh, and the prob-ability that any nerve impulse will cause a muscle action potential is reduced. The edrophonium chloride (Tensilon) test uses a rapid acting and degrading acetylcholine esterase inhibitor. It causes neuromuscular transmission to be increased in the patient. The physician injects the Tensilon and then looks for rapid relief of the symptoms, particularly the eyelids and the diplopia. Other structures labeled in the electron micrograph are: A = nucleus, B = mitochon-dria, C = myofilaments, and D = nerve terminal.

Cardiovascular System, Blood, and Bone Marrow

Questions

150. Vasa vasorum provide a function analogous to that of which one of the following structures?

a. Valves
b. Basal lamina
c. Coronary arteries
d. Endothelial diaphragms
e. Arterioles

151. The cell labeled A in the figure is best described as which of the following?

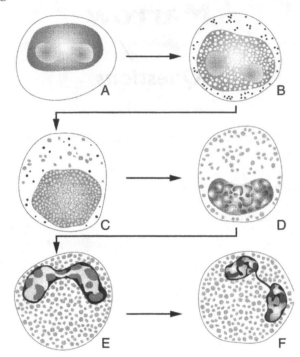

a. Myeloblast
b. Proerythroblast
c. Metamyelocyte
d. Myelocyte
e. Promyelocyte

152. A newborn girl presents with a mutation in the erythropoietin receptor gene which leads to primary familial erythrocytosis (familial polycythemia). During the seventh to ninth months of fetal development, the primary effect was on red blood cell production in which of the following?

a. Liver
b. Yolk sac
c. Spleen
d. Thymus
e. Bone marrow

153. A 64-year-old man presents with splenomegaly, lymphadenopathy, persistent fever, night sweats, and weight loss. Bone marrow aspiration and biopsy are scheduled. Which of the following would be the best place to sample bone marrow?

a. Iliac crest
b. Sternum
c. Scapula
d. Humerus
e. Tibia

154. Organs such as the brain and thymus have a more effective blood barrier because their blood capillaries are of which of the following types?

a. Continuous type with few vesicles
b. Fenestrated type with diaphragms
c. Fenestrated type without diaphragms
d. Discontinuous type with diaphragms
e. Discontinuous type without diaphragms

155. A 62-year-old African American man presents with exercise-induced angina. His serum cholesterol is 277 mg/dL (normal <200), LDL is 157 (normal <100), HDL is 43 (normal >35), and triglycerides 170 (normal <150). His body mass index (BMI) is 34 and his coronary risk ratio is 6.84 (normal <5). On cardiac catheterization, there is occlusion of the left anterior descending and the origin of the right coronary artery. The disease process is initiated by which one of the following?

a. Proliferation of smooth muscle cells
b. Formation of an intimal plaque
c. Intimal thickening through the addition of collagen and elastin with an abnormal pattern of elastin cross-linking
d. Adventitial proliferation
e. Injury to the endothelium

156. A 66-year-old man who was diagnosed with type II diabetes 10 years ago presents with an aching pain in the muscles of his lower extremities. He says the pain is relieved by rest and worsened by resumed physical activity. His lower limbs appear cold, pale, and discolored, and he has a sore on the skin of his left calf. He has a weak tibial pulse on both sides and poor skin filling from capillaries. In this patient, which of the following functions would be primarily affected in the blood vessel from the lower extremity shown in the accompanying transmission electron micrograph?

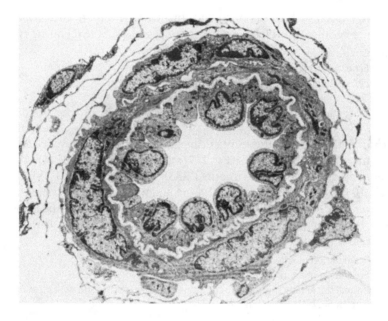

a. Adaptation to systolic pressure
b. Distribution of blood within an organ
c. Blood flow from the aorta to specific organs
d. Return of lymphocytes to the blood
e. Return of venous blood to the heart

157. A 35-year-old woman's physician orders laboratory blood tests. Her fresh blood is drawn and centrifuged in the presence of heparin as an anti-coagulant to obtain a hematocrit. The resulting fractions are which of the following?

a. Serum, packed erythrocytes, and leukocytes
b. Leukocytes, erythrocytes, and serum proteins
c. Plasma, buffy coat, and packed erythrocytes
d. Fibrinogen, platelets, buffy coat, and erythrocytes
e. Albumin, plasma lipoproteins, and erythrocytes

158. A hematologist diagnoses a 34-year-old woman with idiopathic thrombocytopenic purpura (ITP). Which of the following symptoms/characteristics would one expect in this patient?

a. Decreased clotting time
b. Normal blood count
c. Abnormal bruising
d. Hypercoagulation
e. Light menstrual periods

159. A 47-year-old man presents to his family physician complaining of unusual thirst, increased frequency of urination, dizziness, blurred vision, and numbness in his left foot. His BMI is 32. He reports that his lifestyle is sedentary with very rare exercise. His diet consists largely of what he describes as "fast and junk food." A finger stick reading indicates a blood glucose level of 190 mg/dL and two fasting blood sugars are 156 and 166 mg/dL. Over time, which of the following describes the changes that may occur in the structure labeled "A" in the accompanying light micrograph?

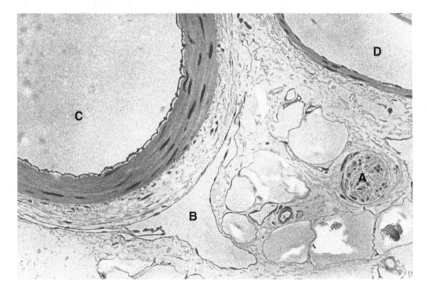

(Micrograph courtesy of Dr. John K. Young.)

a. Loss of β cells
b. Arteriosclerosis
c. Progressive decrease in nerve conduction velocity
d. Altered smooth muscle glucose transporter function
e. Altered lymphatic flow

160. A 42-year-old woman presents to her family physician with dizziness and lightheadedness, shortness of breath after light activity, an uncomfortable tingling, crawling feeling in her legs, and frequent headaches. She describes herself as "always tired and fighting colds." She has pale skin, overall weakness, cold hands and feet, a blue tinge to her sclerae, soreness and inflammation of the tongue, and brittle nails. She reports a craving for ice. She says that her husband and children find her irritable and say that she "gets easily upset by little things." Her hemoglobin is 11.0 g/dL (normal = 11.7-13.8 g/dL), her hematocrit is 33.9% (normal = 36%-46%), and her serum ferritin is 12 g/dL (normal ≥ 15.0 g/dL). What erythrocytic shape and size changes would one expect in her CBC?

a. Microcytic, hypochromatic anemia with smaller mature erythrocytes
b. Macrocytic, hyperchromatic anemia with fewer, larger mature erythrocytes
c. Poikilocytosis and more fragile erythrocytes
d. Spherocytosis
e. No change in erythrocyte size or shape, but a substantial drop in the hematocrit

161. A 43-year-old woman who has suffered from diabetes for 30 years comes into the clinic. Her hematocrit is 21 and she has a reduced RBC count. Her serum creatinine is 3.0 (normal 2.0 or below). She has a negative pregnancy test and is a nonsmoker. Which one of the following would best explain her condition?

a. Decreased hepatic production of erythropoietin leading to decreased numbers of circulating reticulocytes in the bloodstream
b. Increased erythropoietin production by the liver resulting in increased numbers of reticulocytes
c. Decreased renal erythropoietin production leading to reduced red blood cell production
d. Decreased estrogen levels stimulating hepatic production of erythropoietin
e. Decreased estrogen levels directly inhibiting red blood cell production by the bone marrow

162. Which one of the following is a metabolic function of the cells labeled with arrows in the accompanying light micrograph?

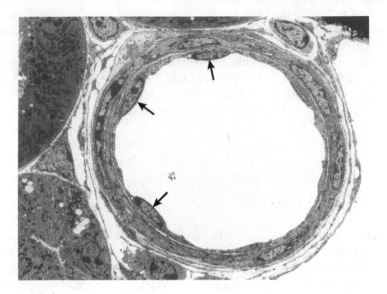

a. Receptors for endothelin
b. Release of serotonin
c. Production of type I collagen
d. Production of type III collagen
e. Synthesis of plasminogen activator
f. Production of thromboxane

163. A research laboratory is studying cardiovascular function. The studies in that laboratory use a "knockout" mouse in which the gene for atrial natriuretic peptide (ANP) is deleted. Which one of the following would one most likely find elevated?

a. ANP levels in the bloodstream
b. Excretion of urine
c. Excretion of sodium
d. Peripheral vasoconstriction
e. Capillary permeability

164. A 43-year-old anatomy professor is working in her garden, pruning rose bushes without gloves. She has a thorn enter the skin of her forefinger. The area later becomes infected and she removes the thorn, but there is still pus remaining at the wound site. Which of the following cells functions in the formation of pus?

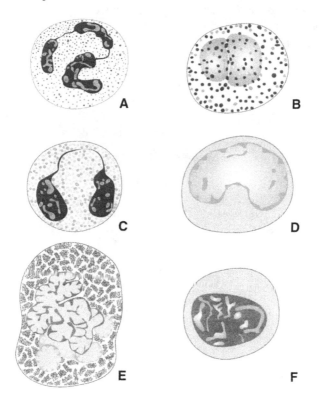

a. A
b. B
c. C
d. D
e. E
f. F

165. A 27-year-old man returns from a climbing trip to Ouray, Colorado. He spent 2 weeks camping with his fellow climbing friends. He is dehydrated and complains that he has been vomiting and has had "foul-smelling" diarrhea since his return from camping. He says that he has noticed several large worms in the vomitus and had a visible worm in his loose stool last week. A stool sample is positive for ova and parasites. How do the structures labeled in the accompanying electron micrograph assist in defending against this condition?

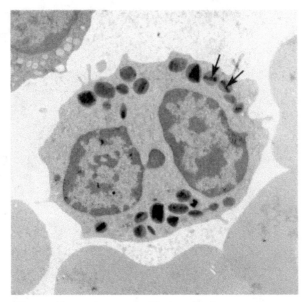

(Electron micrograph courtesy of Dr. Amy Klion.)

a. Phagocytose parasites
b. Release IL-1 which activates antigen presenting cells (APCs) and CD4⁺ lymphocytes
c. Release IL-2 which stimulates the proliferation and activation of B cells and T cells
d. Produce IL-5 which stimulates the production and maturation of eosinophils during inflammation
e. Contain a toxin for parasites

Cardiovascular System, Blood, and Bone Marrow

Answers

150. The answer is c. (*Mescher, pp 190, 192.*) Vasa vasorum are vessels within a vessel and are found primarily in the adventitia of large arteries and veins. They provide nutrition and oxygenated blood to the thick media and adventitia of these vessels, which are unable to obtain nutrition by diffusion from the lumen. Coronary arteries fulfill a similar function for the myocardium (**answers a, b, d, and e**).

151. The answer is a. (*Mescher, pp 217, 219-224. Ross, pp 268, 270-271.*) The first stage in granulopoiesis is the myeloblast (**A**), a large cell with prominent light-staining nucleoli with only a little cytoplasm, generally without granules. The lineage shown in the figure illustrates eosinophilic development in the bone marrow. Basophils may be bilobed or segmented, but with larger and more irregular granules that obscure the nucleus in Wright-stained blood smears. The promyelocyte (**B**) is the next cell in the lineage. It is larger than the myeloblast, nucleoli are less visible, and primary granules are present in the cytoplasm. Granule specificity is attained in the myelocyte with flattening of the nucleus. The eosinophilic myelocyte (**C**) differentiates into the eosinophilic metamyelocyte (**D**) when invagination of the nucleus begins. Further invagination leads to the formation of an eosinophilic band (**E**) and ultimately a mature eosinophil (**F**). An eosinophil has a bilobed nucleus and plays an important role in allergic and parasitic infections (also see Questions 164 and 165). The granules stain with eosinophilic dyes and contain major basic protein, histaminase, peroxidase, and some hydrolytic enzymes. Eosinophils have an affinity for antigen-antibody complexes and, although phagocytic, are not as active against bacteria as neutrophils. The histaminase secreted by eosinophils counteracts the release of histamine from basophils and mast cells, essential in hypersensitivity reactions. B lymphocytes differentiate into antibody-producing plasma cells; T lymphocytes are responsible for cell-mediated responses including graft rejection; and neutrophils are responsible for phagocytosis of bacteria.

152. The answer is e. *(Ross, p 254. Mescher, p 216. Kumar, p 590.)* The bone marrow becomes the predominant hematopoietic site during the 3rd trimester of gestation. The first site of blood cell development (hematopoiesis) is extraembryonic, in the yolk sac **(answer b)**, which produces hemangioblasts, the precursors of the hematopoietic stem cells (HSCs) and primitive erythroblasts from the third week through the second month of gestation. Hepatic erythropoiesis **(answer a)** is active during the second trimester. Whereas, the spleen **(answer c)** is involved specifically in the production of red blood cells (erythropoiesis) from months 2 to 7 of gestation with some activity continuing postnatally. The spleen is a minor extramedullary source of monocytes and lymphocytes throughout life. From the second month of gestation, the lymph nodes produce lymphocytes, and the thymus **(answer d)** is responsible for the education of T cells. Those T lymphocytes are seeded to T-dependent areas, such as the deep cortex of the lymph node and periarteriolar lymphoid sheath of the spleen.

153. The answer is a. *(Kumar, p 590. Ross, p 254. Mescher, pp 216, 219.)* The iliac crest is the best location for bone marrow sampling. The sternum is not a safe place for bone marrow aspiration and biopsy because of possible damage to thoracic structures **(answer b)**. The patient in the vignette suffers from chronic lymphocytic leukemia more common in adults over 60 years old. Hematopoiesis occurs in the flat bones **(answer c)** and other bones in the adult human. Although most bones in the body are involved in hematopoiesis during growth, the marrow of the sternum, ribs, vertebrae, iliac crest, skull, and proximal femora are the primary sites of blood cell development by the time skeletal maturity is achieved. It also occurs in the long bones **(answers d and e)** during development, but in adulthood many of those areas become dominated by yellow marrow containing many fat cells (adipose tissue). The inactive yellow marrow can be reactivated on exposure to the proper stimulus (eg, severe blood loss).

154. The answer is a. *(Young, pp 146, 160, 162. Mescher, pp 154, 236. Ross, pp 423-424. Kierszenbaum, pp 358-360.)* The capillary endothelia in the brain and thymus are continuous, as is the basal lamina. The blood-thymus barrier provides the appropriate microenvironment for education of T cells without exposure to self. The capillaries are further surrounded by perivascular connective tissue and epithelial cells and their basement membrane. In the blood-brain barrier, there is also a continuous endothelium with a basal lamina and an absence of fenestrations. Surrounding the basal lamina in the brain are the foot processes of astrocytes, which form the glia limitans; however, it is important to note that the barrier function of the blood-brain barrier is formed specifically by endothelial cell occluding junctions with many sealing strands. Other capillary endothelia **(answers b → e)** in the body are fenestrated (transcellular openings) or discontinuous (sinusoids). The fenestrae are transcellular openings that occur in many of the visceral capillaries. In hematopoietic organs, there are large gaps in the endothelium, and the capillaries are classified as discontinuous. Diaphragms (thinner cell membrane) are present in some fenestrated capillaries and produce an intermediate level of molecular transit. Diaphragms have a pore-like structure and contain proteoglycans with particularly high concentrations of heparan sulfate. This results in numerous anionic sites that repel anionic proteins. The diaphragms facilitate the passage of water and small molecules dissolved in fluid. Physiologically, the large pores (50-70 nm) of endothelia are represented by pinocytotic vesicles. Intercellular junctions, particularly the tight junctions, function as the small endothelial pores (approximately 10 nm in diameter) observed in physiologic studies. Plasmalemmal vesicles and channels are neutrally charged and rich in galactose and N-acetylglucosamine. Vesicular and channel pathways are required for transport of anionic proteins such as insulin, transferrin, albumin, and low density lipoprotein (LDL).

155. The answer is e. *(Mescher, p 192. Moore, pp 155-158. Kierszenbaum, pp 367-368.)* The site at which coronary arteries become occluded are: first, at the left anterior descending (thus affecting both ventricles anteriorly); second, at the origin of the right coronary artery affecting both the right atrium and ventricle and disrupting cardiac rhythm; and third, the circumflex branch (affecting both left atria and ventricle). Atherosclerosis is initiated by damage to the endothelial cells, which exposes the subjacent connective tissue. The loss of the antithrombogenic endothelium results in aggregation of platelets. Atherosclerosis is one form of arteriosclerosis (hardening of the arteries) that involves deposition of fatty material primarily in the walls of the conducting arteries. The intima and media become infiltrated with lipid. Intimal thickening occurs through the addition of collagen and elastin with an abnormal pattern of elastin cross-linking (answer c). Platelets release mitogenic substances that stimulate proliferation of smooth muscle cells (answer a). The thickening of the intima is also called an atheromatous plaque (answer b) and worsens with repeated damage to the endothelium. It is most dangerous in small vessels, particularly the coronary arteries, where occlusion can result in a myocardial infarction. Atherosclerotic plaques also lead to thrombi and aneurysms. Adventitial proliferation occurs during atherosclerosis, but is not the initiating event (answer d).

156. The answer is b. (*Young, pp 157-159, 163-165. Mescher, pp 193-194, 196. Ross, p 371.*) The blood vessel in the electron micrograph is an arteriole (small artery) involved in intraorgan blood flow. There is only one layer of smooth muscle, but a distinct internal elastic membrane is present.

There is no visible internal elastic membrane in a venule. A capillary lacks smooth muscle and is composed only of a single layer of endothelial cells.

The aorta and large arteries (answer a) contain extensive elastic fibers that permit rapid arterial wall stretch in response to the force of ventricular contraction during systole (120-160 mm Hg) followed by sudden relaxation (60-90 mm Hg) during diastole. Blood is ejected from the left ventricle into the large arteries only during systole; however, blood flow is uniform because of the elasticity of the large, conducting arteries.

The muscular (distributing) arteries regulate blood flow to organs (answer c). Muscular (medium) arteries contain more smooth muscle than the arteriole in the figure and distribute blood to organs. Contraction of muscular arteries is regulated by local factors as well as sympathetic innervation. The degree of contraction regulates blood flow between organs. When the tunica media of the muscular artery is contracted, less blood flow occurs to the organ. In a more relaxed state, there is increased blood flow to the same organ.

The thoracic duct (answer d) returns lymphocytes from the lymphoid compartment to the circulation. The thoracic duct shows complete disorganization in the wall with no distinct media or adventitia. The large veins (answer e), such as the vena cava, that return blood to the heart contain smooth muscle bundles in the adventitia and are also the only vessel in which one sees both circularly and longitudinally arranged smooth muscle in the same vessel.

157. The answer is c. *(Mescher, p 204. Ross, p 248.)* After blood is removed from the body, a clot forms that contains platelets, erythrocytes, leukocytes, and a clear, yellow fluid known as serum. Hematocrit is the volume of erythrocytes per unit volume of blood (eg, 40%-50% in adult human males). When centrifuged with anticoagulants, blood separates into three layers. The uppermost layer is the plasma; the buffy coat is a thin white layer consisting of leukocytes found beneath the plasma; and the packed erythrocyte layer is found at the bottom of the tube.

158. The answer is c. *(Mescher, p 225. Kierszenbaum, pp 173-174. Kumar, pp 667-668.)* ITP is primarily a disease of increased peripheral platelet destruction and/or reduction in platelet production by the bone marrow. The main symptom is bleeding, which can include bruising ("ecchymosis") and tiny red dots on the skin or mucous membranes ("petechiae"). In some instances bleeding from the nose, periodontal ligament ("gums"), urinary or gastrointestinal tracts may occur. Cerebral hemorrhage occurs rarely in ITP. Red and white cell counts are normal, but platelet counts range from 10,000 to 30,000/mL^3 **(answer b)** with 150,000 mL^3 as normal and higher than 100,000 mL^3 is safe.

The reduction in platelets increases clotting time **(answer a)**, decreases coagulation **(answer d)**, and would result in heavier menstrual bleeding **(answer e)**. ITP appears to be an autoimmune disease since most patients have autoantibodies to specific platelet membrane glycoproteins. Acute ITP often follows an acute infection or in response to pharmaceutical administration. It can also occur during pregnancy and in chronic diseases such as hepatitis C, HIV, and lupus.

159. The answer is c. *(Ross, p 395. Mescher, pp 162, 164, 196, 199.)* The photomicrograph shows several types of blood or lymphatic vessels. Frequently, peripheral nerves are found in association with blood vessels (neurovascular bundle). In this section, a small peripheral nerve is labeled **A**. It is characterized by an outer covering of perineurium. The dark nuclei visible within the cross section belong mostly to Schwann cells. Neuronal cell bodies (perikarya) are not found within peripheral nerves. The structure labeled **B** is a small lymphatic vessel. Small lymphatic vessels are characterized by a wall consisting only of an exceedingly thin, single layer of endothelium. The lumen is usually larger than that of comparable venules. As observed in the photomicrograph, valves are also present in lymphatic vessels. A small muscular artery (C) and comparable vein (D) are also present in the field. The patient is diagnosed with diabetic neuropathy.

160. The answer is a. (*Mescher, pp 204-206. Fauci, pp 630-632. Kumar, pp 659-662.*) The patient in the vignette has iron deficiency that leads to anemia with the presence of smaller, pale-staining erythrocytes (microcytic, hypochromatic). Hyperchromatic, macrocytic anemia results from vitamin B_{12} deficiency (**answers b and e**). The presence of spherical rather than biconcave erythrocytes is known as spherocytosis (**answer d**). The RBC membrane undergoes deformation due to the inability of ankyrin to bind spectrin. The shape change results in trapping in the splenic sinusoids and excessive destruction of red blood cells in that organ. Poikilocytosis is the generic term for abnormally shaped erythrocytes (**answer c**). Hereditary elliptocytosis and hereditary poikilocytosis are inherited diseases in which there is RBC membrane fragility and abnormal shape due to spectrin mutations. Mutations in band 3 (anion exchanger 1) result in RBCs that are hyperchromatic with poikilocytosis.

161. The answer is c. (*Fauci, pp, 355-356. Mescher, pp 56, 204-206, 218, 220, 332.*) Normal hematocrit for a woman is 37% to 47%. The most likely cause of anemia is renal failure due to diabetic nephropathy. Diabetes alters glomerular basement membranes, causes glycation of proteins resulting in advanced glycation end-products, and induces glomerular hypertrophy contributing to glomerulosclerosis. Renal insufficiency leads to decreased production of the kidney-derived red blood cell growth factor, erythropoietin (**EPO, answers a and b**). In the initial stages of renal failure EPO production is increased, but as renal damage continues, the peritubular capillary cells that produce EPO are destroyed. Therefore, there are initially increased levels of reticulocytes (immature red blood cells) in the bloodstream, but this is later reversed. Low production of reticulocytes is a hallmark of anemia associated with renal disease. Although the patient may have decreased estrogen levels, estrogen decreases hematocrit (**answers d and e**). Also, women who are pregnant (third trimester) can have slightly decreased hematocrits (37 ± 6 [third trimester women] vs 40 ± 6 [adult women] and 42 ± 6 [postmenopausal women]). However, this patient had a negative pregnancy test. Administration of recombinant EPO is the preferred treatment for anemia caused by advanced renal disease. Generally, EPO is administered if the hematocrit is less than 30%. EPO is synthesized by the peritubular (interstitial) cells of the kidney cortex, stimulates the differentiation of cells from the erythrocyte colony-forming units (E-CFUs), and the differentiation and release of reticulocytes from the bone marrow. CFUs are distinct cell lineages derived from pluripotential stem cells in the bone marrow.

162. The answer is e. *(Kumar, pp 115-118. Kierszenbaum, pp 364, 366-367. Mescher, pp 187-188, 194. Fauci, p 364.)* Endothelial cells synthesize a number of antithrombogenic factors including plasminogen activator and prostacyclin. Prostacyclin functions through cyclic AMP to inhibit thromboxane production by platelets **(answer f)**. Endothelial cells synthesize the basal lamina including type IV collagen. Fibroblasts synthesize collagens type I and III **(answers c and d)**. Serotonin is released from platelets and enteroendocrine cells **(answer b)**. Other endothelial cell functions include: secretion of endothelin (the most potent vasoconstrictor [**answer a**]), plasminogen inhibitor (a coagulant), and nitric oxide (NO), also known as endothelium-derived relaxing factor. Angiotensin-converting enzyme (ACE) on the endothelial cell surface converts angiotensin I to angiotensin II (a potent vasoconstrictor), but also serves as an inactivation enzyme (bradykininase) for bradykinin, a vasodilator. Von Willebrand factor (factor VIII) is found in Weibel-Palade granules localized in the endothelial cells of vessels larger than capillaries. A deficiency of factor VIII leads to decreased platelet aggregation and hemophilia.

163. The answer is d. *(Kierszenbaum, pp 35, 421. Kumar, p 531. Mescher, p 182. Fauci, pp 1743-1748.)* ANP is an important diuretic and natriuretic molecule that is released from the atria in response to atrial stretch and/or endothelin-1 stimulation. In the absence of ANP, peripheral vasoconstriction increases due to the absence of the ANP-induced relaxation of vascular smooth muscle and the increase in aldosterone levels. Aldosterone increases Na^+ permeability of the luminal membrane in the distal renal tubule and the activity of Na^+ pumps. The increased salt causes water retention, expanded blood volume, and elevated blood pressure. ANP would not be expressed in ANP knockout mice **(answer a)**. Excretion of urine (diuresis [**answer b**]) and sodium (natriuresis [**answer c**]), and capillary permeability **(answer e)** all decrease in the absence of ANP. The main targets of ANP are the kidneys and vascular smooth muscle. ANP decreases blood pressure due to a direct relaxation of vascular smooth muscle. In addition, it increases salt and water excretion, enhances capillary permeability, and inhibits the release or action of several hormones, in addition to aldosterone, such as angiotensin II, endothelin, renin, and vasopressin. The natriuretic effect results from a direct inhibition of sodium absorption in the renal collecting duct, increased glomerular filtration rate, and inhibited aldosterone production and secretion. ANP counteracts the renin-angiotensin-aldosterone system. Increased ANP levels are detected in congestive heart failure, chronic renal failure, and in severe essential hypertension.

164. The answer is a. *(Young, pp 49-57. Mescher, pp 206-212.)* Mature neutrophils (also known as polymorphonuclear leukocytes [PMNs]) have 3 to 5 lobes. They phagocytose bacteria. Dead neutrophils are a major constituent of pus.

Neutrophil. The neutrophil **(A)** contains neutrophilic granules. Neutrophils are involved in the acute phase of inflammation and are responsible for the phagocytosis of invading bacteria. Neutrophils contain lysozyme and alkaline phosphatase within their granules. They die soon after phagocytosing bacteria and are added to the pus, which consists of dead neutrophils, serum, and tissue fluids.

Basophil. The basophil **(B)** is about the same size as the neutrophil **(A)** and contains granules of variable size that may obscure the nucleus. The nucleus of the basophil is irregularly lobed with condensed chromatin. Basophils are involved in the attraction of eosinophils to the site of infection. This occurs in parasitic and nonparasitic infections and involves chemoattraction by histamine and eosinophil-chemoattractant factor of anaphylaxis. Basophils are similar in structure and function to the connective tissue mast cell. Basophils are also phagocytic granulocytes, but are involved in inflammation through the release of histamine and heparin. Immunoglobulin E (IgE) produced by plasma cells becomes bound to the cell surface of mast cells and basophils on first exposure. At the time of secondary exposure, the antigen binds to the IgE and stimulates the degranulation of mast cells and basophil granules releasing histamine and heparin. Basophils and mast cells are involved in anaphylactic and immediate **hypersensitivity reactions**.

Eosinophil. The eosinophil **(C)** is bilobed with more regular granules than the basophil **(B)**. Eosinophils have less phagocytic ability than neutrophils and may kill parasites by either phagocytosis or exocytotic release of granules. Eosinophils contain major basic protein, histaminase, acid phosphatase, and other lysosomal enzymes. Eosinophils are essential for the destruction of parasites such as trichinae and schistosomes.

Monocyte. The monocyte (**D**) contains an eccentric nucleus, which is often kidney-shaped. The chromatin generally has a ropelike appearance and, therefore, is less condensed than the chromatin of a lymphocyte (**F**). The monocyte has some phagocytic activity in the blood, but its major role is as a source of macrophages throughout the body including Langerhans cells (skin), microglia (brain), and Kupffer cells (liver).

Megakaryocyte. The megakaryocyte (**E**) is a large cell with a multilobular appearance and is the source of platelets. Megakaryocytes fragment to form the platelets, which are key elements of the blood.

Lymphocyte. The lymphocyte (**F**) is considered an agranular cell with an ovoid nucleus and scanty cytoplasm. The shape and the arrangement of chromatin vary, depending on the classification of the lymphocyte: small, medium, or large. Small and medium are involved in chronic inflammation, whereas large lymphocytes are the source of T and B cells. Lymphocytes are either T or B cells based on their education in the thymus or bone marrow. Plasma cells differentiate from B lymphocytes that undergo mitosis and form a plasma cell and a memory cell after exposure to appropriate antigen. An antigen-presenting cell and a specific subtype of T lymphocyte called a helper T cell are required for B cell differentiation into antibody-producing plasma cells.

165. The answer is e. (*Mescher, pp 206-210. Ross, pp 257-258. Fauci, pp 383, 757, 2029-2030.*) The patient returning from a camping trip most likely has contracted a parasitic infection. The cell in the transmission electron micrograph is an eosinophil. Eosinophil granules contain a number of important substances including histaminase, eosinophil peroxidase, eosinophil cationic protein, and major basic protein (MBP). MBP forms the core of the eosinophilic granules and is a toxin for parasites. MBP binds to and disrupts the membrane of the parasite. The binding is mediated by the Fc receptor. MBP also causes basophils to release histamine. Eosinophils phagocytose parasites, but MBP is not directly involved (**answer a**). IL-1 and IL-2 carry out the functions of activating APCs and stimulating proliferation of B and T cells, respectively. However, the eosinophil does not release IL-1 and IL-2 (**answers b and c**). IL-5 stimulates production and maturation of eosinophils, but is not released by eosinophils (**answer d**).

Lymphoid System and Cellular Immunology

Questions

166. Clonal selection functions to do which one of the following?
a. Create the optimal immune response to one specific antigen
b. Stimulate immunoglobulin class switching
c. Stimulate the production of self-reacting lymphocytes
d. Form specific colony-forming units (CFUs) for erythropoiesis and granulopoiesis in the bone marrow
e. Choose the appropriate homing receptors for lymphocytes

167. Tacrolimus (FK506) is prescribed for a patient who received an allogeneic liver transplant. The mechanism of action of tacrolimus is blockage of signal transduction pathways in which one of the following cells?
a. T lymphocytes
b. Plasma cells
c. Monocytes
d. Eosinophils
e. Mast cells

168. The shortage of human organs for transplant has focused attention on xenotransplantation as a potential solution for obtaining donor organs. Rejection of a pig pancreas transplanted into a human would occur primarily through which one of the following mechanisms?
a. Preformed antibodies recognize carbohydrates on endothelial cells in the graft.
b. T_C lymphocytes recognize dendritic cells in the graft.
c. T_H lymphocytes recognize macrophages in the graft.
d. Plasma cell response to antigens in the β cells of the islets.
e. Hyperacute response of T cells to the pancreatic acinar cells.

169. The organ, shown at low magnification (A) and high magnification (B) is which one of the following?

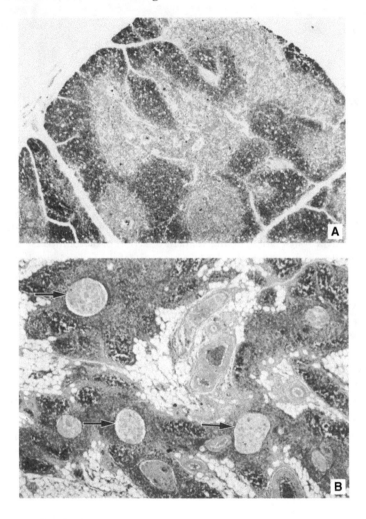

a. A site of antibody production
b. The site of filtration of the lymph and blood
c. Derived embryologically from the third branchial arch
d. The site of production of CD4⁺ and CD8⁺ cells
e. A major site of red blood cell degradation and bilirubin recycling

170. Gene rearrangement of cytotoxic T cells occurs primarily in which one of the following locations?

a. Bone marrow
b. Spleen
c. Germinal centers
d. Thymus
e. Mesenteric lymph nodes

171. Gene products of class II major histocompatibility complex (MHC) present antigenic peptides primarily to which one of the following cells?

a. Helper T cells
b. Cytotoxic T cells
c. Antigen-presenting cells (APCs)
d. B cells
e. Plasma cells

172. Expression of antigen associated with class I MHC molecules is recognized primarily by which of the following cells?

a. B cells
b. CD4+ T lymphocytes
c. CD8+ T lymphocytes
d. Plasma cells
e. Macrophages

173. Interleukin-2 is produced by which one of the following cells?

a. Plasma cells
b. Natural killer cells
c. CD4+ T lymphocytes
d. CD8+ T lymphocytes
e. Macrophages

174. A young boy presents at the pediatric clinic. He weighed 3.5 kg at birth and appeared to be perfectly normal. Through his first 2 years of life, he had persistent otitis media, dry cough, and on one occasion bilateral pneumonia. At 5 months, the boy had oral *Candida albicans*. and a red rash in the diaper area. He was not gaining weight and was admitted to the hospital with tachypnea. His tonsils were observed to be very small. He had hepatomegaly, and cultures of his nasal fluid grew *Pseudomonas aeruginosa*. He also had coarse, harsh breath sounds from both lungs. Blood work showed a white blood cell count = 4800 cells μL^{-1} (normal 5000-10,000 cells μL^{-1}), absolute lymphocyte count = 760 cells μL^{-1} (normal 3000 lymphocytes μL^{-1}). None of his lymphocytes reacted with anti-CD3; 99% of his lymphocytes bound antibody against the B-cell molecule CD20 and 1% were natural killer cells reacting with anti-CD16. His serum contained IgG at a concentration of 30 mg dL^{-1}, IgA at 27 mg dL^{-1}, IgM at 42 mg dL^{-1} (IgG levels are normally 400 mg dL^{-1}; the IgA and IgM levels were at the low end of the normal range for his age). His blood mononuclear cells were completely unresponsive to phytohemagglutinin (PHA), concanavalin A (ConA), and pokeweed mitogen (PWM), as well as to specific antigens to which he had been previously exposed by immunization or infection— tetanus and diphtheria toxoids, and Candida antigen. His B lymphocytes did not react with an antibody to the γ chain of the interleukin-2 receptor (IL-2Rγ).

The accompanying images are low magnification (A) and high magnification (B) photomicrographs. In the case presented above, what would one expect to find immediately surrounding the region labeled with the arrow?

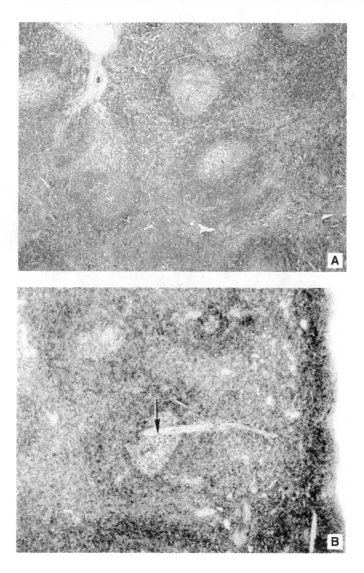

a. Absence of T cells
b. Proliferation of T cells
c. Proliferation of B cells
d. Absence of B cells
e. Absence of APCs

175. A 6-year-old boy is brought to the pediatrics clinic. His mother reports that after her son eats peanut butter he complains of a tingling feeling on the lips and in his mouth. After eating an ice-cream cone at a local dairy he developed an itchy rash with some swelling on his face. He also had some difficulty in swallowing and breathing. This was followed by complaints of "tummy pain" and cramping with diarrhea. During the patient's reaction, the cells in the accompanying micrograph, treated with fluorescein-labeled antihuman immunoglobulin, would most likely be developing in which organ and would be producing which of the following?

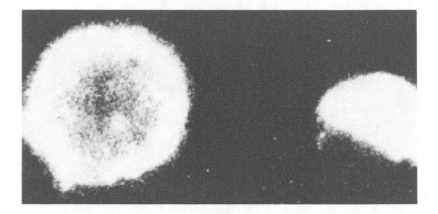

a. Deep cortex of the lymph node, IgE
b. Germinal center of the lymph node, IgE
c. Germinal centers in the lymph node, IgA
d. Skin-associated lymphoid tissue, IgG
e. Periarteriolar lymphoid sheath of the spleen, IgE

176. Which of the following is the primary site of heavy class (or isotype) switching from IgM to IgG?

a. Bone marrow
b. Peripheral blood
c. Germinal centers
d. Thymus
e. Splenic red pulp

177. A 32-year-old woman has a positive tuberculin skin test. Helper T cells assist in which one of the following ways?

a. Autocrine-mediated inhibition of proliferation of helper T cells
b. The down-regulation of IL-2 receptors on helper T cells
c. Secretion of interleukins that promote T cell proliferation
d. Secretion of IL-1
e. Inactivation of macrophages by release of γ-interferon

178. A 27-year-old school teacher "catches" the flu from her students. Which one of the following would occur during the influenza infection?

a. Phagocytosis of virus by CD4⁺ T cells
b. Presentation of antigen by CD4⁺ T cells
c. Killing of virus-infected cells by CD4⁺ T cells
d. Formation of memory T and B cells
e. Killing of virus-infected cells by neutrophils

179. The mechanism for lymphocyte circulation from the lymphoid compartment in the region marked with the asterisk to the blood involves which one of the following?

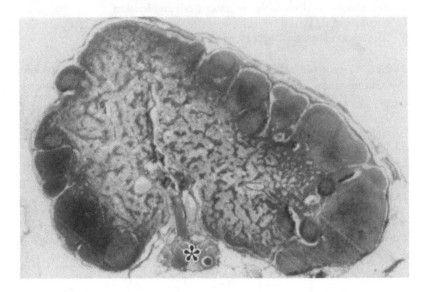

a. Homing receptors on lymphocytes that recognize vascular addressins on high-endothelial venule cells
b. Lymphocyte binding to endothelial integrins followed by passage through endothelial cells lining the high-endothelial postcapillary venules
c. Lymphocyte passage through the zonulae occludentes by diapedesis after dissolution of the junctions by proteolytic enzyme release
d. Lymphocyte passage from the efferent lymphatic vessel to the thoracic duct and subsequently the venous system
e. Passage of plasma cells through the discontinuous sinusoidal wall into the blood

180. Macrophages are directly involved in immune responses in which one of the following ways?

a. Production of IL-2
b. Presentation of antigen
c. Specific killing of tumor cells
d. Production of antibodies
e. Inactivation of helper T cells

181. A police officer in New York receives a vaccine for anthrax. The immunological basis for the vaccine is based on which one of the following facts?

a. The primary response has a longer lag period.
b. The secondary response has a shorter duration.
c. The primary response is primarily an IgM response.
d. The primary response lacks specificity.
e. The primary response generates memory B and T cells.

Lymphoid System and Cellular Immunology

Answers

166. The answer is a. (*Alberts, pp 1544-1545, 1574-1575. Kindt, pp 7, 16-18. Abbas, pp 6, 7f, 249. Parmely, pp 19-20, 21, 49.*) Clonal selection is the immune system's way of fine-tuning the immune response. Clonal selection is the means by which the immune system makes antigen receptor sites (T cells) or antibodies (B cells) more and more specific to create the optimal response to one specific antigen.

In clonal selection, a clone of lymphocytes is committed to respond to a particular antigen. The antigenic determinants, which consist of specific amino acids or monosaccharides, actually induce many clones and a wide variety of humoral and cell-mediated responses. This occurs during the development and maturation of the immune system and is responsible for the specificity of lymphocyte cell surface receptors for antigens. Immunoglobulin class switching **(answer b)** occurs during the maturation of B cells after antigen stimulation. Homing receptor differentiation **(answer e)** is an important part of naïve T- and B-cell maturation in the thymus and bone marrow, respectively. Regulatory T cells (T$_{reg}$) actively suppress activation of the immune system and inhibit pathological self-reactivity and autoimmune disease **(answer c)**. Clonal selection does not lead to formation of CFUs **(answer d)**.

167. The answer is a. (*Abbas, pp 189-190. Kindt, pp 426-434. Parmely, pp 26-28, 205, 206.*) Transplant (acute graft) rejection is mediated by the action of T cells. Helper T (T$_H$) cells recognize peptides associated with MHC antigens from the donor tissue and become activated. Activated T$_H$ cells release interleukin-2 (IL-2) and interferon-γ (IFN-γ), which activate cytotoxic T (T$_C$) cells, B cells, and macrophages. Although all of those cells may be involved in the rejection process **(answers b → e)**, T$_C$ cells are the primary agents of transplant rejection in an acute graft rejection response. This has been confirmed by animal studies; animals deficient in T cells are incapable of rejecting grafts. Tacrolimus (FK506) blocks signal transduction pathways leading to IL-2 production and therefore preventing T cell activation.

168. The answer is a. (*Abbas, p 202. Kindt, pp 434-435. Parmely, p 204.*) Because of the shortage of human organs for transplant, xenotransplantation is considered as the main potential solution for obtaining donor organs. Xenotransplantation induces hyperacute graft rejection since human preformed antibodies recognize [alpha]Gal(1–3)[beta]Gal terminal carbohydrates present on animal endothelial cells in the graft (**answers b → e**). Interestingly, Old World monkeys and humans do not express that xenoantigen on their endothelial cells.

169. The answer is d. (*Abbas, pp 84-86. Kindt, pp 40-41, 245-248. Alberts, pp 1560-1561, 1572-1573, 1581-1583.*) The organ in the photomicrograph is the thymus, which produces CD4$^+$ (helper) and CD8$^+$ (cytotoxic) T cells. It functions in the generation of self/nonself discrimination because self-reactive T cells are deleted and self-MHC-restricted cells are expanded during their education within the thymus. T-cell receptors (TCR) for antigen develop during the education of T cells in the thymus. Those T cells also develop homing receptors for subsequent seeding to T-dependent areas of lymph nodes, spleen, and other lymphoid tissues throughout the body. The thymus can be identified at low magnification (A) from the lobulation with cortex and medulla in each lobule and the absence of germinal centers. At high magnification (B), the presence of Hassall (thymic) corpuscles is an identifying characteristic. Hassall corpuscles contain degenerating epithelial cells in concentric arrays that increase with age and instruct thymic dendritic cells to induce development of regulatory T cells (T_{reg}). The thymus is derived from the third and fourth branchial pouches, not the third branchial arch (**answer c**). Production of memory B cells as well as effector and memory T cells occurs in the secondary lymphoid organs. Production of antibodies is the responsibility of plasma cells, which arise from B lymphocytes and are found in germinal centers in lymph nodes throughout the body as well as in the spleen and tonsils (**answer a**). The lymph nodes filter the lymph and blood (**answer b**). The spleen is the site of erythrocyte degradation and bilirubin recycling (**answer e**).

170. The answer is d. (*Alberts, pp 1570-1571, 1572-1574. Kindt, pp 223-225, 231-235, Abbas, pp 67-70, 74-76. Parmely, pp 64-65.*) T-cell gene rearrangement occurs during the education of T cells in the thymus in fetal and early neonatal development (**answers a → c and e**). The TCR is composed of α and β chains. Each chain contains a variable amino-terminal portion and a constant carboxyl-terminal portion. These chains are encoded for by V, D, J, and C gene segments, which undergo rearrangement during development in the thymus. There are three types of T cells: cytotoxic T cells, T regulatory (T$_r$) cells, and helper T cells. Helper T cells possess the specific cell membrane marker CD4, whereas the regulatory and cytotoxic subgroups have CD8 on their cell surface. T cells require close contact with other cells to perform their cell-mediated function. This is quite different from B cells, where antibodies are secreted into the bloodstream. B-cell gene rearrangement occurs in the bone marrow during B-cell education by a similar process. It must be remembered that TCRs are antibody-like heterodimers. Gene rearrangement in B- and T-cell education involves similar V(D)J recombinations.

171. The answer is a. (*Abbas, pp 10f, 11, 139-141. Alberts, pp 1573-1574. Mescher, pp 232-236. Parmely, pp 84-87.*) Fragments of antigen associated with class II MHC glycoproteins are recognized by helper T cells (**answers b → e**). Activation of helper T cells is required as an early step in the immune response. For B and T$_c$ cells to respond to most antigens, helper T cells are required. However, in the case of some bacterial polysaccharides, B cells respond to the antigens in the absence of helper T cells. The primary cell type for expression of class II MHC is the macrophage or dendritic cell (APCs), but thymic epithelial cells and B cells can also present antigen under appropriate conditions.

172. The answer is c. (*Abbas, p 63f. Alberts, pp 1579-1583. Parmely, pp 72-74.*) Cytotoxic T cells possess the CD8 cell surface marker. CD8$^+$ T cells recognize foreign antigen in association with class I MHC molecules (**answers a, b, d, and e**). Cytotoxic T cells are effective in killing virus-infected cells that express fragments of viral proteins combined with MHC I molecules on their surfaces. In contrast, helper T cells (CD4$^+$) recognize antigen in association with class II MHC molecules. MHC class I is present on the surface of most cells, whereas APCs (including B lymphocytes) and thymic epithelial cells possess MHC class II.

173. The answer is c. (*Abbas, pp 102f, 103, 103f. Kindt, pp 68, 307-312. Mescher, pp 229-236. Parmely, pp 71-72.*) Interleukin-2 (IL-2) is produced by helper T cells (cell surface marker CD4). IL-2 is a cytokine that affects the proliferation and differentiation of other cells (**answers a, b, and d)**

including the proliferation of T and B cells. APCs synthesize interleukin (IL)-1 with helper T cells as the primary target. Helper T cells are greatly diminished during the immunodeficiency that follows AIDS infection. Natural killer (NK) cells comprise about 10% to 15% of circulating lymphocytes. They produce products that kill tumor cells **(answer e)**.

Interleukin-1 (IL-1) plays a critical role in inflammation and in the immune response mediating pathogenetic events. IL-1 is mainly secreted by monocytes and macrophages and binds to T cells that have been activated by exposure to antigenic or mitogenic stimuli. Binding of IL-1 induces activated T cells to produce IL-2. There are two forms of IL-1: keratinocytes secrete IL-1α and monocytes/macrophages secrete IL-1β. IL-1 binds to receptors on activated T cells to induce production and release of IL-2. IL-1 has a wide variety of other effects including induction of chemokine expression (eg, monocyte chemoattractant protein-1), up-regulation of vascular adhesion molecules (eg, selectins) by capillary endothelium, and up-regulation of matrix metalloproteases that degrade the extracellular matrix and degrade IL-1. IL-1 is also required for IFN-γ production. See the figure below that illustrates the role of IL-1 and IL-2 in communication between immune cells.

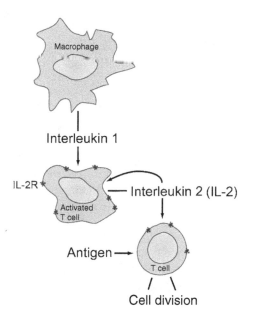

174. The answer is a. (*Young, pp 229, 233. Mescher, pp 245-248. Kindt, pp 29-30, 494-498. Abbas, pp 224-227. Parmely, pp 42, 118, 146, 182.*) The boy in the scenario suffers from severe combined immunodeficiency (SCID) and has no T cells (**answers b → e**). The CD3 antibody recognizes a group of five proteins that are associated with the α and β chains of the TCR. Recognition of antigen-MHC by the TCR-CD3 complex does not require any other molecules. Other "accessory molecules" on T cells (T_H or T_c) and their partner ligands on APCs or target cells provide a "second signal" to stimulate T cells. The region shown is a T-dependent region of the spleen. The photomicrograph shows an area of white pulp with a central artery. The sheath surrounding the central artery is known as the periarterial lymphoid sheath (PALS) and is analogous to the deep cortex (paracortex) of the lymph node or the interfollicular zone of Peyer patches, the other T-dependent regions within lymphoid tissue.

The histologic structure of the spleen includes the presence of a connective tissue capsule with extensions into the parenchyma, forming trabeculae. The parenchyma consists of red pulp, which represents areas of red blood cells, many of which are undergoing degradation and phagocytosis by macrophages lining the sinusoids of the red pulp, and white pulp, which represents lymphocytes involved in the filtration of the blood. The germinal centers within the white pulp are the B-dependent regions of the spleen.

(The case of Martin Causubon is provided courtesy of the Jeffrey Modell Foundation and "The Primary Immunodeficiency Resource Center:" http://www.info4pi.org/patienttopatient/index.cfm?section=patienttopatient&c)

175. The answer is b. (*Abbas, pp 206-209, 133-136. Kindt, pp 372-375. Fauci, pp 2042, 2061-2063. Mescher, pp 90-93. Alberts, pp 1556-1557. Parmely, pp 149-150, 159.*) The patient in the scenario suffers from peanut allergy. Allergic reactions involve IgE produced by plasma cells (shown in the fluorescein-labeled micrograph) in the germinal centers of the lymph nodes or spleen (**answers c and d**). Allergens, like peanut antigen, are originally recognized by TCRs on T_H2 cells. The T_H2 cell produces IL-4 which stimulates B cells to differentiate into plasma cells (like those in the photomicrograph), which synthesize and secrete IgE. IgE binds specifically to the high affinity receptor, Fc epsilon RI, on mast cells and basophils. The presence of IgE primes the mast cell; it is then capable of an allergic response by secreting histamine and heparin when the child is again exposed to the allergen (peanut antigen). Histamine alters vascular permeability leading to edema and in severe cases to anaphylaxis. Differentiation of IgE-plasma cells is regulated by the low affinity IgE receptor, Fc epsilon RII, also known as CD23. Immunoglobulin-producing cells are found in the germinal centers of the white pulp of the spleen and other secondary lymphoid organs (ie, germinal centers in the cortex of the spleen and in the tonsils and lymphoid follicles in the MALT and SALT). B lymphocytes can be identified by the presence of immunoglobulin on their surface membranes and differentiate into antibody-secreting plasma cells under the appropriate conditions. T lymphocytes, on the other hand, do not have readily detectable cell membrane immunoglobulin. The thymus is the site of T-cell education and the deep cortex of the lymph node and the PALS are T-dependent regions (answers a and e).

176. The answer is c. *(Alberts, pp 1562-1568. Kindt, pp 128-130. Abbas, pp 72-73. Parmely, pp 34, 47-48.)* Heavy chain class (or isotype) switching, formerly called immunoglobulin switching, normally occurs in the germinal centers during the maturation of B cells. Synthesis of B-cell antibody begins as IgM inserted into the cell membrane and then switches to membrane-bound IgM and IgD. After antigen stimulation, a switch to surface IgM, IgA, IgG, or IgE occurs, and those antibodies are secreted. Most antibody production occurs in the germinal centers of the lymph nodes, tonsils, and spleen. It occurs to a lesser extent in the bone marrow (answer a), but the bone marrow functions in the education of B cells as well as representing the major site of hematopoiesis in the adult. The thymus is responsible for the education of T cells (answer d). The splenic red pulp is the site of red blood cell breakdown (answer e).

Recognition of antigen by B cells is accomplished by the expression of IgM molecules on the cell surface. Some investigators use the term pre-B cell, or virgin B cell, to distinguish those B cells that have not yet synthesized IgM from those that have synthesized and inserted IgM into their cell membranes. IgD, which is produced later by maturing B cells, also serves as an antigen receptor. Immunoglobulin switching does not occur in peripheral blood (answer b).

177. The answer is c. *(Alberts, pp 1574-1575, 1583-1585. Kindt, p 393. Mescher, pp 229-236, Abbas 119, 287-288.)* In a tuberculin skin test, T-cell proliferation is increased by secretion of interleukins (answer a). An extract of tuberculin (an antigen of lipoprotein composition obtained from the tubercle bacillus) is injected into the skin of a person who has had tuberculosis or has been immunized against tuberculosis. Memory helper T cells react to the tuberculin and secrete IL-2, which up-regulates IL-2 receptors **(answer b)**. IL-2 binding to IL-2 receptors on the same cell is an example of autocrine regulation in which a cell secretes a ligand that binds to a receptor on its own surface. The result of this up-regulation and ligand-receptor binding is an increase in T-cell proliferation. T cell–derived cytokines such as tumor necrosis factor-alpha and -beta (TNF-α and β) induce leukocyte recruitment. Production of gamma-(γ) interferon (γ-IFN) by helper T cells attracts and activates macrophages—monocytes comprise most of the cellular infiltrate. γ-IFN also converts other cells (such as endothelial cells) to APCs by induction of class II MHC expression, which further augments the response. The result of the activity of helper T cells is a dramatic increase in the number of lymphocytes and macrophages at the test site, which produces swelling. IL-1 is synthesized by APCs and macrophages with helper T cells as the targets **(answers d and e)**.

178. The answer is d. *(Abbas, pp 58-62, 90f, 148. Kindt, pp 448-454. Parmely, pp 166-167.)* There are some viruses in which antibody-mediated immunity is critical to prevention/recovery, whereas with others cell-mediated immunity is the key. Therefore, both memory T and memory B cells will be formed. B cells will divide to form a plasma cell and a memory B cell. Activated T cells enlarge to form large lymphocytes and subsequently undergo cell proliferation to form T cells and memory T cells. In those responses, macrophages phagocytose virus **(answer a)**. Cells that become infected with virus can be killed by CD8+ cytotoxic T cells **(answers c and e)**, which can react to the antigen in the presence of MHC class I molecules. T and B cell areas of the spleen and lymph nodes will be involved in the filtration of blood and lymph, respectively. B cell differentiation requires the presence of CD4+ helper T cells and an APC. The APC will phagocytose the virus and present it to helper T cells in the presence of MHC class II molecules **(answer b)**. The B cell also presents antigen during viral infections.

179. The answer is d. *(Mescher, p 243. Ross, pp 410, 412. Abbas, p 254.)* Passage of lymphocytes from the lymphoid compartment of the lymph node to the bloodstream involves passage from the efferent lymphatic vessel to the thoracic duct and eventually into the venous system (at the juncture of the left brachiocephalic and subclavian veins). The region of the lymph node marked with the asterisk in the photomicrograph is the hilus of the lymph node. Passage from the blood to the lymphoid compartment involves specific homing receptors on lymphocytes, which are complementary to addressins on the postcapillary high endothelial venules (HEVs) and explains the specificity of lymphocyte homing **(answer a)**. The cells that line the HEVs permit the selective passage of lymphocytes by diapedesis through the intercellular junctions **(answer c)**. Lymphocytes have specific homing receptors on their cell surfaces that provide entry for mucosal (versus lymph node) seeding. HEVs provide a mechanism for lymphocytes to leave the bloodstream and enter specific areas of the lymph nodes. HEVs are also found in Peyer patches and during inflammation of tissues (eg, the synovium in rheumatoid arthritis). Under normal conditions, HEVs are found in the T-dependent areas, that is, the deep cortex (paracortex) of the lymph nodes and the interfollicular regions of the Peyer patches. T cells are home to T-dependent areas of the lymph nodes, spleen, and Peyer patches. The circulation and recirculation of lymphocytes is a constant process that allows lymphocytes to continuously monitor the presence of antigen. The circulation process also allows augmentation of the immune response to infection. Plasma cells do not enter the bloodstream under normal conditions, but secrete antibodies into the circulation from the medulla of the lymph nodes or the marginal zone of the spleen **(answer e)**. Lymphocytes and other cells (eg, monocytes and neutrophils) that leave the blood never pass through the endothelial cells **(answer b)**.

In the histologic section of a lymph node, there is a distinctive cortex and medulla with a connective tissue capsule. The organ possesses the classic bean shape with a hilus (marked by an asterisk in the figure). Afferent lymphatics enter the lymph node on the convex side, and lymph percolates through the subcapsular, cortical, and medullary sinuses. The medullary sinuses converge on the hilus, where the efferent lymphatic vessel drains the node. The hilus also contains an artery and a vein.

180. The answer is b. *(Alberts, pp 1452, 1594-1595, Mescher, pp 87, 89, 234, 235. Kindt, pp 65-68, 263-264. Abbas, p 13. Parmely, pp 4t, 22, 84-87, 130.)* Macrophages are a group of monocyte-derived phagocytic cells that present antigen and synthesize IL-1 **(answer a)**. Macrophages arise from the bone marrow (monocytes) and include the Kupffer cells of the liver, Langerhans cells of the skin, and microglia of the central nervous system. Antigen presentation is the process by which macrophages, dendritic cells, and B cells phagocytose antigen and partially degrade the antigen in the endosomal system. Certain portions of the antigen are returned to the cell surface in combination with type II MHC as a complex. IL-1 activates the helper T cell (answer e). Although macrophages may be required for the differentiation of plasma cells from B cells, they are not directly involved in antibody production (answer d). Also note, B cells can present antigen in addition to the more traditional APCs. Natural killer cells and cytotoxic T cells carry out tumor specific killing of tumor cells (answer c).

181. The answer is e. (*Kindt, pp 289-290, 481-484. Alberts, p 1546. Abbas, pp 169f, 169-170. Parmely, pp 170-171.*) The goal of all vaccines is to promote a primary immune reaction so that when the organism is again exposed to the antigen, a much stronger secondary immune response will be elicited. Any subsequent immune response to an antigen is called a secondary response. A secondary immune response is more rapid, of longer duration, and more intense than the primary immune response (answers a, b, and d). The secondary response is more specific to the invading antigen because of the generation of memory cells produced during the primary response. The design of an immunizing vaccine hinges on the specificity and cross-reactivity of antigen and receptor. Vaccines are more effective and long-lived when live attenuated virus is used to develop the vaccine. Vaccines developed to inactivated virus are not as effective. Live attenuated virus undergoes limited replication in the host cells resulting in a strong, site-specific response to the antigen. Anthrax vaccine is made to inactivated virus and requires boosters at yearly intervals. The primary immune response involves primarily IgM while the secondary response predominantly involves IgG antibodies (answer c). Humoral immunity and cell-mediated immunity involve retention of immunologic memory through memory B and T cells, respectively. A secondary immune response may involve memory T cells, helper cells, macrophages, and memory B cells. The proliferation of either T or B cells during the first exposure to antigen results in the production of memory cells. Specificity is retained. For example, the introduction of a different (new) antigen induces a primary rather than a secondary response. However, exposure to an antigen again will produce a secondary immune response.

Respiratory System

Questions

182. A 52-year-old man, who has smoked two packs of cigarettes per day for the past 38 years, presents with diminished breath sounds detected by auscultation accompanied by faint high-pitched rhonchi at the end of each expiration and a hyperresonant percussion note. He is afebrile. In addition, he shows discomfort during breathing and is using extra effort to involve accessory muscles to lift the sternum. The diminished lung sounds in this patient are primarily due to which cellular events?

a. Monocytic infiltration leading to collagenase destruction of bronchiolar connective tissue support
b. Neutrophilic infiltration leading to destruction of bronchiolar and septal elastic fibers
c. Monocytic infiltration leading to breakdown of the bronchiolar smooth muscle
d. Neutrophilic infiltration leading to excess production of antiprotease activity in the lung parenchyma
e. Monocytic infiltration leading to excess production of antiprotease activity in the lung parenchyma

183. A 43-year-old man who has smoked a pack of cigarettes a day for two decades presents with cough, sputum production, and wheezing. Symptoms were initially intermittent and diagnosed as asthma. He now complains of dyspnea that first occurred only with strenuous exertion, but now occurs even with mild activities. Tachypnea, scalene and intercostal muscle retraction, and tripod position are noted on physical examination. Liver enzymes are elevated and a liver biopsy shows fibrosis and cirrhosis. Which one of the following is the portion of the respiratory system that is the initial target of the disease in this patient?

a. Respiratory bronchiole
b. Alveolar duct and alveolus
c. Terminal bronchiole
d. Bronchiole
e. Segmental bronchi
f. Intrapulmonary bronchi

184. A 72-year-old man presents to the emergency department after experiencing 4 days of extreme shortness of breath. He has been unable to sleep "normally" lying down in his bed. He had a myocardial infarction at the age of 63 and bypass surgery was performed at that time. He reports that his breathlessness began with strenuous exercise and now even occurs during short walks. He has a nonproductive cough and ankle swelling (3 + pitting edema). His blood pressure is 160/90, his pulse is 130 and irregular, and his respiration is 32 and labored. On chest examination, scattered bilateral rhonchi are detected along with crackles and wheezes and pleural effusion. He has elevated neck veins and abdominojugular reflux. A very strong S3 sound is detected. If bronchioalveolar lavage were completed on this patient, which one of the following cells would one expect to find that is characteristic of this patient's disease?

a. Type I pneumocytes containing hemosiderin granules
b. Type II pneumocytes containing surfactant
c. Macrophages containing hemosiderin granules
d. Erythrocytes
e. Fibroblasts containing type I procollagen
f. Neutrophils containing hemosiderin granules

185. A 4-month-old infant is brought to the emergency department by his parents because he has been suffering from a chronic cough and diarrhea for about a week. They report that their son "wheezes" more than normal for a child with a cold. In the emergency department the physician notes an ear infection and salt crystals are present on the boy's skin. Chest auscultation reveals the presence of rhonchi in the right upper lobe of the lung. He has a positive sweat test and is diagnosed with cystic fibrosis (CF). Genetic analysis detects the ΔF508 mutation. Which one of the following mechanisms explains why the boy in this vignette has increased levels of chloride in his sweat, but does not secrete chloride properly in the pancreas, lungs, and salivary glands?

a. Cystic fibrosis transmembrane conductance regulator (CFTR) is only abnormally inserted into the membrane of cells lining the airways.
b. CFTR is only abnormally inserted into the cell membrane in the sweat ducts.
c. CFTR regulates the epithelial Na^+ channel (ENaC) only in the cells lining the airways and gastrointestinal (GI) glands.
d. The cells of the sweat duct fail to resorb NaCl while in the airway there is decreased Cl^- secretion and increased water and Na^+ resorption.
e. The CFTR is located on the basal surface of the cells lining the airways and GI glands and on the apical surface in the sweat ducts.

186. After 35 weeks of gestation, a 5 lb 5 oz female infant is born to a 30-year-old gravida 2, para 2 (G2P2) woman. The infant has rapid and labored breathing that is viewed as transient tachypnea of the newborn. The infant's 1- and 5-min APGAR scores are 8 and 9, respectively. She has respiratory distress, with a normal pulse and no heart murmurs. She is transported to the neonatal intensive care unit with worsening tachypnea. In this infant, the cell labeled with the arrows fails to do which one of the following?

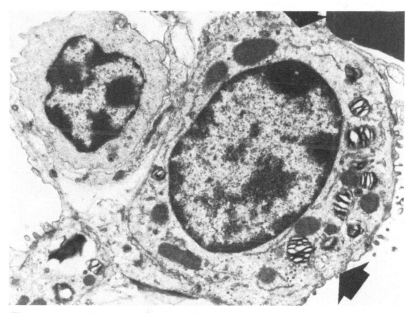

(Electron micrograph courtesy of Dr. Kuen-Shan Hung.)

a. Form during gestation
b. Proliferate sufficiently during gestation
c. Differentiate sufficiently during gestation
d. Produce sufficient amniotic fluid
e. Form its basal lamina resulting in an incomplete blood-air barrier

187. A teenage girl presents in the emergency room with paroxysms of dyspnea, cough, and wheezing. Her parents indicate that she has had these "attacks" during the past winter, and that they have worsened and become more frequent during the spring allergy season. Which of the following cell types and their location is correctly matched to a function it may perform in this patient's disease?

a. Cilia in alveoli, enhanced mucociliary transport
b. Plasma cells in bronchus-associated lymphoid tissue (BALT), bronchoconstriction
c. Eosinophils in BALT, bronchodilation
d. Goblet cells in bronchioles, hyposecretion
e. Mast cells in BALT, edema

188. A 62-year-old man presents with tremor, rigidity, bradykinesia, gait disturbance, and anosmia. Decreased function in the region highlighted by the arrow occurs early in this patient's disease. Signal transduction in the epithelium of that region differs from that in rod cells stimulated by light in which of the following ways?

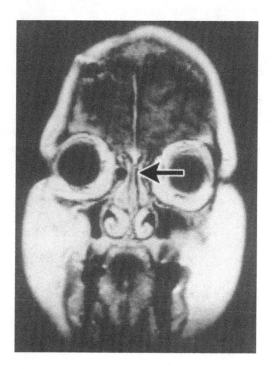

a. Sodium influx into receptor cells
b. Involvement of specific G proteins
c. Stimulation of a cyclic nucleotide
d. Stimulation leading to depolarization
e. Bypass of the protein kinase system

189. A 28-year-old man is diagnosed with a testicular germ cell tumor. The tumor is surgically removed and he begins chemotherapy with cisplatin, etoposide, and bleomycin. Bleomycin chemotherapy is known to affect the alveolar-capillary wall. Which one of the following best describes the structural site of those effects?

a. Fused basal laminae of epithelial and endothelial cells
b. Alveolar pores of Kohn
c. Alveolar macrophages in the alveoli
d. Type II pneumocytes linked by junctional complexes
e. Smooth muscle cells of the pulmonary arteries and veins

190. A 62-year-old woman presents with fever, cough, and malaise that have lasted for 6 days. She had a kidney transplant 5 years ago, and is receiving prednisone, cyclosporine, and azathioprine for posttransplant immunosuppression. Her chest x-ray shows multiple nodular opacities. Major defense mechanisms of the respiratory system suppressed in this patient include which one of the following?

a. Phagocytic activity of type II pneumocytes to ingest microorganisms
b. Cell specific killing by type I pneumocytes
c. Alveolar mucociliary action for clearance of microorganisms
d. IgA activation of complement in the alveolar fluid
e. IgM and IgG activation of complement in the alveolar fluid

191. A 56-year-old man presents to his family medicine physician. He is a 41 year pack/day smoker. He reports that he has had a "typical smoker's cough" for years; however, the morning cough has turned into a chronic productive cough with hemoptysis. He has dyspnea, chest pain, cachexia, and increasing dysphonia. He has been treated for 4 respiratory infections in the past 18 months. Examination of the sputum reveals the presence of malignant cells confirmed by fine needle aspiration. Imaging reveals a tumor that is 3 cm in greatest dimension, surrounded by lung parenchyma. Bronchoscopic evaluation reveals a cavitary lesion of a proximal bronchus. Surgical resection is completed and the pathologist classifies the tumor as a T1, N2, M0 non–small-cell lung cancer, specifically a squamous cell carcinoma. Tumor vascularity assessed by bronchial arteriography and immunocytochemistry indicates a highly vascular tumor with many microvessels. Vascularity of the tumor is inhibited by up-regulation of which of the following?

a. Vascular endothelial growth factor (VEGF)
b. Platelet-derived growth factor (PDGF)
c. Extracellular matrix synthesis
d. Endostatin
e. Periendothelial cell recruitment and proliferation

Respiratory System

Answers

182. The answer is b. (*Mescher, p 314. Kumar, pp 684-687. Fauci, pp 1639-1640.*) The patient is diagnosed with emphysema, in which neutrophils enter the lung parenchyma and secrete elevated levels of elastase, leading to the destruction of the bronchiolar and alveolar septal elastic tissue support **(answers a, c, d, and e)**. The destruction of the elasticity in emphysema leads to diminished breath sounds. This is coupled with faint high-pitched rhonchi at the end of expiration and a hyperresonant percussion note. The rhonchi are adventitious (not normally present) sounds that may be high pitched, generally because of bronchospasm, or low pitched, generally because of the presence of airway secretions. Emphysema is a disease characterized by parenchymal tissue destruction and, therefore, is not associated with adventitious breath sounds. However, because most emphysema is due to cigarette smoking, there is almost always some degree of chronic bronchitis, and therefore, rhonchi can be auscultated.

There are genetic and environmental causes of emphysema. The environmental causes include smoking and air pollution, whereas deficiency in α_1-antitrypsin (antiprotease) activity is the genetic cause of the disease. The balance between normal elastase-elastin production and protease-antiprotease activity is altered in emphysema. Persons with a deficiency in α_1-antitrypsin activity lack sufficient antiprotease activity to counteract neutrophil-derived elastase. When there is an increase in the entry and activation of neutrophils in the alveolar space, more elastase is released, and elastic structures are destroyed. In smoking, there is an increase in the number of neutrophils and macrophages in alveoli and increased elastase activity from neutrophils and macrophages. Those changes are coupled with a decrease in anti-elastase activity because of oxidants in cigarette smoke and antioxidants released from the increased numbers of neutrophils. The increased protease activity causes breakdown of the alveolar walls and dissolution of elastin in the bronchiolar walls. The loss of tethering of the bronchioles to the lung parenchyma leads to their collapse. The bronchioles, unlike the trachea and bronchi, do not contain hyaline cartilage. A relatively thick layer of smooth muscle is found in the bronchioles, but the bronchioles are tethered to the lung parenchyma by elastic tissue, which plays a key role in the stretch and recoil of the lungs during inhalation and exhalation.

183. The answer is b. *(Fauci, pp 1636-1638. Kumar, pp 717-720. Ross, pp 623-625.)* The patient in the vignette has α_1-antitrypsin deficiency which initially targets the alveolar duct and alveolus causing distension of the peripheral structures. Later in the disease process there is extension to the respiratory bronchiole. This form of emphysema is known as panacinar (panlobular); "pan" refers to damage to the entire acinus. In contrast, centriacinar emphysema targets the respiratory bronchiole **(answer a)**. Emphysema disturbs the balance between protease and anti-protease activity in the lung. The absence of protease activity in α_1-antitrypsin deficiency leaves neutrophil elastase capable of digesting the lung parenchyma. The terminal bronchiole **(answer c)**, bronchiole **(answer d)**, and bronchi **(answers e and f)** are not the targets of either form of emphysema. Smoking aggravates panacinar emphysema causing a decade of acceleration of the onset of major symptoms.

184. The answer is c. *(Kumar, p 535. Mescher, p 313.)* The alveolar macrophage containing hemosiderin granules has been called the "congestive heart failure cell." The presence of large numbers of those cells, containing hemosiderin granules, is an indicator of edematous lung changes. During congestive heart failure, edema results in micro-hemorrhages and leakage of erythrocytes into the alveoli. Transferrin and hemoglobin are also present in the edematous fluid released from the capillaries. These two products are phagocytosed by alveolar macrophages, which convert those products to hemosiderin.

185. The answer is d. *(Kumar, pp 465-468. Fauci, pp 1632-1633.)* In CF patients, the sweat glands produce a normal secretion, but the duct cells with defective CFTR cannot resorb the NaCl. In the airway, CF patients have decreased Cl⁻ secretion and increased Na⁺ and water resorption leading to dehydration of the mucus layer coating epithelial cells, defective mucociliary action, and mucus plugging of the airways. CFTR lacks an exit code and is degraded in the endoplasmic reticulum of both airways, GI gland duct cells, and sweat duct cells **(answers a and b)**.

CFTR regulates multiple ion channels including the ENaC found on the apical surface of sweat duct, airway, and exocrine duct cells **(answers c and e)**. The ENaC is inhibited by normal functioning CFTR. In the airways of CF patients, ENaC activity increases markedly augmenting sodium transport across the apical surface. The opposite occurs in the sweat ducts where ENaC activity decreases as a result of CFTR mutations; therefore, a luminal fluid containing high sodium chloride is formed.

186. The answer is c. *(Mescher, pp 308, 311. 312 313. Kumar, pp 678, 680-682. Moore and Persaud, p 207.)* Differentiation of type II pneumocytes (shown in the electron micrograph) occurs late in gestation and is, therefore, incomplete at birth in premature infants **(answers a, b, d, and e)**. Those newborn "premies" have a deficiency of surfactant because of the immaturity of the type II pneumocytes. The deficiency of surfactant inhibits normal expansion of the alveoli and results in idiopathic respiratory distress syndrome ([RDS]; hyaline membrane disease). The lecithin/sphingomyelin ratio is a test that can be performed on a sample of amniotic fluid obtained by amniocentesis. It is used to determine whether the type II pneumocytes are mature and are synthesizing and secreting surfactant. Maternally administered glucocorticoids may be used to induce surfactant production prior to birth, and exogenous surfactant may be given intratracheally to premature infants to reduce the severity of RDS.

The surfactant is produced by type II pneumocytes in the lung and is stored in the form of lamellar bodies (the whorls seen in the electron micrograph). Surfactant consists of an aqueous layer, or hypophase, that contains proteins and mucopolysaccharides. That layer is covered by a functional layer of phospholipid that consists predominantly of dipalmitoyl phosphatidylcholine (lecithin). The release of lamellar bodies by exocytosis is followed by their general unraveling to form tubulomyelin figures. The tubulomyelin consists of a crisscross lipid bilayer that covers the type II pneumocytes. Surfactant-associated proteins (SAP) stabilize surfactant, activate surfactant recycling, enhance surfactant-induced reduction of surface tension, and possess antiviral and antibacterial activities. Turnover occurs by both endocytosis (type I and II pneumocytes) and phagocytosis (macrophages); 90% of surfactant is recycled.

The blood-air barrier is formed by the type I pneumocyte, the capillary endothelial cell, and their fused basal laminae.

G2P2 refers to two pregnancies and two children.

187. The answer is e. *(Kumar, pp 688-691. Fauci, pp 1596, 1601-1602. Mescher, p 305.)* The teenage patient is suffering from an asthmatic attack, probably allergen-induced. Mast cells are a key player in this airway disease. Mast cells in the bronchioles are stimulated to release histamine and heparin that induce the contraction of smooth bronchiolar muscle (bronchoconstriction, [answers b and c]) and edema in the wall. If the bronchoconstriction is chronic, the long-term result is thickening of the bronchiolar musculature. There are no cilia in the alveoli (answer a). Alveolar macrophages (dust cells) ingest particulate matter that enters the alveoli. Hypersecretion of viscous mucus from goblet cells in the bronchi (not bronchioles) can obstruct the airway (answer d). Eosinophils, neutrophils, lymphocytes, and macrophages signal to each other through a complex cytokine network using a variety of mediators: bradykinin, leukotrienes, and prostaglandins, which enhance bronchoconstriction, vascular congestion, and edema. The airway epithelium responds to those mediators. Eosinophils (answer c) release proteins that destroy the airway epithelium (releasing Creola bodies—rounded balls of sloughed off ciliated columnar epithelial cells). T lymphocytes are also present in more severe "attacks" and, along with B lymphocytes, may play a role in the initiation of allergic asthma. T lymphocytes also release cytokines that activate cell-mediated immunity pathways.

188. The answer is d. (*Alberts, pp 866-867, 1268. Mescher, 300-302.*) The region shown on the MRI is the olfactory area lined by the olfactory epithelium. Decreased olfactory function is among the first signs of idiopathic Parkinson disease. The response of rod cells to light causes hyperpolarization, whereas olfactory stimuli result in depolarization (answers a → c, e). The olfactory epithelium and rod cells are two examples of signal transduction that bypass a protein kinase system. In the case of the olfactory epithelium, an odorant molecule binds to an odor-specific transmembrane receptor found on the modified cilia at the apical surface. The binding activates an odorant-specific G protein, G_{olf}, which binds GTP. (For summary of G proteins, see High-Yield Facts, Table 6.) The resulting dissociation of the α-subunit stimulates adenylate cyclase to produce cyclic AMP (cAMP). cAMP directly stimulates the opening of the cation channels on the membrane of the bipolar olfactory receptor cells, leading to Na^+ influx. The resulting membrane depolarization is transmitted from the modified cilia to the olfactory vesicle through the neuron to the basal axon. Axonal processes traverse the lamina propria as the olfactory nerve and pass through the cribriform plate of the ethmoid to terminate in the olfactory bulb. In the case of the rod, the cyclic nucleotide involved is cGMP.

189. The answer is a. (*Mescher, pp 310, 312.*) Oxygen moving from the alveolar air to the capillary blood and carbon dioxide diffusing in the opposite direction pass through a three-component blood-air barrier. This barrier consists of type I pneumocytes, endothelial cells, and their fused basal laminae. Pulmonary capillaries are sometimes in direct contact with the alveolar wall, whereas in other locations, the alveolar wall and capillaries are separated by cells and extracellular fibers. The areas of direct contact are the location of gas exchange, whereas the other areas represent sites of fluid exchange between the interstitium and air spaces. Macrophages are present for the phagocytosis of debris and surfactant **(answer c)**. The pores of Kohn are connections from one alveolus to another **(answer b)**, and macrophages travel through these passageways. The pores normally equalize air pressure between alveoli and can, in the disease state, provide collateral circulation of air in the event that a bronchiole is blocked. However, they also provide a passageway for the spread of bacteria. Type II pneumocytes **(answer d)** and smooth muscle cells **(answer e)** are not part of the minimal-blood-air barrier.

190. The answer is e. (*Kumar, pp 63-64, 678-679.*) IgM and IgG are serum antibodies present in the alveolar fluid that activate complement by the classic pathway. In that pathway, fixation of C1 to antibody combined with antigen leads to activation of C3b, which binds to bacterial cell walls and enhances opsonization. Neutrophils and macrophages have C3b receptors that facilitate the opsonization. IgG also functions as an opsonin. The type II pneumocytes resorb as well as secrete surfactant and surfactant-associated proteins that have some antiviral and antibacterial function, but they do not ingest microorganisms **(answer a)**. CD8+ T cells carry out cell-specific killing **(answer b)**. Mucociliary action is a critical component of the immune function of the respiratory system, but clearance occurs in the bronchioles → bronchi → trachea as part of the mucociliary apparatus. Microorganisms are entrapped in mucus and then cilia propel them toward the oropharynx. Microorganisms phagocytosed in the alveoli need to be transported to the bronchioles in order to ride on the mucociliary escalator **(answer c)**. IgA functions to prevent attachment of microorganisms to the epithelium, particularly in the upper respiratory tract **(answer d)**.

Overall defense mechanisms of the respiratory system include nasal clearance of material, which occurs through sneezing, whereas other material may be swept into the nasopharynx and subsequently swallowed. The mucociliary action within the trachea and bronchi is often called the mucociliary, or tracheobronchial, escalator. At the distal end of the system, the alveolar macrophages phagocytose foreign material and secrete and respond to an array of cytokines. Neutrophils are attracted by chemokines and factors derived from macrophages and other cells and phagocytose bacteria.

In the bronchi, there is extensive associated lymphoid tissue (BALT), which is analogous to the mucosa-associated lymphoid tissue (MALT) of the gut (GALT) and the skin-associated lymphoid tissue (SALT). There are B- and T-cell areas throughout the BALT. The B cells are precursors of plasma cells and synthesize immunoglobulins such as IgA associated with the bronchial secretion. Helper T cells recognize foreign antigen in association with class II major histocompatibility complex (MHC) molecules. Cytotoxic T cells recognize fragments of antigen (specifically viral fragments) on the surface of viral-infected cells in association with class I MHC. Antigen-presenting cells (ie, alveolar macrophages) also function in a similar fashion to those found elsewhere in the body; they present antigen to helper T cells in conjunction with class II MHC.

191. The answer is d. (*Kumar, p 99-102. Lobov, pp 11205-11210*). Angiostatin and endostatin are cleavage products of plasminogen and type XVIII collagen, respectively and function as anti-angiogenic peptides. VEGF **(answer a)** stimulates the recruitment and growth of endothelial cells through the VEGF-R located on endothelial cell precursors as well as endothelial cells. PDGF recruits smooth muscle cells **(answer b)** and transforming growth factor-beta (TGF-β) stimulates and stabilizes extracellular matrix production. Recruitment and proliferation of periendothelial cells **(answer e)**, smooth muscle cells, pericytes, and fibroblasts are required for development and maturation of new blood vessels. The angiopoietins (Ang) 1 and 2 bind their receptor, Tie2, a receptor tyrosine kinase which regulates endothelial cell proliferative status. Ang 1 binds Tie2 leading to periendothelial cell recruitment and therefore vascular maturation.

Ang 2 is found in organs of the female reproductive tract and blocks Ang 1 effects when VEGF is absent. The result is regression of the blood vessel. Ang 2 in the presence of VEGF leads to loosening of the surrounding cells permitting multiplication of endothelial cells and angiogenesis.

Integumentary System

192. A 43-year-old woman presents with a cyst on her labia majora with foul-smelling drainage. She says the drainage occurs spontaneously and recently the cyst has enlarged and become painful. The cyst is associated with the structure in the photomicrograph delineated by the arrow. Which one of the following is the mechanism of secretion normally used by this structure?

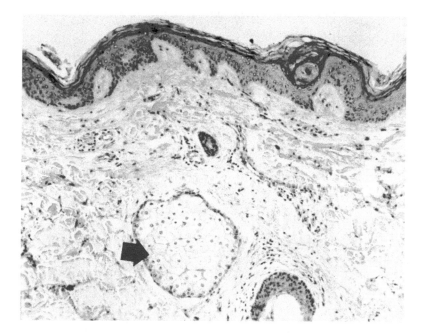

   a. Holocrine
   b. Merocrine
   c. Apocrine
   d. Endocrine
   e. Autocrine

193. A 64-year-old woman, who has always been proud of her suntanned, healthy look, is referred to a dermatologist with a firm, blue-violet, painless, 1.5 cm lump within the skin. The lump is fixed, cannot be moved, and has grown very rapidly over the past few weeks. The mass is removed; the diagnosis is a Merkel cell carcinoma. Merkel cells are modified epidermal cells that function primarily in which of the following?

a. Phagocytosis
b. Expression of Fc, Ia, and C3 receptors
c. Detection of texture and shape during active touch
d. Detection of transient vibratory stimuli
e. Two-point discrimination

194. The layer at the tip of the pointer is which one of the following?

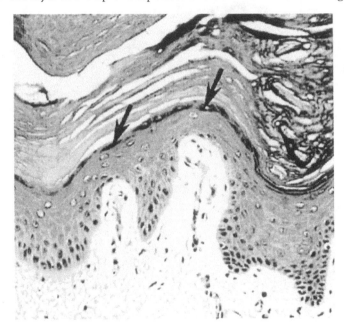

a. Proliferative zone of the vaginal epithelium
b. Proliferative zone of the epidermis
c. Source of the granules that form part of the water impermeability barrier of the skin
d. Layer of the epidermis that shows prominent desmosomes and is the target of autoantibodies in pemphigus
e. Source of new cells following a dermal wound

195. A 37-year-old woman presents with a suspected Schwannoma. The radiology report reads as follows: "a soft tissue mass to the right of L1 at the level of the L1 to L2 neural foramen. The mass cannot be differentiated from the L1 nerve root and extends into the neural foramen such that it has a 'dumbbell' configuration with components lateral to the neural foramen, a waist in the foramen itself, and a component within the spinal canal to the right of the thecal sac." The neurologist applies the base of a vibrating 128 cps tuning fork to the skin overlying the patient's right and left thighs and asks her to describe the sensation. She asks the patient to close her eyes and then to tell her whether the tuning fork is vibrating or not. Vibration sense is impaired on the right side. Tests for pain and temperature indicate impairment on the left side. Using the tuning fork, the neurologist is primarily testing the function of which of the following sensory receptors?

a. Ruffini endings
b. Pacinian corpuscle
c. Meissner corpuscle
d. Merkel corpuscle
e. Free nerve endings

196. A woman presents with blisters on her back and buttocks (Figure A). She has autoantibodies to one of the cadherins that is distributed as shown in Figure B. The cause of this disease is disruption of which one of the following?

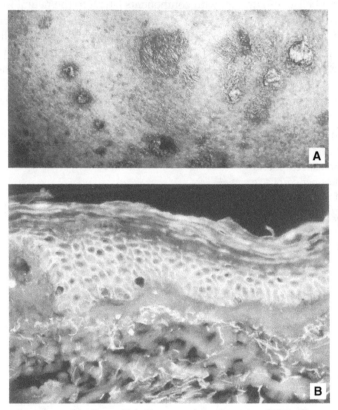

(Micrograph courtesy of Dr. Kristin M. Leiferman and the University of Utah, Department of Dermatology site:http://uuhsc.utah.edu/derm/.)

a. Macula adherens
b. Hemidesmosome
c. Gap junction
d. Zonula occludens
e. Connections between the lamina densa and lamina rarae in the basal lamina

197. A first-year medical student presents with patches of raised red skin covered by a flaky white buildup on her knees and elbows. The patches enlarge and become itchy with a burning sensation immediately before and during major exams in the first year of medical school. A biopsy from her skin is shown below. Which one of the following is the underlying cause of this disorder?

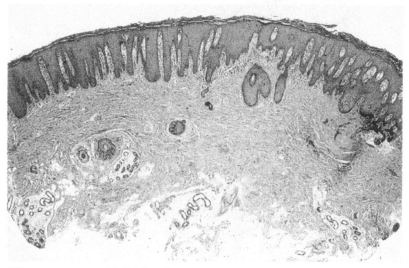

(Micrograph courtesy of Dr. Wolfram Sterry.)

a. A longer keratinocyte cell cycle
b. Autoantibodies to desmoglein 1
c. Autoantibodies to the bullous pemphigoid antigens (BPAG)
d. Mutations in keratins 5 and 14
e. Mutations in laminin subunits
f. Production of cytokines by infiltrating inflammatory cells

198. A 52-year-old woman presents with severe blistering over her buttocks. Analysis of sera with immunofluorescence demonstrates autoantibodies localized as shown in the accompanying photomicrograph. A biopsy indicates extensive inflammatory infiltrates with numerous eosinophils present. The underlying cell biological mechanism most likely involves an abnormality in which one of the following structures?

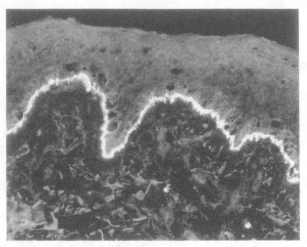

(Micrograph courtesy of Dr. Kristin M. Leiferman and the University of Utah, Department of Dermatology site: http://uuhsc.utah.edu/derm/.)

a. Macula adherens
b. Hemidesmosomes
c. Gap junctions
d. Zonula occludens
e. Zonula adherens

199. A boy is born with blonde hair, blue eyes, and a very fair complexion; dramatically lighter features than both of his parents. A phenylketonuria (PKU) test is positive. The boy's lighter skin and hair is most likely due to which one of the following?

a. Fewer melanocytes differentiating from the neural crest
b. Reduced proliferation of melanocytes in the basal layer of the epidermis
c. Elevated levels of tyrosinase in melanocytes
d. Deficiency in tyrosine in keratinocytes throughout the epidermis
e. Competitive inhibition of phenylalanine for tyrosinase in melanocytes

Integumentary System

Answers

192. The answer is a. (*Young, pp 175, 178. Mescher, pp 78-79, 316-319, 329.*) The cyst in the vignette is an epidermoid or sebaceous cyst and the gland shown in the photomicrograph is a sebaceous gland, located in the dermis and associated with a hair follicle. Secretion from sebaceous glands is classified as holocrine (ie, shedding of the disintegrated cell along with sebum into the hair follicle). Blockage of sebaceous gland ducts, presumably from injury, infection or irritation, results in cyst formation. Sebaceous cysts are prone to infection and can have foul-smelling drainage with inflammation and pain. The lesion usually consists of an enlarged sebaceous gland with numerous lobules grouped around a centrally located sebaceous duct, which has become obstructed causing the cyst. The photomicrograph represents a microscopic section obtained from thin skin. The presence of sebaceous glands/hair follicles identifies the section as thin skin. Sebaceous glands and hair follicles are not found in thick skin. Another difference between thick and thin skin is the virtual absence of the stratum lucidum in thin skin. There are two types of sweat glands: merocrine and apocrine. The merocrine glands release their secretion through exocytosis with conservation of membrane (**answer b**). In anal, areolar, and axillary regions, sweat glands are apocrine (**answer c**); the apical part of the cell is released with the secretion. Endocrine secretion occurs into the blood (**answer d**); autocrine secretion is self-stimulation (**answer e**). For example, activated T cells stimulate their own proliferation by secreting IL-2 and synthesizing IL-2 receptors that bind the IL-2.

193. The answer is e. (*Mescher, pp 232, 233, 316, 320-321, 323-324.*) The Merkel cell is a neuroendocrine cell. It is a modified keratinocyte found in areas in which fine tactile sensation is critical, such as the fingertips. A Merkel cell is associated with an unmyelinated nerve ending, forming a Merkel corpuscle (disk), essential for two-point discrimination: the ability to discriminate two closely placed points as separate. Two-point discrimination is dependent on the size of receptive fields and the density of Merkel corpuscles. Langerhans cells function in phagocytosis (**answer a**), antigen presentation (APCs), cytokine production, and expression of Fc, Ia, and C3 receptors (answer b). They phagocytose epidermal antigens and present them in association with class II MHC molecules to a helper T cell. Meissner corpuscles detect texture and shape during active touch and are found in the thick skin of the digits (answer c). Transient vibratory stimuli are detected by Pacinian corpuscles (answer d). Merkel cell carcinoma is a rare tumor that is rapidly increasing in incidence.

194. The answer is c. (*Mescher, pp 316-320. Kumar, pp 1256-1257.*) The cells labeled with the arrows contain numerous keratohyalin granules and are located in the stratum granulosum. These cells also produce lamellar granules, which form a bidirectional lipid bilayer barrier to penetration of substances. The skin or integument is composed of an epithelial layer (epidermis) and underlying connective tissue (dermis). The epidermis consists of four to five strata (from the basement membrane to the skin surface): stratum basale, stratum spinosum, stratum granulosum, stratum lucidum, and stratum corneum. The basal layer contains most of the mitotic cells **(answers a and b)** and is attached to the basement membrane with hemidesmosomes. The stratum spinosum contains cells, with numerous cytoplasmic tonofilaments and intercellular desmosomes **(answer d)**. The stratum basale + stratum spinosum = stratum Malpighii. Those layers are hyperproliferative in psoriasis. Normally, gradual replacement occurs in the epidermis; new cells are produced in the stratum basale, and migration toward the surface occurs as they gradually differentiate. The stratum lucidum is a translucent layer typical of thick skin. The stratum corneum contains as many as 20 layers of flattened cells.

In deep wounds, new epithelial cells are obtained from the epithelium of the hair follicles and sweat glands located in the dermis **(answer e)**.

195. The answer is b. (*Costanzo, pp 71, 74-76. Mescher, pp 316, 320-321, 323-325. Ross, pp 452-455, 472-473.*) The Pacinian corpuscle is the primary sensory receptor for vibratory sensation. The Ruffini endings are the simplest encapsulated receptor and are associated with collagen fibers **(answer a)**. Mechanical stress results in displacement of the collagen fibers and stimulation of the receptor. The Meissner and Merkel corpuscles respond to texture and two-point discrimination, respectively **(answers c and d)**. Free nerve endings detect light pressure and touch **(answer e)**. In the vignette, the Schwannoma (a nerve sheath tumor arising from Schwann cells) results in impairment of proprioception (position sense) and vibratory sense ipsilaterally while pain and temperature are impaired contralaterally. It is compressing the spinal cord from its lateral or anterolateral aspect causing impairment of pain and temperature sensation on the contralateral side to the Schwannoma, with weakness, spasticity, and loss of proprioception and vibratory sense on the ipsilateral side to the tumor. Damage to the antero-lateral system (ALS; spinothalamic tract) of the spinal cord causes impairment or loss of pain and temperature sensation *contralateral* to the lesion, and damage to the corticospinal tract in the spinal cord (lateral corticospinal tract; LCST) results in upper motor neuron syndrome *ipsilateral* to the lesion. This is classical Brown-Séquard syndrome.

196. The answer is a. (*Alberts, p 1144. Fauci, pp 303, 311-313. Kumar, pp 1192-1195.*) In pemphigus, autoantibodies to desmogleins (a member of the cadherin protein family) result in disruption of the macula adherens or desmosomes. The desmogleins are the transmembrane linker proteins of the desmosome. Specific desmogleins are the target of the autoantibodies in different forms of the disease. Cadherins are Ca^{2+}-dependent transmembrane-linker molecules essential for cell-cell contact, so their disturbance in pemphigus leads to severe blistering of the skin because of disrupted cell-cell interactions early in the differentiation of the keratinocyte (epidermal cell) and excessive fluid loss. Hemidesmosomes (**answer b**) contain different proteins than desmosomes and are not affected in pemphigus. Therefore, the basal layer of the epidermis remains attached to the basal lamina in pemphigus. In contrast, in bullous pemphigoid (BP), antigens develop that are specific for the hemidesmosomes. In that disease the entire epithelium separates from the basal lamina. For more details on junctional complexes (**answers c, d, and e**), see Table 8 in the High-Yield Facts section and the answer for Question 198.

197. The answer is f. (*Kierszenbaum, pp 15, 35-36. Fauci, pp 309-313, 328, 2469. Kumar, pp 1190-1196, 1198.*) Psoriasis is a chronic disease that affects both the epidermis and dermis of the skin. There is hyperplasia of the epidermis and abnormal microcirculation in the dermis as venules predominate in the capillaries resulting in increased extravasation of inflammatory cells. Thus, the underlying cause is the infiltration of inflammatory cells into the dermis with further migration of neutrophils into the epidermis. Those inflammatory cells release cytokines that induce an inflammatory response. There is hyperplasia of the epidermis as keratinocytes traverse the cell cycle in a shorter period of time (**answer a**). Autoantibodies to desmoglein 1 (**answer b**) are the cause of pemphigus foliaceus and autoantibodies to the BPAG are the cause of bullous pemphigoid (answer c). Mutations in keratins 5 and 14 result in epidermolysis bullosa a group of inherited bullous disorders characterized by blister formation in response to mechanical trauma (answer d). Mutations in laminin 5 subunits cause junctional epidermolysis bullosa (answer e).

198. The answer is b. (Kierszenbaum, pp 35-36, 338. Fauci, pp 335, 338. Kumar, pp 1195-1196.) The patient is suffering from bullous pemphigoid in which BP antigens are produced to proteins specific to the hemidesmosomes. The immunofluorescence image shows specific labeling of the epidermal-dermal interface. Therefore, the entire epidermis separates from the basal lamina in contrast to pemphigus in which the desmosomes disaggregate due to antibodies to the desmogleins causing a disruption of the macula adherens (desmosomes [answer a]) in the stratum spinosum. The gap junction (answer c) is a communicating junction; the zonula occludens (answer d) prevents material from flowing between cells; and the zonula adherens (answer e) is a belt-like component of the junctional complex that links to the actin cytoskeleton. Below is a helpful "memory grid" to remind you of the components of the junctional complexes and their attachments to the cell. You can move down or across, but not diagonally.

MEMORY GRID*			
	Cadherins	**Integrins**	
Actin	Adhesion Belts	Focal Adhesions	No Plaque
Intermediate Filaments	Desmosomes	Hemidesmosomes	Plaque
	Cell to Cell	Cell to Matrix	

*No fair going diagonally!
(Table courtesy of Dr Ronal R. MacGregor.)

199. The answer is e. (Kumar, pp 463-464. Fauci, pp 2470-2471.) In patients with PKU, there is a diffuse pigmentary dilution due to elevated levels of L-phenylalanine resulting from a deficiency in the enzyme L-phenylalanine hydroxylase that converts L-phenylalanine to L-tyrosine. The high levels of phenylalanine provide competitive inhibition for tyrosinase (answers c and d). The characteristic blonde hair of PKU can undergo darkening when the patient is on a low-phenylalanine diet. The number of melanocytes that differentiate from the neural crest would be normal (answer a). Melanocytes do not proliferate (answer b).

Gastrointestinal Tract and Glands

Questions

200. A 50-year-old woman presents to the family medicine clinic. She admits to drinking a six-pack of beer each day with a little more intake on weekends. Laboratory tests show elevated alanine aminotransferase/serum glutamic pyruvic transaminase (ALT/SGPT) and aspartate aminotransferase/serum glutamic oxaloacetic transaminase (AST/SGOT). Her sclerae appear jaundiced and her serum bilirubin is 2.5 mg/dL (normal 0.3-1.9 mg/dL). A biopsy of her liver shows eosinophilic intracytoplasmic inclusions (Mallory bodies) derived from intermediate filament proteins. What is the most likely source of Mallory bodies?

a. Hepatic stellate cells
b. Kupffer cells
c. Vimentin
d. Keratin
e. Desmin

201. The resting parietal cell does not secrete acid for which one of the following reasons?

a. The Na⁺, K⁺-ATPase is inserted into the apical membrane.
b. The chloride channel of the apical plasma membrane is closed.
c. The H⁺, K⁺-ATPase is sequestered in tubulovesicles.
d. Carbonic anhydrase is not produced.
e. Histamine receptors are uncoupled from their second messengers.

202. A 52-year-old man is diagnosed with a carcinoid after an appendectomy. The cell of origin in the carcinoid differs from goblet cells in which of the following ways?

a. The direction of release of secretion
b. The use of exocytosis for release of secretory product from the cell
c. Their presence in the small and large intestine
d. Their origin from a crypt stem cell
e. Secretion by a regulated pathway

203. In regard to the enteroendocrine cells and the cells composing the enteric nervous system of the gut, which of the following applies to both types of cells?

a. They are derived from neural crest
b. They secrete similar peptides
c. They are essential for the intrinsic rhythmicity of the gut
d. They are turned over rapidly
e. They are found only in the small intestine

204. A 17-year-old with counterfeit identification has a piercing done at a local tattoo/piercing establishment. She chooses to have a stainless steel barbell inserted in the piercing through the anterior two-thirds of her tongue. There is damage to the structures shown in the associated photomicrograph. Primary afferents from those structures travel through which of the following cranial nerves?

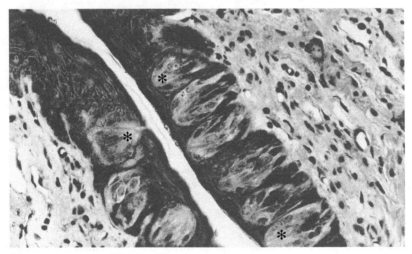

(Micrograph courtesy of Dr. John K. Young.)

a. V
b. VII
c. IX
d. X
e. XII

205. Hirschsprung disease and Chagas disease result in disturbance of intestinal motility. The site of this disruption is most likely which of the layers on the accompanying micrograph?

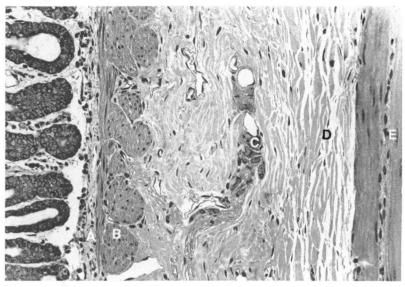

(Micrograph courtesy of Dr. John K. Young.)

a. Layer A
b. Layer B
c. Layer C
d. Layer D
e. Layer E

206. A 48-year-old woman presents to the allergy and rheumatology clinic with itching eyes, dryness of the mouth, difficulty swallowing, loss of sense of taste, hoarseness, fatigue, and swollen parotid glands. She reports increasing joint pain over the past 2 years. She complains of frequent mouth sores. Laboratory tests show a positive antinuclear antibody (ANA) and rheumatoid factor (RF) levels of 70 U/mL (normal levels less than 60 U/mL) by the nephelometric method. A parotid gland biopsy shows inflammatory infiltrates in the interlobular connective tissue with damage to acinar cells and striated ducts. In this case, resorption of which of the following will be most altered by destruction of the striated ducts?

a. Na^+
b. K^+
c. HCO_3^-
d. Cl^-
e. Ca^{2+}

207. Which of the following is the primary regulator of salivary secretion?

a. Antidiuretic hormone
b. Autonomic nervous system
c. Aldosterone
d. Cholecystokinin
e. Secretin

208. A young child presents with hepatomegaly and renomegaly, failure to thrive, stunted growth, and hypoglycemia. A deficiency in glucose 6-phosphatase is identified and the diagnosis of von Gierke disease is made. In the liver, the structures labeled with the arrows in the accompanying transmission electron micrograph accumulate during this disease. What are the labeled structures?

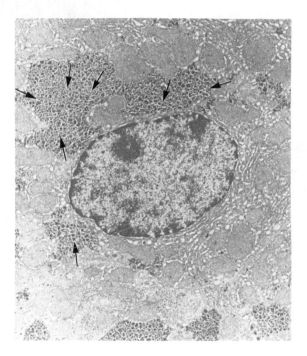

a. Chylomicra
b. Glycogen
c. Mitochondria
d. Peptide-containing secretory granules
e. Ribosomes

209. The branching structures highlighted by the arrows in the scanning electron micrograph below (taken from the region between two adjacent hepatocytes) are involved in which of the following?

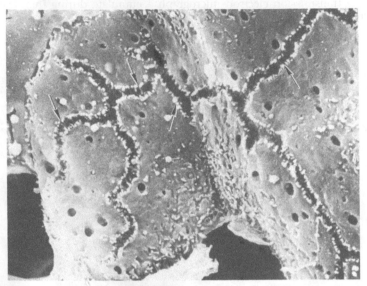

(Electron micrograph courtesy of Dr. Kuen-Shan Hung and Karen Grantham, KUMC Electron Microscopy Center.)

a. Communication between the hepatocytes
b. Preventing flow between adjacent hepatocytes
c. Bile flow
d. Blood flow
e. Spot welds between hepatocytes

210. In the photomicrograph of a plastic-embedded, thin section shown below, which of the following is the structure labeled A?

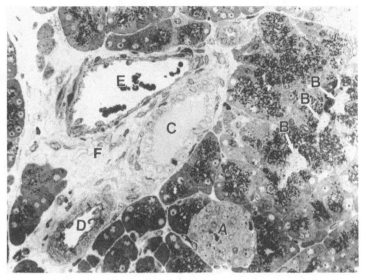

(Micrograph courtesy of Eileen Roach.)

a. A parasympathetic ganglion
b. A cluster of hepatocytes
c. A serous acinus
d. An intralobular duct
e. An islet of Langerhans

211. A pathologist views the following tissues (A and B) in a biopsy. She determines that the tissues are normal. The presence of both of these tissues indicates that the sample was taken from the region of the junction between which of the following?

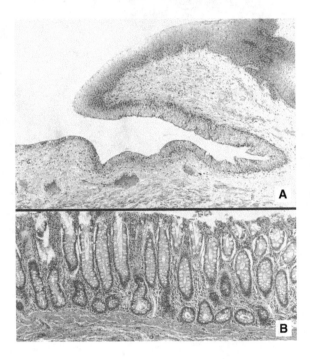

a. Anal canal and rectum
b. Esophagus and stomach
c. Skin of the face and mucous epithelium of the lip
d. Stomach and duodenum
e. Vagina and cervix

212. A 52-year-old woman with a provisional diagnosis of celiac disease presents with bouts of diarrhea and extreme fatigue. Verification was sought through performance of esophagogastroduodenoscopy to obtain small bowel biopsies. Biopsies of the region shown in the accompanying light micrograph disclose hyperplasia of the structures labeled with the asterisks. The labeled structures produce which of the following?

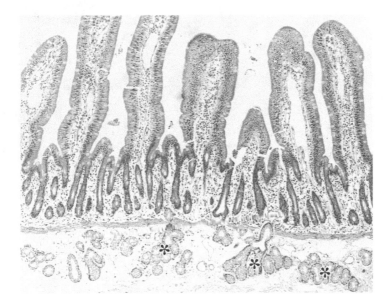

a. Acid
b. Mucus and HCO_3^-
c. Pepsinogen
d. Lysozyme
e. Enterokinase

213. Inflammation in the organ shown in the photomicrograph may result in referred pain to which of the following areas?

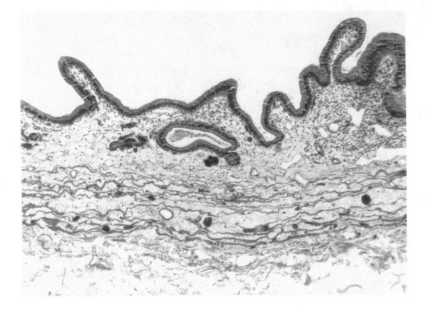

a. Top of the right shoulder
b. Neck
c. Spine between the scapulae
d. Groin
e. Umbilical region

214. The asterisk-labeled cells in the center of the transmission electron micrograph below function in which one of the following processes?

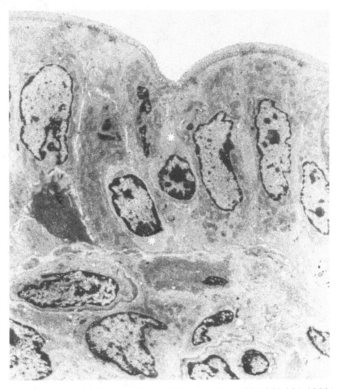

(Reproduced with permission, from McKenzie, Klein, Am. J. Anat. 164: 175-186, 1982.)

a. Immune defense mechanisms
b. Mucus secretion
c. Heparin and histamine secretion and release
d. Endocrine secretion
e. Regulation of the flora of the small bowel
f. Absorption of nutrients from the lumen of the small bowel

215. In hemolytic jaundice, the structure labeled with the arrow in the accompanying photomicrograph will contain which one of the following?

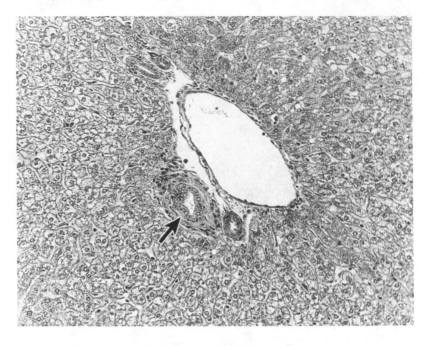

a. Elevated urobilinogen levels
b. Elevated bilirubin levels
c. Decreased urobilinogen levels
d. Decreased bilirubin levels
e. Elevated numbers of lymphocytes undergoing diapedesis

216. A 4-day-old newborn weighing 7 lb 6 oz is brought to the emergency room by his parents. The examining emergency room physician notes that his skin and sclerae are icteric. A blood test indicates elevated unconjugated bilirubin in the serum. The elevated bilirubin levels in this patient are most likely the result of which one of the following?

a. Deficiency of enzymes regulating bilirubin solubility
b. Hepatocellular proliferation
c. Decreased destruction of red blood cells
d. Dilation of the common bile duct
e. Increased hepatocyte uptake of bilirubin

217. A 42-year-old woman (5 ft 3 in, 170 lb) complains of sudden onset of severe pain in the right upper abdomen "under the ribs" accompanied by sweating, nausea, and a feeling of imminent collapse. The pain lasts for about 2 hours and then persists as a dull ache. When seen several hours later, she has normal bowel sounds, is tender throughout the abdomen, especially in the right upper quadrant, and is faintly icteric. She has noticed her urine is darker than usual but has not passed stool recently. She recalls occasional episodes of "indigestion" referred to the right upper abdomen and radiating to the shoulder. This has occurred especially after eating fried foods or after eating a meal following a long period of fasting. She has no fever but is anxious and tachycardic. The test results available are a blood count and blood chemistry including liver enzymes, alkaline phosphatase, and bilirubin. She has a WBC of 10,000. Her cellular hepatic enzymes are: AST/SGOT = 52 (normal 3-33) and ALT/SGPT = 70 (normal 4-44), alkaline phosphatase = 300 (normal 17-91), bilirubin = 6.3 (normal 0.2-1.0). Which one of the following is the most probable diagnosis?

a. Hepatitis A
b. Hepatitis B
c. Carcinoma of the head of the pancreas
d. Gallstone obstructing common bile duct
e. Biliary cirrhosis

218. A 14-month-old girl is brought to the pediatric dentistry clinic because her erupted deciduous teeth are opalescent with fractures and chips in the surface. X-rays reveal bulb-shaped crowns and thin roots. Structure D on the diagram is abnormally large in her teeth. The structure labeled "B" on the diagram is prepared for histology and shows disoriented, irregular, widely-spaced tubules with wide vascular channels. Which one of the following applies to the layer labeled "B"?

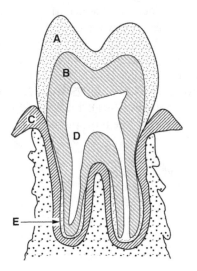

a. It has a composition similar to that of bone and is produced by cells similar in appearance to osteocytes.
b. It is formed on a noncollagenous matrix that is resorbed on mineralization by the same cells that secreted it.
c. It contains abundant nerves, blood vessels, and loose connective tissue.
d. It consists of mineralized collagen secreted by cells derived from neural crest.
e. It is the site of inflammation in diabetic patients and is sensitive to deficiency in vitamin C.

219. A 39-year-old woman presents with dyspnea, fatigue, pallor, tachycardia, anosmia, and diarrhea. Laboratory results are: hematocrit 32% (normal 36.1%-44.3%), MCV 102 fL ([normal 78-98 fL]), 0.3 % reticulocytes (normal 0.5%-2.0%), 95 pg/mL vitamin B_{12} (normal 200-900 pg/mL), and an abnormal stage I of the Schilling test. Autoantibodies are detected to a cell type that is found in a region shown in the accompanying diagram. In which region would those cells be found?

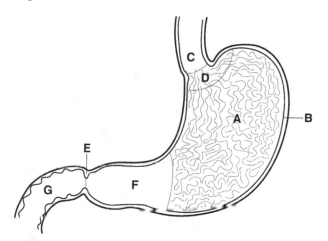

a. A
b. B
c. C
d. D
e. E
f. F
g. G

220. A 43-year-old man who recently returned from a trip to rural Peru presents with severe watery diarrhea, vomiting, and dehydration. He also has marked leg cramps and has lost 8 lb since his return from the trip. Fecal culture is positive for *Vibrio cholerae*. How does this bacterium exert its effect?

a. Activation of enterokinase on the brush border of epithelial cells
b. Activation of cholecystokinin effects on pancreatic secretion
c. Closure of chloride channels in the enterocyte cell membrane
d. Inhibition of cyclic AMP in the enterocytes
e. ADP-ribosylation of G_s of the GTP-binding protein in enterocytes

221. A 35-year-old man visits his family medicine physician complaining of bloating, a sense of urgency, cramping abdominal pain, meteorism, and diarrhea with excessive flatulence several hours after ingestion of milk or dairy products. He says that he has always enjoyed milk and dairy products without any problems, but now eating them causes him abdominal distress. In this disorder, the area shown by the arrows would most likely have a decrease in which one of the following?

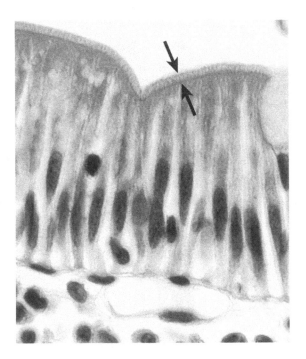

a. Specific disaccharidase activity
b. Glucose/galactose transporter activity
c. Passive diffusion of monosaccharides
d. Uptake of triglycerides by endocytosis
e. Active transport of glycerol

Gastrointestinal Tract and Glands

Answers

200. The answer is d. (*Ross, p 63. Kumar, pp 858.*) Mallory bodies are derived from keratin intermediate filaments within hepatocytes. Hepatic stellate cells (**answer a**) secrete the collagen that replaces normal liver parenchyma in cirrhosis. Kupffer cells (**answer b**) are the macrophages of the liver. Vimentin (**answer c**) is the intermediate filament protein found in cells of mesenchymal origin; the liver and hepatocytes are epithelial in origin. Desmin (**answer e**) is the intermediate filament protein associated with muscle. ALT/SGPT and AST/SGOT are hepatic aminotransferases; when their blood levels are elevated, it is indicative of liver damage.

201. The answer is c. (*Johnson, pp 1123-1124. Mescher, pp 264, 266-269. Ross, pp 528-530.*) In the resting parietal cell, the proton pump (H^+, K^+ ATPase) is found in the tubulovesicle membranes that are located intracellularly (**answer a**). The sequestration of the proton pump in intracellular tubulovesicles in the resting state prohibits secretion. On activation of the parietal cell through Ca^{2+} and diacylglycerol second messengers, the tubulovesicle membranes fuse with the plasma membrane by exocytosis. Histamine (**answer e**), along with gastrin and acetylcholine, activate the parietal cell. Na^+, K^+-ATPase located in the basal membrane, and the chloride channel (**answer b**) of the apical plasma membrane maintain the appropriate ionic gradients to facilitate acid secretion. Carbonic anhydrase, a cytoplasmic enzyme, catalyzes the formation of carbonic acid (H_2CO_3) from carbon dioxide, which is the source of protons in the parietal cell and other cell types, such as the osteoclast, that also depend on a proton pump (**answer d**). After dissipation of the stimulus (ie, gastrin, acetylcholine, or histamine) or exposure to an H_2 blocker, the parietal cell returns to the resting state by recycling (endocytosis) of membrane to reform the tubulovesicular arrangement within the cytoplasm.

202. The answer is a. (*Mescher, pp 83, 264-266, 268-269, 275. Kumar, pp 787-789, 828.*) Carcinoid tumors arise from enteroendocrine cells.

Enteroendocrine cells release peptides from their basal surface (domain) while goblet cells secrete mucus from their apical surface (domain). The goblet cells are unicellular mucus-secreting glands analogous to the enteroendocrine cells that are unicellular endocrine glands. Enteroendocrine cells secrete into the bloodstream (endocrine function) or into the local area to affect nearby cells (paracrine function). The enteroendocrine cells may be identified by their staining response to silver or chromium stains, hence the older terms argentaffin and enterochromaffin, respectively. Examination of such preparations indicates that the enteroendocrine cells are rare compared with other mucosal cell types, including the mucous cells. Enteroendocrine and goblet cells release granules by a regulated exocytotic secretion **(answer b)**. Both cells are formed by stem cells in crypt base of both the small and large intestinal glands ([of Lieberkühn] **answers c and d)**.

203. The answer is b. *(Kierszenbaum, pp 464, 468, 478. Mescher, pp 249, 268, 275. Ross, pp 521, 530, 534.)* The enteroendocrine cells and the enteric (intrinsic) nervous system secrete similar peptides and are found throughout the gastrointestinal tract **(answer e)**. Enteroendocrine cells are derived from the same stem cell as other epithelial cell types and originate embryonically from the endoderm. These cells turn over at a slower rate than other epithelial cell types. In contrast, the cells that compose the enteric nervous system are neurons, derived from neural crest **(answer a)**. There is little cell replacement except in the glial populations **(answer d)**. The enteric nervous system, particularly the myenteric (or Auerbach) plexus, is responsible for the intrinsic rhythmicity of the gut and peristalsis **(answer c)**. The enteroendocrine cells function in local paracrine regulation of the mucosa (eg, acid secretion in the stomach, mucosal growth, small intestinal secretion, and turnover).

204. The answer is b. *(Kierszenbaum, pp 430-431. Avery, pp 285-287. Moore, pp 938-941.)* Piercing of the tongue can result in complaints of pain, numbness, and loss of taste when eating. The loss of taste is associated with damage to the taste buds, which are shown in the photomicrograph. Taste buds in the anterior two-thirds of the tongue as described in the vignette in this question are innervated by the VII (facial) cranial nerve, specifically the chorda tympani. The V (trigeminal) cranial nerve **(answer a)** is responsible for transmitting general sensation from the anterior two-thirds of the tongue. The taste buds from the posterior one-third of the tongue are innervated by the IX (glossopharyngeal) cranial nerve (answer c). The X (vagus) cranial nerve (answer d) innervates taste buds on the epiglottis and palate. The XII (hypoglossal) cranial nerve innervates the intrinsic musculature of the tongue (answer e).

205. The answer is e. (*Sadler, pp 231, 323. Mescher, p 251.*) Hirschsprung disease (congenital megacolon) and Chagas disease have different etiologies, but both inhibit intestinal motility by affecting the myenteric (Auerbach) plexus located between the layers of the muscularis externa (layer E) in the figure. The submucosal (Meissner) plexus is more involved in regulation of lumenal size and, therefore, will affect defecation, but will be less involved in peristalsis. Vascular smooth muscle, the muscularis mucosa, and enteroendocrine cells do not play a major role in the regulation of peristalsis, which is observed even after removal of the gut and placement in a nutrient solution. Hirschsprung disease, also known as aganglionic megacolon, results from failure of normal migration of neural crest cells to the colon, resulting in an aganglionic segment. Although both the myenteric and submucosal plexuses are affected, the primary regulator of intrinsic gut rhythmicity is the myenteric plexus. Chagas disease is caused by the protozoan *Trypanosoma cruzi*. Severe infection results in extensive damage to the myenteric neurons.

The wall of the GI tract contains four layers: mucosa, submucosa, muscularis externa, and serosa. The structure labeled A in the photomicrograph is the lamina propria, a loose connective tissue layer immediately beneath the epithelium. The last part of the mucosa is a double layer of smooth muscle cells (layer B) comprising the muscularis mucosa. In the photomicrograph, an inner circular and outer longitudinal layer of smooth muscle cells is discernible. A thick layer of dense irregular connective tissue, the submucosa (layer D), separates the muscularis mucosa from the muscularis externa. The structure labeled C is a nest of parasympathetic postganglionic neurons forming part of Meissner plexus. The muscularis externa (layer E) generally consists of inner circular and outer longitudinal layers of smooth-muscle cells. Slight variations in these components occur in specific organs of the GI tract. The respiratory, urinary, integumentary, and reproductive systems differ from the gastrointestinal system in their epithelia and arrangement of underlying tissues.

206. The answer is a. (*Avery, pp 306-310. Costanzo, p 344.*) The woman in the scenario suffers from Sjögren syndrome, which like other autoimmune

diseases (presence of ANA and RF), is much more common in women than men. The striated ducts resorb Na^+ and secrete K^+ (**answer b**) from the isotonic saliva converting it to a hypotonic state. Na^+-independent chloride-bicarbonate anion exchangers appear to be involved in these processes by generating ion fluxes into the salivary secretion. The striated duct is the primary region for electrolyte transport in the salivary gland duct system. The primary secretion produced by the acinar cells is comprised of amylase, mucus, and ions in the same concentrations as those of the extracellular fluid. In the duct system, Na^+ is actively absorbed from the lumen of the ducts, Cl^- is passively absorbed (although the tight junctions between striated duct cells inhibit Cl^- from following Na^+ [**answer d**]). HCO_3^- is secreted (**answer c**); Ca^{2+} transport is not a factor (**answer e**). The result is a hypotonic sodium and chloride concentration and a hypertonic potassium concentration.

207. The answer is b. (*Costanzo, pp 342-344.*) The autonomic nervous system is the primary regulator of salivary gland function in contradistinction to the pancreas, which is regulated primarily by hormones (cholecystokinin and secretin [**answers d and e**]). Parasympathetic fibers carry neural signals that originate in the salivatory nuclei of the medulla and pons. The sympathetic nervous system originates from the superior cervical ganglion of the sympathetic chain and stimulates acinar enzyme production. Elevated aldosterone levels affect the amount and ionic concentration of the saliva, resulting in decreased NaCl secretion and increased K^+ concentration (**answer c**). Cholecystokinin (pancreozymin) and secretin are the hormones that regulate acinar and ductal secretions, respectively, in the exocrine pancreas. Antidiuretic hormone can modulate salivary gland production, but does not have a major role in regulation (**answer a**).

208. The answer is b. (*Young, p 24. Mescher, pp 3, 25-28, 46, 76, 110-111.*) The disease described in the scenario is type I (hepatorenal, von Gierke) glycogenosis (glycogen storage disease) caused by a defect in glucose-6-phosphatase, resulting in accumulation of glucose 6-phosphate and glycogen in the liver. The cytoplasmic inclusions labeled with the arrows in the transmission electron micrograph are glycogen. The hepatocyte, under the regulation of insulin and glucagon, stores glucose in its polymerized form of glycogen. In electron micrographs, glycogen appears as scattered dark particles with an approximate diameter of 15-25 nm. Lipid droplets appear as spherical, homogeneous structures of varying density and diameter, although their diameter is considerably larger than that of the glycogen granules. Ribosomes **(answer e)** are found on the rough endoplasmic reticulum or as free structures, in which case they are not found in clusters like glycogen. Mitochondria **(answer c)** contain distinctive cristae and are much larger (0.5-1.0 μm in diameter) than glycogen. Chylomicra **(answer a)** are located at the basal surface of the hepatocytes and are less dense than glycogen. Secretory granules **(answer d)** would also show polarity in their location.

209. The answer is c. *(Mescher, pp 291, 293.)* The bile canaliculi are labeled with arrows in the scanning electron micrograph. They comprise the space between the lateral surfaces of adjacent hepatocytes and transport bile (not blood [**answer d**]) toward the bile ducts. Microvilli line the bile canaliculi and are visible protruding into the lumen. The membranes between the cells are connected by tight (zonulae occludentes) and gap junctions **(answer a)**, neither of which are visible in the photomicrograph. The zonulae occludentes prevent material from passing between the hepatocytes **(answer b)**. Desmosomes, when present between cells, function as spot welds **(answer e)**.

210. The answer is e. *(Young, pp 342-343 Mescher, pp 285-286, 359-360, 364.)* The organ in the photomicrograph is the pancreas, and the cells labeled are the islets of Langerhans. The pancreas functions as both an exocrine (secretion of pancreatic juice) and endocrine (secretion of insulin and glucagon) gland. The islets **(A)** have a heterogeneous distribution within the pancreas (ie, they decrease from the tail to the head of the gland) and may be used to distinguish the pancreas from the parotid gland. The submandibular and sublingual glands can be ruled out because of the purely serous nature of the acini within the exocrine portion of the gland. The centroacinar cells **(B)** are modified intralobular duct cells, specifically from the intercalated duct, and are present in the lumen of each acinus. The duct **(C)** can be distinguished by the presence of a cuboidal epithelium, the absence of blood and blood cells from the lumen, and the absence of a characteristic vascular wall. A pancreatic artery **(D)** and a vein **(E)** are shown within the interlobular connective tissue **(F)**.

211. The answer is a. *(Mescher, pp 263, 270, 279-280, 405, 407-408.)* Photomicrographs A and B show two distinctly different types of epithelium: stratified squamous epithelium of the anus (top panel) and crypts (without villi) of the rectum (lower panel). The anus has anal valves and an absence of the muscularis mucosa. The esophageal-cardiac junction also represents a junction between stratified squamous and simple columnar epithelium, but the cardiac portion of the stomach forms the mucus-secreting cardiac glands with no goblet cells (**answer b**). The junction of the stomach (pylorus) and duodenum represents the juncture of two simple columnar epithelia, the pylorus containing the short (compared with fundus) pyloric glands and the duodenum with crypts and villi as well as the submucosal Brunner glands (**answer d**). Skin is keratinized (**answer c**). The cervical mucosa contains extensive cervical glands, and the vaginal epithelium is keratinized. In vagina and cervix, the GI tract pattern of alternating layers: epithelium, connective tissue (CT), muscle, CT, muscle, CT is not present (**answer e**).

212. The answer is b. (*Young, p 275. Mescher, pp 263, 269, 271, 276.*) The patient in the scenario is suffering from celiac disease, an allergic response to gliadin. The result is villous atrophy and crypt and Brunner gland (the structures labeled with the asterisks in the photomicrograph) hyperplasia. The presence of the mucus and bicarbonate (HCO_3^-) secreting Brunner glands in the submucosal layer of the small intestine are an identifying feature of the duodenum. The Brunner gland secretions function to neutralize the acidic pH of the stomach and establish the appropriate pH for function of the enzymes in the pancreatic juice. Parietal cells are unique to the stomach and synthesize acid (**answer a**) and intrinsic factor (required for vitamin B_{12} absorption from the small intestine). Chief cells in the fundic glands produce pepsinogen (**answer c**) that is activated by acid to form pepsin. Paneth cells in the base of the crypts make lysozyme (**answer d**) and modulate the flora of the small intestine. Enterokinase (**answer e**) is made by the duodenal mucosa and is instrumental in the conversion of pancreatic zymogens to their active form (eg, trypsinogen to trypsin).

213. The answer is a. (*Young, p 298. Mescher, p 297. Moore, pp 159, 257, 259-260, 287, 297, 373.*) The photomicrograph illustrates the structure of the gallbladder that stores and concentrates the bile. Gallbladder inflammation can lead to pain referred to the top of the right shoulder. Diaphragmatic pain may be felt in the neck (**answer b**), stomach pain may refer to the spine between the scapulae (**answer c**), kidney pain may be felt in the groin area (**answer d**), and intestinal dysfunction may be felt in the middle or low back. Umbilical pain is typically referred from the appendix (**answer e**).

Although the fingerlike extensions of the gallbladder resemble villi, they represent changes that occur in the mucosa with increasing age. The thinness of the wall is the notable characteristic of the gallbladder. Bile is synthesized by hepatocytes and transported from the liver to the gallbladder, where it is stored and concentrated.

214. The answer is a. (*Mescher, pp 90-93, 270, 272, 274, 275.*) The transmission electron micrograph is taken from the small intestinal epithelium. Intraepithelial lymphocytes (labeled with the asterisks) are lymphocytes that have crossed the basal lamina. The intraepithelial lymphocytes may respond to antigen in the lumen of the small bowel. In the Peyer's patches of the ileum lymphocytes in the lamina propria may respond to antigen that has been sampled from the lumen and transported by M cells in the Peyer patches. Enterocytes are the absorptive cells of the gut and possess numerous microvilli on their apical surfaces (**answer f**). Goblet cells synthesize and secrete mucins (**answer b**). Paneth cells and enteroendocrine cells contain granules, but secrete lysozyme (regulation of flora [**answer e**]) and endocrine peptides (**answer d**), respectively. Mast cells synthesize and secrete histamine and heparin (**answer c**).

215. The answer is b. (*Fauci, pp 261-263. 1927-1931. Costanzo, pp 356-358. Young, pp 288-295. Kumar, pp 839-843. Mescher, pp 289, 292.*) The structure labeled with the arrow is a bile duct and would contain elevated levels of bilirubin following hemolytic jaundice (**answers a and d**). Hemolytic jaundice is associated predominantly with unconjugated hyperbilirubinemia. The overproduction of bilirubin occurs because of accelerated intravascular erythrocyte destruction or resorption of a large hematoma. When hepatic uptake and excretion of urobilinogen are impaired or the production of bilirubin is greatly increased (eg, with hemolysis), daily urinary urobilinogen excretion may increase significantly. In contrast, cholestasis (arrested flow of bile due to obstruction of the bile ducts [intrahepatic]) or extrahepatic biliary obstruction interferes with the intestinal phase of bilirubin metabolism and leads to significantly decreased production and urinary excretion of urobilinogen (**answer c**). Diapedesis of lymphocytes across the endothelium of the postcapillary high endothelial venules of lymphoid organs (eg, lymph nodes) increases during inflammation (**answer e**).

Bile is formed by the hepatocytes and is released into bile canaliculi, which are located between the lateral surfaces of adjacent hepatocytes. The direction of flow is from the hepatocytes toward the bile duct, which drains bile from the liver on its path to the gallbladder, where the bile is stored and concentrated. The hepatic artery and hepatic portal vein (shown in the photomicrograph) plus the bile duct comprise the portal triad. Blood flows from the triad (hepatic artery, portal vein, and bile duct) toward the central vein, whereas bile flows in the opposite direction toward the triad.

Bile is synthesized by hepatocytes using the smooth endoplasmic reticulum (SER) and consists of bile acids and bilirubin. Bile acids are 90% recycled from the distal small and large intestinal lumen and 10% newly synthesized by conjugation of cholic acid, glycine, and taurine in the SER. Bilirubin is the breakdown product of hemoglobin derived from the action of Kupffer cells in hepatic sinusoids and other macrophages, particularly those lining the sinusoids of the spleen where degradation of RBCs is prominent.

216. The answer is a. (*Mescher, p 294. Fauci, pp 1928-1930. Kumar, pp 839-843.*) Commonly, initial low levels of glucuronyl transferase in the underdeveloped smooth endoplasmic reticulum of hepatocytes in the newborn, result in jaundice (neonatal unconjugated hyperbilirubinemia); less commonly, this enzyme is genetically lacking (**answers b → e**). The neonatal small intestinal epithelium also has an increased capacity for absorption of unconjugated bilirubin, which contributes to the elevated serum levels.

Bilirubin, a product of iron-free heme, is liberated during the destruction of old erythrocytes by the mononuclear macrophages of the spleen and, to a lesser extent, of the liver and bone marrow. The hepatic portal system brings splenic bilirubin to the liver, where it is made soluble for excretion by conjugation with glucuronic acid. Increased plasma levels of bilirubin (hyperbilirubinemia) result from increased bilirubin turnover, impaired uptake of bilirubin, or decreased conjugation of bilirubin. Increased bilirubin turnover occurs in Dubin-Johnson and Rotor syndromes, in which there is impairment of the transfer and excretion of bilirubin glucuronide into the bile canaliculi. In Gilbert syndrome, there is impaired uptake of bilirubin into the hepatocyte and a defect in glucuronyl transferase. In Crigler-Najjar syndrome, a defect in glucuronyl transferase occurs in the neonate.

The ability of mature hepatocytes to take up and conjugate bilirubin may be exceeded by abnormal increases in erythrocyte destruction (hemolytic jaundice) or by hepatocellular damage (functional jaundice), such as in hepatitis. Finally, obstruction of the duct system between the liver and duodenum (usually of the common bile duct in the adult and rarely from aplasia of the duct system in infants) results in a backup of bilirubin (obstructive jaundice, see Question and Answer 217).

217. The answer is d. *(Fauci, pp 1919-1920, 1999. Kumar, pp 882-886. Mescher, pp 294, 296.)* The pattern of elevated liver enzymes, alkaline phosphatase, and bilirubin are consistent with obstructive jaundice (see table below [answers a → c, e]). The presence of pain (in the right upper quadrant radiating to the shoulder) after eating a meal consisting of fried foods makes gallstones the most probable diagnosis. Similar pain often occurs in those patients when they have not eaten for long periods of time and then eat a large meal. The pain is caused by the obstruction of the cystic duct or common bile duct that produces increased lumenal pressure within the bile vessels, which cannot be compensated for by cholecystokinin-induced contractions. The pain usually lasts for one to four hours as a steady, aching feeling. A mnemonic device for gallstones is 4F (F, F, F, F): female, forty, fat, and fertile.

Enzyme	Obstructive	Parenchymal
Liver enzymes (AST and ALT)	↑	↑↑↑
Alkaline phosphatase	↑↑↑	↑
Bilirubin	↑↑↑	↑↑↑

218. The answer is d. *(Mescher, p 256. Kumar, p 740. Fauci, pp 2463-2464.)* The patient in the scenario suffers from type II dentinogenesis imperfecta, an autosomal dominant disorder caused by mutation in the *DSPP* gene. The result is defective dentin, discoloration of the translucent teeth (blue-gray or yellow-brown color). These teeth are weaker than normal, making them prone to rapid decay, wear, breakage, and loss. Type II dentinogenesis imperfecta occurs about 1 in 6000 to 8000 births. Type I occurs in conjunction with osteogenesis imperfecta with mutations in type I collagen; children with type I have typical blue sclerae with defects in bone and dentin.

The structure labeled **B** is dentin, which consists of mineralized collagen synthesized by odontoblasts. Odontoblasts are derived from the neural crest. The pulp of a mature tooth (labeled **D** in the diagram) consists primarily of loose connective tissue rich in vessels and nerves. Odontoblasts lie at the edge of the pulp cavity and secrete collagen and other molecules, which mineralize to become dentin **(B)**. Mineralization of the matrix occurs around the odontoblast processes and forms dentinal tubules. Ameloblasts, which are ectodermal derivatives, lay down an organic matrix and secrete enamel, initially onto the surface of the dentin. As hydroxyapatite crystals form at the apices of ameloblast (Tomes') processes, rods of enamel grow peripherally, and the ameloblasts resorb the organic matrix so that the enamel layer **(A)** is almost entirely mineral. It contains unique proteins such as the amelogenins and enamelins, but no collagen.

On eruption of the tooth, enamel deposition is complete and the ameloblasts are shed. Cementum **(E)** has a composition similar to that of bone, is produced by cells similar in appearance to osteocytes, and covers the dentin of the root. The periodontal ligament **(C)** consists of coarse collagenous fibers running between the alveolar bone and the cementum of the tooth and separates the tooth from the alveolar socket. Although the periodontal ligament suspends and supports each tooth, the ligament permits physiologic movement within the limits provided by the elasticity of the tissue. It is a site of inflammation in diabetic patients and is affected in scurvy (recall the image of the 18th century British sailor).

219. The answer is a. (*Young, pp 268-272. Mescher, p 264. Kumar, pp 655-658.*) The woman in the scenario suffers from pernicious anemia resulting from autoantibodies to the parietal cells that synthesize intrinsic factor as well as HCl. The abnormal stage I Schilling test is indicative of a deficiency in intrinsic factor. Chief cells and parietal cells are found in the fundus **(region A)**. Chief cells synthesize pepsinogen. The gastric (fundic) glands contain mucous cells, chief cells, and parietal cells. Intrinsic factor is required for absorption of vitamin B_{12} from the small intestine. The diagram shows the anatomic relationship between the esophagus, stomach, and duodenum. The esophagus **(C)** joins the stomach in the cardiac region **(D)**. The pylorus **(F)** contains shorter glands with deeper pits than those of the fundus and body. Those glands contain more mucous cells and many gastrin-secreting enteroendocrine cells. Food entering the pylorus stimulates the release of gastrin that stimulates HCl production by the parietal cells. The pylorus connects with the duodenum **(G)**, which contains the mucus and bicarbonate-neutralizing secretion of the Brunner glands. The wall of the stomach consists of the mucosa (epithelium, lamina propria, and muscularis mucosa), submucosa, muscularis externa, and serosa **(B)** lined by a mesothelium.

220. The answer is e. *(Fauci, pp 739, 814, 970. Kierszenbaum, pp 466-468. Alberts, pp 629, 906, 1492, 1493, 1504.)* Cholera toxin causes secretory diarrhea through the ADP-ribosylation of G_s of the GTP-binding protein, which leads to elevated cyclic AMP and the opening of the chloride channel **(answers c and d)**. The exit of chloride through the open channels is followed by the passage of sodium and water. The result can be dehydration, which can be offset by intravenous feeding or oral rehydration therapy. Pancreatic secretion is regulated by hormones. Secretin regulates ductal secretion, whereas cholecystokinin **(answer b)** regulates the release of enzymes (amylase, lipase, DNAse, RNase, and the other enzymes that compose the pancreatic juice). A number of pancreatic secretions are released into the pancreatic duct system as zymogens (inactive precursors). They are activated only when they arrive in the small intestinal lumen. Enterokinase, a brush-border enterocyte enzyme, converts trypsinogen to trypsin **(answer a)**. Trypsin and enterokinase are responsible for the activation of chymotrypsinogen, proelastase, and procarboxypeptidase A and B to their active forms: chymotrypsin, elastase, and carboxypeptidase A and B. These hormones are not related to cholera-induced diarrhea.

221. The answer is a. *(Fauci, pp 1872-1876. Kierszenbaum, pp 465-467. Kumar, pp 794, 797. Ross, pp 538-539.)* The area shown in the photomicrograph is the glycocalyx (brush border consisting of microvilli) of the small intestinal epithelium. It is the location of the brush-border enzymes including lactase. The patient in the scenario is diagnosed with lactase deficiency which often has an adult onset since lactase activity decreases after childhood. The absence of lactase or reduced lactase activity results in passage of undigested lactose into the colon. Colonic bacteria carry out fermentation of the lactose to organic acids and hydrogen. The bloating, cramping, and abdominal pain are due to the breakdown of lactose and production of the hydrogen gas. The microvilli are also the site of the glucose/galactose transporter **(answers b and c)**. However, the glucose/galactose transporter is not the site of the deficiency in lactose intolerance. Other brush-border enzymes include the other monosaccharidases and enterokinase, which are important for cleavage of pancreatic zymogens (eg, trypsinogen) to their active form.

Digestion of lipids occurs through the action of bile (from the liver and bile duct) and lipase (from the pancreas). Bile serves to emulsify the lipid to form micelles, whereas lipase breaks down the lipid from triglycerides to fatty acids, glycerol, and monoglycerides (answers d and e). Those three breakdown products diffuse freely across the microvilli to enter the apical portion of the enterocyte by passive diffusion. Triglycerides are resynthesized in the SER. Proteins are synthesized in the RER and are combined with sugar and lipid portions in the Golgi to form glycoproteins and lipoproteins. Those two types of molecules form the coverings of the triglyceride cores of the chylomicra. The chylomicra are released at the basolateral membranes by exocytosis into the lacteals. From the lacteals, the chylomicra travel into the cisterna chyli and eventually into the venous system by way of the thoracic duct. Digestion of fat occurs to a greater extent in the duodenum and jejunum than in the ileum.

Sugars are broken down by amylase in the oral cavity, with continued digestion by brush-border monosaccharidases. Proteins are broken down by pepsinogen in the stomach with continued breakdown in the small intestine by the enzymes of the pancreatic juice (eg, trypsin, chymotrypsin, and carboxypeptidases). The products of protein digestion are amino acids that are actively transported by transporters also located in the brush border.

Endocrine Glands

Questions

222. The adrenal cortex influences the secretion of the adrenal medulla by which one of the following mechanisms?

a. Secretion of aldosterone into the intra-adrenal circulation
b. Secretion of glucocorticoids into the intra-adrenal circulation
c. Autonomic neural connections
d. Secretion of monoamine oxidase into the portal circulation
e. Secretion of androgens into the intrarenal circulation

223. A pheochromocytoma is a common tumor of the adrenal medulla. In the presence of this tumor, which one of the following symptoms would most likely be observed?

a. Hypotension
b. Hypoglycemia
c. Hirsutism
d. Decreased metabolic rate
e. Paroxysms

224. Which one of the following applies to the gland shown in the photomicrograph (A) and labeled with the arrow in the MRI (B) below?

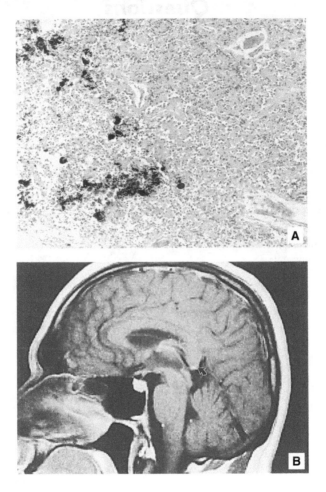

a. It arises as an outgrowth of the midbrain.
b. It influences the rhythmicity of other endocrine organs.
c. It contains many melanocytes.
d. It is innervated by preganglionic sympathetic fibers.
e. It secretes melanocyte-stimulating hormone (MSH).

225. During the physical examination of a newborn child, it is observed that the genitalia are female, but masculinized. The genotype is determined to be 46,XX. Which one of the following is the most likely cause of this condition?

a. Androgen insensitivity
b. Decreased blood ACTH levels
c. Atrophy of the zona reticularis
d. A defect in the cortisol pathway
e. Hypersecretion of vasopressin

226. A 33-year-old woman visits the office of her general internist. Her chief complaint is nervousness that has increased over the past 6 weeks. She is atypically "easy to anger" and often cries for little or no apparent reason. She has lost 22 lb since her last office visit 9 months ago and has not changed her diet. She describes herself as always "hot." Her eyes protrude and appear red and inflamed, and she describes them as feeling "dry." Examination reveals asthenia, tachycardia, pretibial myxedema, and a tremor in her right arm. A biopsy of the organ shown below shows an increase in lymphoid cells. An array of tests is completed. To which of the following would you expect to detect autoantibodies within this organ?

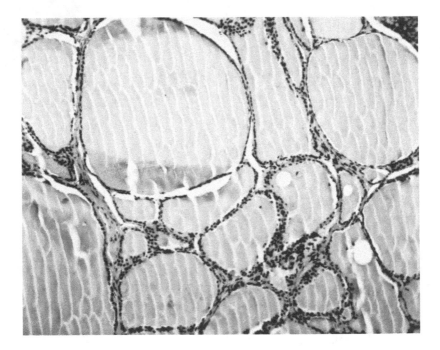

a. C cells
b. Parathyroid principal cells
c. Thyrotropin-releasing factor receptors
d. Thyroglobulin and thyroid peroxidase
e. TSH receptors

227. A 45-year-old woman, who works as a corporate executive, presents with the primary complaint of "always being tired." She comments that she has been tired for 4 months even though she is sleeping more. She complains of being unable to finish household chores and "dragging at work." She indicates that she is often constipated and is intolerant to cold. She is continuously turning the thermostats in the house and work to higher temperatures, to the dismay of family members and coworkers, respectively. She also complains that her skin is very dry; use of lotions and creams have not helped the dryness. A biopsy of the organ shown in Question 226 indicates dense lymphocytic infiltration with germinal centers throughout the parenchyma. A battery of tests is carried out. Which one of the following lab results would be most likely in this patient?

a. Elevated TSH levels in the serum
b. Elevated T_3 and T_4 levels in the serum
c. Autoantibodies to the thyroid hormone receptor
d. Elevated calcitonin levels
e. Elevated glucocorticoid levels

228. Which one of the following cells or parts of the pituitary are derived embryologically from neuroectoderm?

a. Gonadotrophs
b. Pars intermedia
c. Pars tuberalis
d. Herring bodies
e. Lactotrophs

229. A pituitary adenoma is likely to result in which one of the following?

a. Cushing syndrome
b. Deficiency in T_3 and T_4
c. Diabetes insipidus
d. Osteoporosis
e. Stunted growth or dwarfism

230. A tumor in the specific region denoted by the asterisks will most likely cause which one of the following?

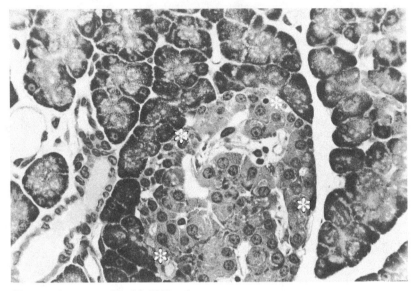

(Micrograph courtesy of Dr. John K. Young)

a. Diabetes
b. Hypoglycemia
c. Elevated blood pressure
d. Decreased blood pressure
e. Increased bone resorption

231. A 30-year-old woman presents with progressive, chronic fatigue, muscle weakness, and loss of appetite, with a 15-lb weight loss since her last visit. She "craves salty foods" when she is able to eat. She is often nauseous and vomits after eating. Her bowel movements are loose with frequent diarrhea. Her blood pressure is low and she becomes dizzy when standing. It is the middle of winter and she has a healthy tan, most visible in her skin folds and at her elbows, knees and, knuckles. She is "irritable and depressed," with very irregular menstrual periods and no "hot flashes." Which one of the following would occur in the regions of a biopsy specimen labeled in the accompanying photomicrographs at low (A) and high magnification (B)?

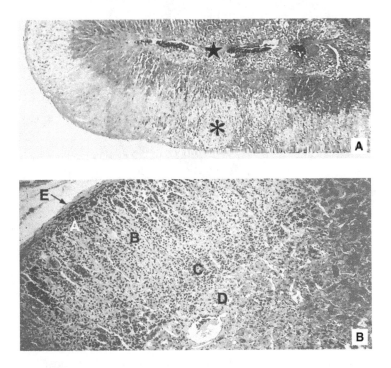

a. Hypertrophy of zone A only
b. Hypertrophy of zones A, B, and C only
c. Hypotrophy of zones A, B, and C only
d. Hypotrophy of zones A, B, C, and D only
e. Hypertrophy of zones A and B only

232. The region labeled C is not a good candidate for transplantation compared with other endocrine glands for which one of the following reasons?

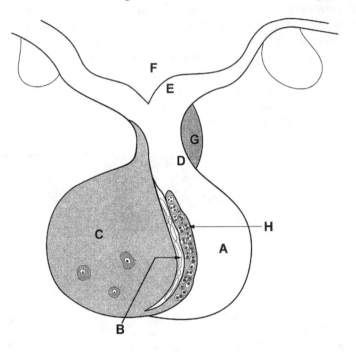

a. More severe rejection of neurally-related tissue occurs compared with other endocrine organs.
b. Its hormonal source is unavailable after its axonal connections to the hypothalamus are disrupted.
c. It lacks function when separated from the hypothalamo-hypophyseal portal system.
d. Neogenesis of blood vessels will not occur at the transplant site.
e. The vascular wall of the superior hypophyseal arteries is unique.

233. Measuring T_3 levels does not necessarily accurately depict the thyroid's ability to secrete T_3 for which one of the following reasons?

a. T_3 is bound to thyroid-hormone binding proteins.
b. The liver and kidney convert T_4 to T_3 peripherally.
c. T_3 and T_4 are regulated by two different anterior pituitary hormones.
d. Thyrotrophs produce T_3.
e. T_4 and T_3 immunoassays cross-react in immunoassays.

Endocrine Glands

Answers

222. The answer is b. (*Mescher, pp 355, 357-358, 406. Kierszenbaum, pp 554-558. Ross, pp 709-710.*) Metabolism in the adrenal medulla is regulated by glucocorticoids because they induce the enzyme phenylethanolamine-N-methyltransferase, which catalyzes the methylation of norepinephrine to epinephrine. Most of the blood supply entering the medulla passes through the cortex. Glucocorticoids synthesized in the zona fasciculata of the adrenal are released into the sinusoids and enter the medulla **(answers a and e).** The adrenal gland is not usually considered a classic portal system although there are similarities. Monoamine oxidase is a mitochondrial enzyme that regulates the storage of catecholamines in peripheral sympathetic nerve endings **(answers c and d).** The adrenal gland functions as two separate glands. The adrenal cortex is derived from mesoderm and the adrenal medulla from neural crest. The blood supply to the adrenal is derived from three adrenal arteries: (1) the superior adrenal (suprarenal) from the inferior phrenic, (2) the middle adrenal from the aorta, and (3) the inferior adrenal from the renal artery.

223. The answer is e. (*Fauci, pp 2269-2271. Mescher, p 358. Kumar, pp 1159-1161.*) Patients with a pheochromocytoma often have paroxysms that are the hallmark of this tumor. These are seizure-like catecholamine-induced attacks that include headache, profuse sweating, palpitations, and overall anxiety. Pheochromocytoma is a common tumor of the adrenal medulla that leads to excess release of norepinephrine (noradrenaline) and epinephrine (adrenaline), which cause hypertension and hyperglycemia **(answers a and b).** Vasoconstriction of arterioles occurs in conjunction with the increased blood pressure. Hirsutism is due to the action of the androgen, dihydrotestosterone, that acts on the hair follicle to produce terminal hair **(answer c).** Markedly elevated plasma catecholamine levels are known to increase metabolic rate **(answer d).**

224. The answer is b. (*Mescher, pp 367, 369-370. Kumar, p 1163.*) The photomicrograph and the MRI illustrate the structure of the pineal gland, or epiphysis cerebri, which arises as an outgrowth of the diencephalon (answer a). The pinealocytes secrete melatonin in response to the light-dark cycle and influence the rhythmicity of other endocrine organs. In a sense, the pineal, therefore, functions as a biologic clock. The pineal contains two main cell types: pinealocytes and neuroglia (the latter appear to be modified astrocytes [answer c]). The pineal is innervated by postganglionic sympathetic fibers in a fashion similar to other glands in the head and neck region (eg, salivary glands). The adrenal medulla is innervated by preganglionic sympathetic fibers (answer d). Corticotrophs in the anterior pituitary produce MSH. The pineal does not contain melanocytes or secrete MSH (answer e). There are age-related changes in the pineal in which the number of concretions and the degree of calcification of the "brain sand" increase. The pineal can be identified and used as a landmark in radiologic procedures by its calcification.

225. The answer is d. *(Sadler, pp 258-259. Kumar, pp 1152-1154. Moore and Persaud, p 262.)* The newborn described is genotypically female and is diagnosed with adrenogenital syndrome, also known as congenital virilizing hyperplasia or female pseudohermaphroditism, in which there is a deficiency in the pathway that leads to cortisol synthesis. The inability to synthesize cortisol in turn leads to production of high levels of ACTH and ACTH-releasing factor from the hypothalamus (answer b). The result is hypertrophy of the fetal adrenal cortex, which is a critical fetal endocrine organ that produces dehydroepiandrosterone. The excessive production of androgens by the fetal adrenal leads to masculinization of the female genitalia. Increased secretion of cortisol cannot occur because of the metabolic defect in this pathway; therefore, negative feedback control is not functional. The fetal cortex is part of maternal-fetoplacental unit because dehydroepiandrosterone is used by the placenta to produce estradiol. The fetal adrenal cortex involutes following birth, causing an overall reduction in the size of the adrenal. The adult cortex (zona glomerulosa, zona fasciculata, and zona reticularis) replaces the fetal adrenal cortex. The zona fasciculata and zona reticularis produce androgens after birth (answer c). Vasopressin ([AVP] also known as antidiuretic hormone [ADH]) is released by the posterior pituitary and regulates fluid balance. ADH increases the permeability of the collecting duct through an aquaporin-mediated mechanism (answer e). Androgen insensitivity is the cause of testicular feminization and is not a factor in the adrenogenital syndrome (answer a).

226. The answer is e. (*Mescher, pp 361-365. Kumar, pp 1114-1116. Moore and Persaud, pp 169, 173-176, 195.*) The patient is suffering from Graves disease, an autoimmune disease that occurs much more frequently in women than in men. Graves disease accounts for approximately 85% of diagnosed hyperthyroidism. Patients with Graves disease produce autoantibodies to TSH receptors. CD8⁺ T cells are also generated against the TSH receptors, leading to their destruction. The result is an increase in TSH produced by the anterior pituitary with a concomitant increase in thyroid hormone production (T_4 [tetraiodothyronine, thyroxine] and T_3 [tetraiodothyronine]) from the thyroid. The elevated thyroid hormone secretion leads to the nervousness, weight loss, and extreme mood changes experienced by the patient.

The thyroid gland, shown in the photomicrograph, is most often confused histologically with lactating mammary gland, which differs from the thyroid in the presence of an elaborate duct system. The thyroid is composed of follicles filled with colloidal material and surrounded by follicular cells that vary in height from low cuboidal to columnar epithelium. The C cells (also known as interfollicular or parafollicular cells) are clear and found outside the follicular cells. The "C" cells synthesize calcitonin and are derived embryologically from the ultimobranchial bodies (fourth and possibly fifth pair of branchial pouches). Calcitonin decreases elevated serum calcium levels by transiently inhibiting osteoclastic activity through receptors on osteoclasts. In Graves disease there are no autoantibodies to the C cells **(answer a)**. Destruction of C cells would lead to an absence of calcitonin and high serum calcium levels. Autoantibodies to principal cells of the parathyroid **(answer b)** would lead to decreased serum calcium levels as parathyroid hormone (PTH) synthesis and secretion would be reduced. PTH increases osteoclastic resorption and also stimulates Ca^{2+} uptake from the gut and Ca^{2+} reabsorption by the kidneys. The thyroid gland is under the direct regulation of TSH (thyrotropin) production by the anterior pituitary, which in turn is regulated by TSH-releasing factor (TSH-RF) released from the hypothalamus. TSH-RF is transported by the hypothalamic-hypophyseal (pituitary)-portal system to the anterior pituitary. Autoantibodies to TSH-RF **(answer c)** would result in elevated TSH and T_3 and T_4, but the receptors would be located in the anterior pituitary on thyrotrophs. Autoantibodies to thyroglobulin and thyroid peroxidase result in Hashimoto thyroiditis **(answer d** [see Question 227]**)**.

Asthenia is loss of strength and tachycardia is accelerated heart rate. Pretibial myxedema presents as an orange-peel-like rash on the shins in some patients with Graves disease.

The thyroid follicular epithelial cells import iodide and amino acids from the capillary lumen. The follicular cells synthesize thyroglobulin from amino acids. When iodide enters the follicular cells, it undergoes oxidation. Thyroglobulin is iodinated while in the colloid, and iodinated thyroglobulin (not the thyroid hormones) is the storage product in the thyroid colloid. The thyroid follicular cells process iodinated thyroglobulin, and the activity of lysosomes breaks down the colloid to form thyroxine (T_4), triiodothyronine (T_3), diiodotyrosine (DIT), and monoiodotyrosine (MIT). Most of the secretion of the human thyroid gland is composed of thyroxine, although triiodothyronine is more potent.

227. The answer is a. (*Fauci, pp 2230-2232. Greenspan, pp 60, 71-72, 264-266. Kierszenbaum, p 504. Kumar, pp 1111-1113.*) The patient is diagnosed with Hashimoto thyroiditis in which there is extensive lymphocytic infiltration of the thyroid gland. Autoantibodies develop to thyroglobulin and thyroid peroxidase, an iodine transporter and/or the TSH receptor. In cases where there are autoantibodies to TSH receptor, the TSH receptor activity is blocked, resulting in hypothyroidism compared to the hyperthyroidism, which occurs in Graves disease (see Question 226). The antibodies react with a different epitope on the receptor, resulting in the different overall effect. $CD8^+$ T cells are also directed against that site. T_3 and T_4 levels may be elevated early in the disease **(answer b)** process due to disruption of the follicles and release of hormones; however, the overall effect is hypothyroidism. Destruction of thyroid hormone receptors **(answer c)** would lead to hyperthyroidism. Calcitonin is secreted by the C cells in the thyroid and is not affected by the thyroiditis **(answer d)**. Glucocorticoid levels are not elevated **(answer e)**.

228. The answer is d. (*Sadler, pp 34, 308-310. Mescher, pp 348-354.*) The neurohypophysis containing the Herring bodies is formed from neuroectoderm as an extension of the developing diencephalon. The pars nervosa consists of pituicytes (supportive glia) and the Herring bodies, dilated axons that originate in the supraoptic and paraventricular nuclei. These nuclei produce oxytocin and vasopressin that are stored in the Herring bodies.

Overall, the pituitary gland (hypophysis cerebri) is formed from two types of ectoderm. An outgrowth of the oral ectoderm, Rathke pouch, forms the structures that compose the adenohypophysis: pars distalis, pars intermedia, and pars tuberalis **(answers b and c)**. The pars distalis includes the classic histologic cell types: chromophils (acidophils and basophils) and chromophobes (acidophils and basophils that are depleted of secretory product). Acidophils include: lactotrophs (prolactin), somatotrophs (growth hormone); basophils include: corticotrophs (ACTH, α-lipotropin, β-MSH, and α-endorphin), thyrotrophs (TSH), and gonadotrophs (FSH and LH [**answers a and e**]). The pars intermedia is also formed from the oral ectoderm, is rudimentary in humans, and may produce preproopiomelanocortic peptide. The pars tuberalis forms a collar around the pituitary stalk and is also derived from the oral ectoderm. The pars nervosa (including Herring bodies) and the remainder of the pituitary stalk (infundibular stem and median eminence) are formed from a downgrowth of the diencephalon. The posterior pituitary (pars nervosa and stalk) retains this close relationship with the brain (ie, hypothalamus) throughout life.

229. The answer is a. *(Mescher, pp 351-353, 415-416. Kumar, pp 1100-1105.)* Pituitary adenomas are anterior pituitary specific. A corticotroph adenoma would cause increased levels of ACTH and stimulate excessive production of corticosteroids from the adrenal cortex (Cushing syndrome). LH- and FSH-producing gonadotroph-adenomas occur, but tend to result in hypogonadism. Somatotropic tumors produce GH and cause giantism (**answer e**). Prolactinomas are the most common form of pituitary adenoma resulting in infertility, galactorrhea (excessive production of milk), and amenorrhea. Diabetes insipidus (**answer c**) is caused by absence of vasopressin (arginine vasopressin [AVP]), leading to excretion of a large quantity of dilute fluid (hypotonic polyuria). Overproduction of PTH leads to osteoporotic changes, but PTH is not regulated by the anterior pituitary (**answer d**). The thyroid secretes T_3 and T_4 (**answer b**), regulated by TSH from thyrotrophs in the anterior pituitary.

230. The answer is a. *(Mescher, p 359. Costanzo, pp 355, 421. Kumar, p 1147. Fauci, p 2355.)* A tumor of the glucagon secreting alpha (α) or A cells delineated with the asterisks results in hyperglycemia and diabetes (**answers b → e**). This photomicrograph shows both exocrine and endocrine portions of the pancreas. Pancreatic exocrine tissue is found throughout the pancreas with round aggregations of lighter staining cells forming the islets of Langerhans. There are several endocrine cell types within the islets. The more numerous (70% of total) B or β cells are centrally located and secrete insulin that is secreted after a meal and results in a lowering of blood sugar. The smaller population of A or α cells located at the periphery of the islet (*) secrete glucagon. Glucagon is secreted in response to low blood sugar and raises blood sugar levels. A glucagonoma produces excessive amounts of glucagon that results in hyperglycemia and diabetes. The interaction of β and α cells is based on the blood supply. Blood entering the islet initially bypasses the α cells. The result is that blood reaching the α cells already contains insulin, which regulates glucagon production. The absence of normal glucagon regulation by insulin is a further complication in type I diabetes in which insulin is not produced. Other cell types (D [δ] and F) are variable in location and secrete somatostatin and pancreatic polypeptide, respectively. Somatostatin regulates insulin and glucagon release, whereas pancreatic polypeptide appears to regulate exocrine protein and bicarbonate secretion. The exocrine portion of the pancreas consists of acinar and ductal cells. The acinar cells are pyramidal in shape and possess a very basophilic basal cytoplasm, indicating the presence of abundant rough ER and an acidophilic apical cytoplasm due to the presence of numerous secretory (zymogen) granules.

Other tumors of the islets of Langerhans include insulinomas in which elevated levels of insulin are secreted into the bloodstream. The result is hypoglycemia as blood sugar levels drop. Insulin removes sugar from the blood and, in the liver, either stores it as glycogen or metabolizes it through glycolysis. Insulin inhibits glycogen phosphorylase (which catalyzes the breakdown of glycogen to form glucose) and activates glycogen synthase in both muscle and liver resulting in increased storage of glycogen.

231. The answer is c. *(Fauci, p 2262. Mescher, pp 361, 362. Kumar, pp 1155-1157.)* The woman in the scenario suffers from Addison disease, in which there is a progressive destruction (hypotrophy) of the adrenal cortex (zones A, B, and C). The result in the patient is asthenia (lack of strength, overall weakness, and fatigue), anorexia, nausea, vomiting, weight loss, hypotension, and low blood sugar. The hyperpigmentation results from elevated ACTH stimulation of melanocytes. The photomicrographs show the histology of the adrenal gland figure A (cortex [*] and medulla [– ★ –]), which releases stress-related hormones (ie, glucocorticoids and catecholamines [norepinephrine and epinephrine]). The adrenal cortex originates from the intermediate mesoderm, whereas the adrenal medulla forms from neural crest. Adrenocortical cells are under the influence of corticotrophs in the anterior pituitary. Adrenocortical cells import cholesterol and acetate and produce the hormones shown in High-Yield Facts, Table 13. The zona glomerulosa (A) is found immediately beneath the capsule (E) and is followed by the zona fasciculata (B) and zona reticularis (C) as one moves toward the medulla (D). However, in all zones the cells do not store appreciable quantities of hormones, there is an absence of secretory granules, and the steroid hormones are released by diffusion through the plasma membrane without use of the exocytotic process used by most glands, including the adrenal medulla. The cells of the adrenal medulla (D) may be considered as modified postganglionic sympathetic neurons. Adrenal medullary cells synthesize and secrete norepinephrine, epinephrine, and enkephalins in response to stimulation of preganglionic sympathetic fibers that travel through the abdomen in the splanchnic nerves and innervate the gland. The adrenal cortical hormones are viewed as essential for life because of their regulation of metabolism.

232. The answer is c. (*Young, pp 328-332. Moore and Persaud, pp 399, 401. Mescher, pp 348-351. Sadler, p 308.*) The region of the pituitary labeled C is the pars distalis also known as the anterior lobe, which contains corticotrophs, thyrotrophs, lactotrophs, and gonadotrophs that synthesize trophic hormones which regulate other endocrine organs. The anterior pituitary is unique in that it depends on the presence of the hypothalamo-hypophyseal portal system. Releasing and inhibitory factors are transported from the cell bodies in the hypothalamus along axons into the median eminence, where the secretion is released into a primary capillary plexus. The hypothalamo-hypophyseal portal system carries blood from the primary plexus to the secondary plexus, which comprises the sinusoids of the pars distalis. That system brings the hypothalamic hormones into close proximity with the appropriate cell types in the pars distalis. For example, CTH-RF (corticotropin-releasing factor, CRH) is synthesized in the hypothalamus, released into the primary capillary plexus in the median eminence, and subsequently carried in the portal system to the secondary capillary plexus, where it interacts with corticotrophs in the pars distalis. The pars nervosa is the neurally connected portion of the pituitary and contains the dilated axons of hypothalamic cell bodies that produce vasopressin and oxytocin.

The region labeled **A** is the posterior pituitary that stores oxytocin and vasopressin in dilated axonal terminals. Overall, the pituitary is derived from the ectoderm of the oral cavity (Rathke pouch) and the floor of the diencephalon. The anterior (**C**) and intermediate (**H**) lobes and pars tuberalis

(G) are derived from the oral cavity, whereas the remainder of the pituitary (pars nervosa [A] and the pituitary stalk [D]) is derived from a neuroepithelial origin. The cleft of Rathke pouch (B) represents the lumen of the structure formed originally from the oral cavity. The pars distalis (C) contains acidophils and basophils regulated by stimulatory and inhibitory hormones produced by the hypothalamus. In the pars nervosa (A), the major cell type present is the pituicyte, a supportive glial cell. Axons that originate in the supraoptic and paraventricular nuclei of the hypothalamus descend into the pars nervosa. Oxytocin regulates the milk ejection reflex and vasopressin [AVP], also known as antidiuretic hormone [ADH], regulates collecting duct permeability. Those 2 hormones are stored in dilated endings in the pars nervosa called Herring bodies. Those secretions are, therefore, synthesized in the hypothalamus and stored in the pars nervosa. Structure E is the median eminence; F represents the cavity of the third ventricle.

233. The answer is b. *(Fauci, pp 2215-2216. Kumar, pp 1107-1109.)* T_4 (thyroxine) is the primary serum thyroid hormone and is produced only by the thyroid gland. In contrast, only about 20% of T_3 (triiodothyronine) is produced by the thyroid gland. T_3 is formed in the liver and kidney by the action of a specific enzyme, 5'-deiodinase that converts T_4 to T_3. That enzyme also converts T_4 to metabolically inactive thyroid hormone, rT_3 (reverse T_3). T_3 is three to five times more physiologically active than T_4. Both T_4 and T_3 are bound to thyroxine-binding globulin (TBG), transthyretin, and albumin **(answer a)**, with only about 1% of free circulating hormone. Levels of available binding proteins affect measurable levels of total T_4 and T_3. When those binding proteins are found in high concentrations, total T_4 and T_3 levels are also high, but free T_4 and T_3 values remain normal. The free fractions of T_4 and T_3 are responsible for the feedback mechanism at the level of the hypothalamus and the thyrotrophs in the anterior pituitary. T_3 and T_4 are regulated by TSH from the thyrotrophs **(answers c and d)**. There is some cross-reactivity of all immunoassays **(answer e)**, but that is not the reason for the possible inaccuracy of extrapolating from serum T_3 levels to thyroid function.

Reproductive Systems

Questions

234. Elevated estrogen levels during the menstrual cycle result in which one of the following physiological changes?

a. Decreased LH levels
b. Down-regulated follicle-stimulating hormone (FSH) receptors on granulosa cells
c. Increased FSH levels
d. Increased ciliation of the epithelial cells of the oviduct
e. Decreased synthesis and storage of glycogen in the vaginal epithelium

235. A biopsy is reviewed by a pathologist. She diagnoses the tumor as originating from the cell delineated with the star. The tumor would most likely produce which one of the following?

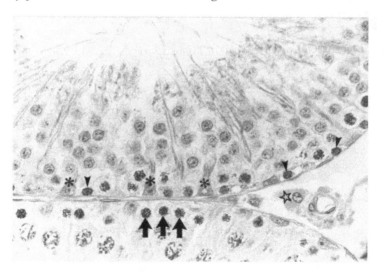

a. Calcitonin
b. Progesterone
c. Androgens
d. FSH
e. Parathyroid hormone

236. The structure or structures labeled B in the photomicrograph from the reproductive system below is which one of the following?

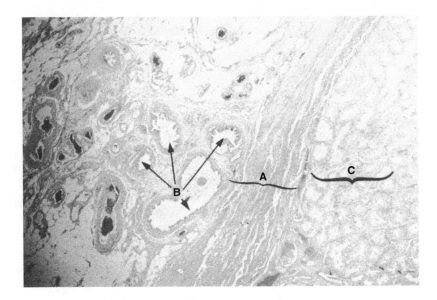

a. Rete testis
b. Efferent ductules
c. Seminiferous tubules
d. Vas deferens
e. Oviduct

237. Which one of the following best describes the function of the organ from the reproductive system shown below?

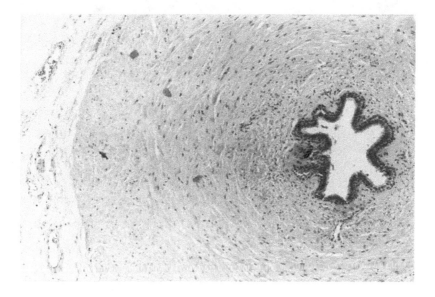

a. Passage of urine and sperm in the male
b. Passage of urine from the urethra to the vestibule in the female
c. Passage of urine from the bladder to the urethrae in males and females
d. Passage of sperm from the epididymis to the urethra
e. Storage of sperm and absorption of fluid

238. What organ is pictured below?

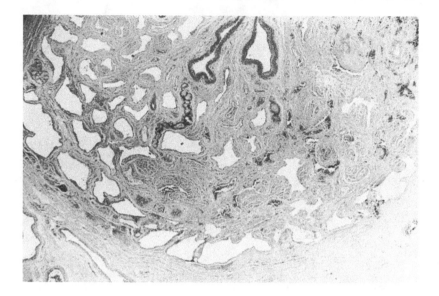

a. Female urethra
b. Male urethra
c. Oviduct
d. Ureter
e. Seminal vesicle

239. Malignancies most frequently arise from which portion of the organ shown in the photomicrograph below?

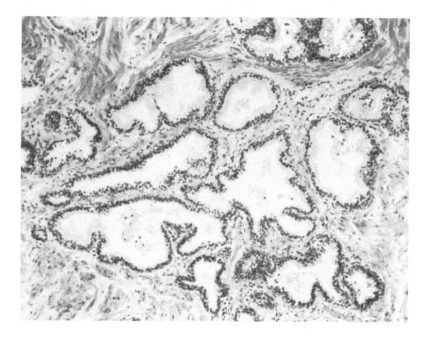

a. Lactiferous duct
b. Periurethral glands
c. Outer peripheral glands
d. Germ cells
e. Mammary alveoli

240. The organ shown in this photomicrograph is responsible for production of which of the following?

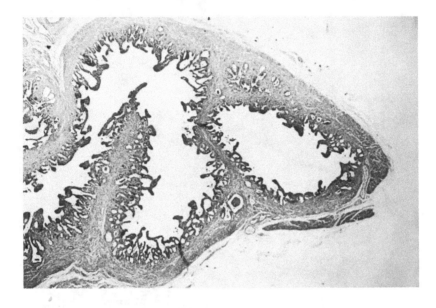

a. Spermine and fibrolysin
b. T_3 and T_4
c. Proteins that coagulate semen
d. Acid phosphatase
e. Milk

241. The organ in the photomicrograph performs which of the following functions?

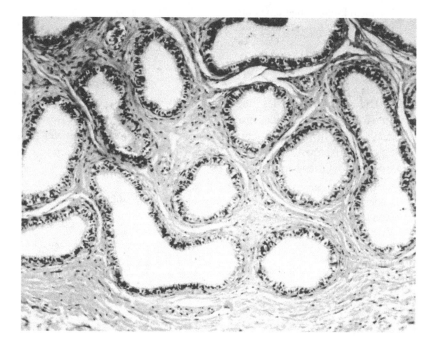

a. The site of spermiogenesis
b. Production of fructose and prostaglandins
c. Phagocytosis of sperm
d. The site of implantation
e. The site of milk production

242. Which of the following is independent of testosterone or other androgens?

a. Secretion from the prostatic epithelium
b. The function of the prostatic glands
c. Development of the penis from an indifferent phallus
d. Spermatogenesis
e. Fetal testis development from an indifferent gonad

243. A 26-year-old woman is in her last trimester of a normal pregnancy. Synthesis of milk by her mammary glands specifically requires which of the following?

a. Oxytocin from the neurohypophysis
b. Prolactin from the corpus luteum
c. The influence of vasopressin
d. Placental lactogen
e. Neurohumoral reflexes

244. The urologist may describe the reattachment of a severed vas deferens (vasovasostomy) as successful, more than 90% of the time. However, it is unsuccessful from the patients' point of view since a much lower percentage of those men can father a child. The difference in success rate is due to which of the following?

a. Spermatogonia are exposed to humoral factors.
b. Genetic recombination in haploid sperm creates novel antigens.
c. Cryptorchid testes are often incapable of producing fertile sperm.
d. Vasectomy prevents phagocytosis of sperm by macrophages.
e. Sperm coated with autoimmune antibodies are unable to fertilize an egg.

245. A 29-year-old woman is trying to become pregnant. She presents with irregular menstrual cycles and heavy, prolonged, irregular uterine bleeding, and undergoes an endometrial biopsy. The biopsy has the appearance shown in the photomicrograph below. Which of the following is characteristic of this stage of the menstrual cycle?

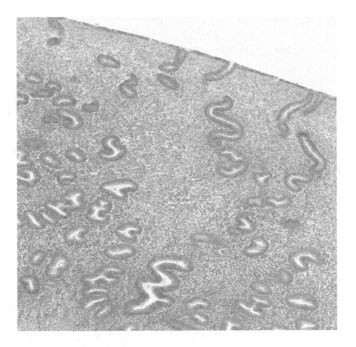

a. It precedes ovulation.
b. It depends on progesterone secretion by the corpus luteum.
c. It coincides with the development of ovarian follicles.
d. It coincides with a rapid drop in estrogen levels.
e. It produces ischemia and necrosis of the stratum functionale.

246. The low pH in the vagina is maintained by which of the following?

a. A proton pump similar to that of parietal cells and osteoclasts
b. Acid secretion derived from intracellular carbonic acid
c. Secretion of lactic acid by the stratified squamous epithelium
d. Bacterial metabolism of glycogen to form lactic acid
e. Synthesis and accumulation of acid hydrolases in the epithelium

247. A 33-year-old woman with an average menstrual cycle of 28 days comes in for a routine Pap smear. It has been 35 days since the start of her last menstrual period, and a vaginal smear reveals clumps of basophilic cells. As her physician, you suspect which of the following?

a. She will begin menstruating in a few days.
b. She will ovulate within a few days.
c. Her serum progesterone levels are very low.
d. There are detectable levels of hCG in her serum and urine.
e. She is undergoing menopause.

248. If the hormone necessary for maintenance of the structure in the photomicrograph below were absent 12 to 14 days after ovulation in a human female, which of the following would be the result?

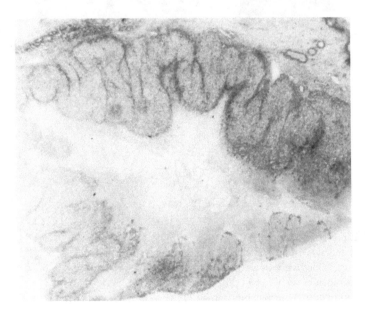

a. The absence of the structure
b. The absence of muscularization
c. Maintenance of the uterine epithelium for implantation beyond 14 days after ovulation
d. Pregnancy
e. The formation of a corpus albicans from the structure

249. A 23-year-old woman has regular menstrual periods. Which of the following pairings of hormonal change and function best describes the response of the structure labeled "A" in the accompanying diagram as this woman enters menses?

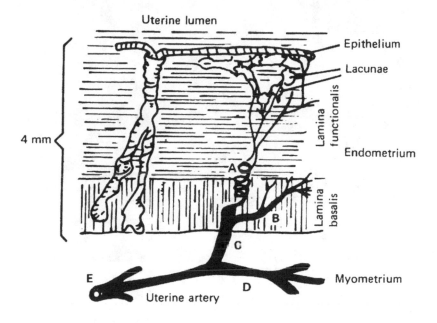

a. Reduced progesterone, continuous dilation
b. Reduced progesterone, continuous contraction
c. Reduced progesterone, spasmodic contraction
d. Reduced estrogen, continuous dilation
e. Reduced estrogen, continuous contraction
f. Reduced estrogen, spasmodic contraction

250. Cells in the layers labeled A and C in the figure below secrete plasminogen activator and collagenase that is required for which of the following?

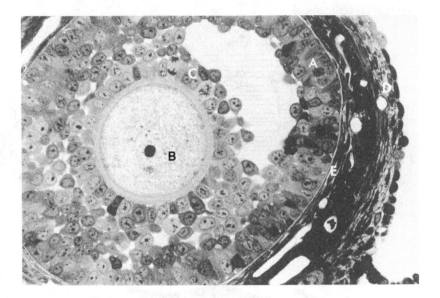

a. Dissolution of the zona pellucida to facilitate sperm penetration
b. pH regulation within the antral cavity
c. Breakdown of the basement membrane between the thecal and granulosa layers, facilitating ovulation
d. Diffusion of androgens between the thecal and granulosa cells
e. Facilitation of follicular atresia through breakdown of the basement membrane between the theca interna and externa

251. Secretions from the organ shown below carry out which of the following functions?

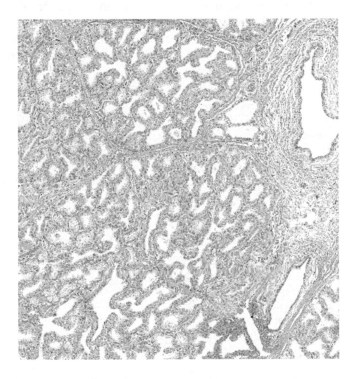

a. Regulation of metabolism
b. Transfer of maternal antibodies to the suckling neonate
c. Removal of waste products during gestation
d. Facilitate clotting of ejaculated semen in the female
e. Enhancement of sperm function

Questions 252 to 254

A 31-year-old woman has been diagnosed with pelvic inflammatory disease (PID) and treated with antibiotics several times in the last decade. She is recently married and wants to become pregnant. She comes to the Reproduction, Endocrine, and Infertility Division of the Obstetrics and Gynecology Department because she and her husband have been unable to conceive.

252. What is the most likely cause of the couple's infertility?

a. Occlusion of the fallopian tubes
b. Apoptosis of ovarian follicular cells
c. Apoptosis of oocytes
d. Inflammation of the uterine wall
e. Vaginitis
f. Ovarian stromal fibrosis leading to lack of nutritive support for the oocytes
g. Altered cervical mucus
h. Low sperm count

253. Which of the following assisted reproductive procedures would be the best technique for overcoming this couple's infertility problem?

a. Gamete intrafallopian transfer (GIFT)
b. Zygote intrafallopian transfer (ZIFT)
c. Tubal embryo transfer (TET)
d. In vitro fertilization (IVF)
e. Clomiphene citrate treatment followed by intercourse
f. Gonadotropin treatment followed by intercourse

254. If the woman conceives "naturally" following multiple episodes of PID which is the most likely complication of that pregnancy?

a. Spontaneous abortion
b. Chorioamnionitis
c. Ectopic pregnancy
d. Multiple pregnancies
e. Molar pregnancy (hydatidiform mole)

Reproductive Systems

Answers

234. The answer is d. (*Mescher, p 400. Costanzo, pp 452-454. Kierszenbaum, pp 624-628.*) Estrogen levels increase during the maturation of ovarian follicles, which results in a concomitant increase in ciliation and height of the oviductal lining cells. Increases in the number of cilia serve to facilitate movement of the ovum. Increased estrogen levels also decrease FSH levels and cause an LH surge (**answers a and c**). Elevated estrogen levels result in increased secretion of lytic enzymes, prostaglandins, plasminogen activator, and collagenase to facilitate the rupture of the ovarian wall and the release of the ovum and the attached corona radiata. Following ovulation, during the luteal phase of the cycle, the theca and granulosa cells are transformed into the corpus luteum under the influence of LH. Ovulation occurs near the middle of the menstrual cycle and is associated with an increase in basal body temperature that appears to be indirectly regulated by elevated estrogen levels, with IL-1 functioning as the endogenous pyrogen. Estrogen also up-regulates FSH receptors on granulosa cell membranes and enhances synthesis and storage of glycogen in the vaginal epithelium (**answers b and e**).

235. The answer is c. (*Young, pp 348-349, 353. Mescher, pp 371, 380.*) The cell marked with a star is a Leydig cell (ie, interstitial cell) and is regulated by luteinizing hormone (LH), formerly known as interstitial cell–stimulating hormone (ICSH), secreted by gonadotrophs in the anterior pituitary. Leydig cells are located between seminiferous tubules and are responsible for the production of testosterone. The Leydig cells normally synthesize and release testosterone in response to LH that is produced by gonadotrophs in the anterior pituitary. Leydig cell tumors develop in males between 20 and 60 years of age and produce androgens, estrogens, and sometimes glucocorticoids. Calcitonin is synthesized by C cells in the thyroid (**answer a**). Progesterone (**answer b**) is synthesized by corpora lutea under the influence of LH. FSH plays a key physiological role in both males (spermatogenesis) and females (regulation of follicular growth), and is produced and released by gonadotrophs in the anterior pituitary (**answer d**). FSH stimulates the maturation of ovarian follicles. FSH treatment of humans results in development of more than the usual number of mature follicles and an increased number of mature gametes. FSH is also critical for sperm production. It supports the function of Sertoli cells, which serve a nutritive role in sperm cell maturation. Parathyroid hormone (answer e) is synthesized and released from the principal cells of the parathyroid gland.

Sertoli cells (*) function in a nutritive and supportive role somewhat analogous to the glial cells of the CNS. The Sertoli cells produce inhibin, which feeds back on the anterior pituitary and hypothalamus to regulate FSH release. Testosterone binds to androgen-binding protein (ABP), which is synthesized by the Sertoli cells. Testosterone is necessary for maintenance of spermatogenesis as well as the male ducts and accessory glands. ABP is regulated by FSH, testosterone, and inhibin. Sertoli cells have extensive tight (occluding) junctions between them that form the blood-testis barrier. Sertoli cells communicate with adjacent cells through gap junctions and extend from outside the blood-testis barrier (basal portion) to luminal (apical portion). During spermatogenesis, preleptotene spermatocytes cross from the basal to the adluminal compartment across the zonula occludens between adjacent Sertoli cells. Each Sertoli cell is, therefore, associated with multiple spermatogenic cells.

The testis is composed of seminiferous tubules containing a number of spermatogenic cells undergoing spermatogenesis and spermiogenesis. The cells labeled with the arrowheads are spermatogonia, the derivatives of the embryonic primordial germ cells. Those cells comprise the basal layer and undergo mitosis (spermatocytogenesis) to form primary spermatocytes, which have distinctive clumped or coarse chromatin (marked by arrows). Secondary spermatocytes are formed during the first meiotic division and exist for only a short period of time because there is no lag period before entry into the second meiotic division that results in the formation of spermatids. The spermatids begin as round structures and elongate with the formation of the flagellum. This last part of seminiferous tubule function is the differentiation of sperm from spermatids (spermiogenesis) and is complete with the release of mature sperm into the lumen of the tubule.

236. The answer is b. (*Young, pp 353-355, Mescher, 380-381.*) The photomicrograph is taken from an area that shows the ductuli efferentes (efferent ductules, **B**), with their distinctive wavy epithelium in which adjoining cells are tall (ciliated) and short (nonciliated). Also shown are the seminiferous tubules (C) and the mediastinum testis containing the rete testis (A). Sperm leave the seminiferous tubules through short tubuli recti into the straight tubules of the rete testis, which subsequently drain into the efferent ductules. For the vas deferens, see answer to Question 237.

237. The answer is d. *(Young, pp 353-355. Mescher, pp 381-383.)* The organ shown in the figure is the vas deferens (ductus deferens). The vas deferens conducts sperm from the epididymis to the urethra. The thick muscular wall is unique in the presence of an inner longitudinal, a middle circular, and an outer longitudinal layer of smooth muscle. The ureter has two thin layers of muscle: inner longitudinal and outer circular **(answer c)**. The male and female urethra contain extensive vascular channels **(answers a and b)**. The epididymis consists of a connective tissue stroma and stores sperm, resorbs fluid, and produces sperm maturation factors **(answer e)**.

238. The answer is b. *(Young, pp 357-358. Mescher, p 387.)* The photomicrograph shows the histology of the male (penile) urethra. It possesses a primarily pseudostratified columnar type of epithelium. The glands of Littré that produce mucus are also observed in the section. Glands of Littré are not present within the oviduct **(answer c)**, ureter **(answer d)**, and the seminal vesicle **(answer e)**. The thick-walled arteries of the penile and cavernous sinuses of penile erectile tissue are also a distinguishing feature of this organ. Helicine arteries supply the sinuses. Action of the parasympathetic nervous system mediates the dilation of these vessels during erection. The female urethra **(answer a)** is surrounded by less erectile tissue.

239. The answer is c. *(Young, pp 355-357. Mescher, pp 383-386. Kumar, pp 993-997. Fauci, pp 593-595.)* The photomicrograph is from the prostate. Seventy percent of carcinomas of the prostate arise from the main (external gland), also known as the outer (peripheral) glands **(answer b)**. The prostate consists of three parts: (1) a small mucosal (inner periurethral) gland, (2) a transition zone that consists of a submucosal (outer periurethral) gland, and (3) a peripheral portion known as the main or external gland. Because of the peripheral location, most prostatic carcinomas (primarily adenocarcinomas) remain undiagnosed until the later symptoms of back pain or blockage of the urethra are detected. Digital rectal examination can identify some tumors earlier. Benign prostatic hypertrophy, also known as benign nodular hyperplasia, occurs in the mucosal and submucosal glands, which are rarely sites of carcinoma. Benign hyperplasia causes urethral obstruction in its early stages because of its location in the mucosal and submucosal glands surrounding the urethra. The main gland is sensitive to androgens, whereas the periurethral glands are sensitive to androgens and estrogens. Acid phosphatase and prostatic-specific antigen (PSA) levels are used in the diagnosis of prostatic carcinoma and its metastasis.

Carcinoma of the breast occurs in about 1 of 10 females in the United States. By definition, a carcinoma is ductal in origin (answers a and e). Carcinoma of the breast metastasizes to the brain, lungs, and bones. The easy access of tumor cells to the extensive axillary blood supply and lymphatic drainage facilitates the spread of the cancer into the blood and lymph supplies. Self-examination and mammography are urged in an attempt to increase early diagnosis, which has reduced mortality of this disease.

Germ cell tumors (answer d) of the testes (testicular neoplasms) are classified as seminomas (germinomas) of pure germ cells and more heterogeneous cell types (eg, teratomas and embryonal carcinomas).

240. The answer is c. *(Young, pp 354-356. Mescher, pp 383-384.)* The organ shown in the light micrograph is the seminal vesicle that produces fructose, ascorbic acid, prostaglandins, and proteins responsible for coagulation of the semen. The seminal vesicle produces about 50% of the seminal fluid on a volume basis and comprises most of the ejaculate. The wall consists of smooth muscle and the mucosa of anastomosing "villus-like" folds. In comparison, the prostate is composed of 15 to 30 tubuloalveolar glands surrounded by fibromuscular tissue with concretions in the lumina. The prostate secretes a thin, opalescent fluid that contributes primarily to the first part of the ejaculate and includes acid phosphatase (answer d), spermine (a polyamine), fibrolysin (answer a), amylase, and zinc. Spermine oxidation results in the musky odor of semen, and fibrolysin is responsible for the liquefaction of semen after ejaculation. Acid phosphatase and prostatic-specific antigen are important for the diagnosis of metastases. The thyroid synthesizes T_3 and T_4 (answer b); the lactating mammary gland produces milk (answer e).

241. The answer is c. *(Young, pp 353-357. Mescher, p 382.)* The figure is a light micrograph of the epididymis which functions in the storage, maturation, and phagocytosis of sperm. In addition, the epididymis is involved in the absorption of testicular fluid and the secretion of glycoproteins involved in the inhibition of capacitation. The epithelium of the epididymis is pseudostratified with stereocilia (long microvilli), and the wall contains extensive connective tissue. The seminal vesicle **(answer b)** produces fructose and prostaglandins and contains a thick smooth muscle layer. Sperm are often found in the lumina. Spermiogenesis occurs in the testes **(answer a)**. Milk production occurs in the lactating mammary gland **(answer e)**, which contains alveoli and lactiferous ducts. Implantation occurs in the uterus **(answer d)**, which is lined by a simple columnar epithelium with endometrial glands that differ in arrangement, depending on the phase of the cycle (long and straight in the proliferative phase and S-shaped in the secretory phase). The myometrium, composed of smooth muscle, is hormone-sensitive and undergoes both hypertrophy and hyperplasia during pregnancy and atrophy after menopause, resulting in a shrinking of the uterus in postmenopausal women.

242. The answer is e. *(Kierszenbaum, p 573. Sadler, pp 246-248. Moore and Persaud, pp 263-266.)* The development of the testis from an indifferent gonad depends on the presence of the testis-determining factor, a gene on the short arm of the Y chromosome. During fetal development, the production of androgens by the developing testis results in masculinization of the indifferent gonadal ducts and the indifferent genitalia **(answer c)**. In the absence of androgens, female genitalia and female ducts (vagina, oviducts, and uterus) develop. In the mature male, testosterone is required for the initiation and maintenance of spermatogenesis as well as the structural and functional integrity of the accessory glands and ducts of the male reproductive system **(answers a, b, and d)**. Testosterone is bound to ABP, which is synthesized by the Sertoli cells under the influence of FSH. ABP is important for both the storage and delivery of androgens in the male ducts and accessory glands.

243. The answer is d. *(Mescher, pp 409-411. Kierszenbaum, pp 530, 651-654, 659. Strauss, pp 307-310.)* The mammary gland enlarges during pregnancy in response to several hormones, including prolactin synthesized by the anterior pituitary (not by the corpus luteum [**answer b**]), estrogen and progesterone synthesized by the corpus luteum, and placental lactogen. The alveoli at the end of the duct system respond to those hormones by cell proliferation, which increases the size of the mammary glands. Growth continues throughout pregnancy; however, secretion is most notable late in pregnancy. Milk is synthesized in the alveoli and is stored in their lumina before passage through the lactiferous ducts to the nipples. Secretion of milk lipids occurs by an apocrine mechanism whereby some apical cytoplasm is included with the secretory product. In comparison, milk proteins, such as the caseins, are secreted by exocytosis. Oxytocin is required for the release of milk from the mammary gland through the action of the myoepithelial cells that surround the alveoli and proximal (closer to the alveolus) portions of the duct system. Oxytocin is not required for milk synthesis (answer a). Arginine Vasopressin (AVP, antidiuretic hormone [ADH]) binds to receptors in the collecting tubules of the kidney and promotes resorption of water into the circulation (answer c). AVP stimulates water resorption by stimulating insertion of aquaporins (water channels) into the membranes of kidney tubules. Those channels transport solute-free water through collecting duct cells and into the blood, leading to a decrease in plasma osmolarity and an increased osmolarity of the urine. Neurohumoral reflexes are involved in the suckling-milk ejection response (answer e).

244. The answer is e. *(Fauci, pp 2332-2333. Moore, p 381.)* Attempts to counteract or repair the effects of a vasectomy (vasovasostomy) are often unsuccessful because of the development of antisperm antibodies. This lack of success occurs despite the fact that 90% of the patients undergoing vasovasostomy have sperm return to the ejaculate. In the case of vasectomy, sperm that have leaked from the male reproductive tract are viewed as foreign by immune surveillance and antibodies develop. The phagocytosis of sperm by macrophages plays a role in the development of antisperm antibodies that occurs following the ligation or removal of a segment of the vas deferens (answer d). Sperm are immunologically foreign because of a number of factors.

Spermatogenesis begins at puberty long after the development of self-recognition in the immune system (answer b). The blood-testis barrier protects developing sperm from exposure to systemic factors (answer a). The basal compartment containing the spermatogonia and preleptotene spermatocytes is exposed to plasma; however, the adluminal compartment, which contains primary and secondary spermatocytes, spermatids, and testicular sperm, prevents those antigens from entering the blood. The inability of cryptorchid testes to produce fertile sperm is related to the higher temperature in the abdomen than in the normal scrotal location (answer c).

245. The answer is b. *(Ross, p 787. Young, pp 369-373. Mescher, pp 397-403. Kierszenbaum, pp 626-629.)* The secretory phase of the menstrual cycle, shown in the photomicrograph, depends on progesterone secretion and follows the proliferative (follicular) phase. The menstrual phase occurs after the secretory phase. During the follicular phase (approximately days 4-16), estrogen produced by the ovaries drives cell proliferation in the base of endometrial glands and the uterine stroma. The proliferative phase culminates with ovulation **(answer a and c)**. The secretory phase (approximately days 16-25) is characterized by high progesterone levels from the corpus luteum, a tortuous appearance of the uterine glands, and apocrine secretion by the gland cells. During this phase, maximum endometrial thickness occurs. The menstrual phase (approximately days 26-30) is characterized by decreased glandular secretion and eventual glandular degeneration because of decreased production of both progesterone and estrogen by the theca lutein cells **(answer d)**. Contraction of coiled arteries and arterioles leads to ischemia and necrosis of the stratum functionale **(answer e)**. The events of the menstrual cycle are shown in High-Yield Facts, Figure 13.

246. The answer is d. *(Young, p 377. Mescher, p 408. Kierszenbaum, pp 630-632, 634.)* The low (4.0) pH of the vagina is maintained by bacterial metabolism of glycogen to form lactic acid **(answers a → c, e)**. The vagina is characterized by a stratified squamous epithelium that contains large accumulations of glycogen. Glycogen is released into the vaginal lumen and is subsequently metabolized to lactic acid by commensal lactobacilli. The low pH inhibits growth of a variety of microorganisms, but not sexually transmitted pathogens, such as *Trichomonas vaginalis*. Treatment for vaginal infections usually includes acidified carriers to reestablish a more acidic pH like that usually seen in mid-menstrual cycle.

247. The answer is d. *(Kierszenbaum, p 631. Young, p 377. Mescher, pp 407-408. Strauss, pp 262-270.)* The patient described in this question is probably pregnant. The delay in menstruation coupled with the presence of basophilic cells in a vaginal smear are clues. Ovulation is the midpoint of the cycle and should be more than a few days away **(answers a and b)**. She is relatively young for the onset of menopause and there are no other symptoms **(answer e)**. The vaginal epithelium varies little with the normal menstrual cycle. Exfoliative cytology can be used to diagnose cancer and to determine if the epithelium is under stimulation of estrogen and progesterone. The presence of basophilic cells in the smear with the Pap-staining method would indicate the presence of both estrogen and progesterone **(answer c)**. The data suggest the maintenance of the corpus luteum (ie, pregnancy).

248. The answer is e. (*Ross, pp 781-782. Young, pp 365, 366. Mescher, pp 393-394, 396. Kierszenbaum, pp 620-623.*) The structure in the photomicrograph is a corpus luteum. In the absence of the hormones necessary for maintenance of the corpus luteum (luteinizing hormone [LH] or human chorionic gonadotropin [hCG]), the corpus luteum regresses to form a corpus albicans, which consists primarily of fibrous connective tissue. Without LH or hCG, the uterine epithelium, which has undergone glandular proliferation in preparation for implantation, collapses and degenerates as part of menstruation (**answers a → d**). The corpus luteum forms from the granulosa and theca layers of the follicle following ovulation. The luteal phase is the second half of the menstrual period and follows the follicular phase during which follicles mature. The corpus luteum synthesizes progesterone in response to high LH levels. In each reproductive cycle, the production of LH stimulates development and maintenance of the corpus luteum, which is well formed by 12 to 14 days following ovulation. In the case of fertilization and subsequent implantation, the corpus luteum of pregnancy is maintained by hCG which is produced by the embryo.

249. The answer is c. (*Young, pp 369-376. Ross, p 791. Mescher, p 401.*) The spiral arteries of the endometrium (**A**) depend on specific estrogen/progesterone ratios for their development during the menstrual cycle. They pass through the basalis layer of the endometrium into the functional zone, and their distal ends are subject to degeneration with each menses. Specifically, it is the reduction in progesterone that induces spasmodic contractions leading to ischemia and the sloughing off of the stratum functionalis (**answers a, b, d, and e**). The basal layer is not affected because basal straight arteries provide independent blood supply to the area.

The straight arteries (**B**) are not subject to these hormonal changes. In the proliferative phase, the endometrium is only 1- to 3-mm thick, and the glands are straight, with the spiral arteries only slightly coiled. The diagram of the early secretory phase, which accompanies the question, shows an edematous endometrium that is 4-mm thick, with glands that are large, beginning to sacculate in the deeper mucosa, and coiled for their entire length. In the late secretory phase, the endometrium becomes 6- to 7-mm thick.

250. The answer is c. (*Young, pp 360-366. Kierszenbaum, pp 615-619, 633-634. Mescher, pp 389-392.*) The cells labeled **A** and **C** in the photomicrograph of the Graafian follicle are granulosa cells that produce plasminogen activator and collagenase. Those molecules, along with plasmin and prostaglandins, facilitate the rupture of the ovarian follicle, leading to ovulation. The increase in LH in midcycle induces production of collagenase and plasminogen activator. Those proteases facilitate ovulation by initiating connective tissue remodeling, including the breakdown of the basement membrane between thecal and granulosa layers. Connective tissue remodeling is involved in the process of follicular atresia. That process occurs throughout life and involves the death of follicular cells as well as oocytes, but there is no basement membrane between the theca interna and externa. In fact, there is an absence of a clear delineation between the theca interna and externa. Development of ovarian follicles begins with a primordial follicle that consists of flattened follicular cells surrounding a primary oocyte. During the follicular phase, those cells undergo mitosis to form multiple granulosa layers (primary follicle) in response to elevated levels of FSH and LH from the anterior pituitary. A glycoproteinaceous coat surrounds the oocyte and is called the zona pellucida. The connective tissue around the follicle differentiates into two layers: theca externa (**D**) and theca interna (**E**). The theca externa is closest to the ovarian stroma and consists of a highly vascular connective tissue. The theca interna synthesizes androgens (eg, androstenedione) in response to LH. Androgens are converted to estradiol by the action of an aromatase enzyme synthesized by the granulosa cells under the influence of FSH. Increased levels of estrogen from the ovary feed back to decrease FSH secretion from gonadotrophs in the anterior pituitary. *Liquor folliculi* is produced by the granulosa cells and is secreted between the cells. When cavities are first formed by the development of follicular fluid between the cells, the follicle is called secondary. When the antrum is completely formed, the follicle is called a mature (Graafian) follicle, and the antrum is completely filled with liquor folliculi. The granulosa cells form two structures. The corona radiata (**C**) represents those granulosa cells that remain attached to the zona pellucida. The cumulus oophorus (not labeled) represents those granulosa cells that surround the oocyte (**B**) and connect it to the wall. Structure **A** is the membrana granulosa.

251. The answer is b. (*Kumar, pp 1066-1067. Mescher, pp 409-411.*) Lactating mammary gland is shown in the photomicrograph. It synthesizes milk including antibodies from IgA secreting plasma cells in the connective tissue of the gland. The lactating mammary gland differs histologically from the thyroid gland **(answer a)** in the presence of lactiferous ducts for exocrine secretion compared to the endocrine secretion of the thyroid. The placenta removes waste products during gestation **(answer c)**; secretions from the seminal vesicle (fructose, prostaglandins, and other proteins **[answer d]**) facilitate clotting of ejaculated semen; and prostatic secretions (zinc, citric acid, antibiotic-like molecules, and enzymes) enhance sperm function **(answer e)**.

252. The answer is a. *(Fauci, pp 829, 831.)* PID often leads to scarring of the oviducts (fallopian or uterine tubes). As a result, sperm cannot reach the oocyte and a zygote cannot reach the uterine cavity for implantation **(answers b → h)**.

253. The answer is d. *(Sadler p 40.)* IVF is the best possible method for assisted reproductive technology (ART) in the case of this couple. GIFT and ZIFT place the gametes (GIFT) or zygote (ZIFT), respectively in the Fallopian tubes, the site of the structural problem **(answers a and b)**. TET is an ART synonym for ZIFT **(answer c)**. Drugs such as Clomid or gonadotropin treatment are effective when the ovary is the source of the infertility **(answers e and f)**. IVF usually requires gonadotropin treatment.

254. The answer is c. *(Fauci, pp 829, 831. Sadler, p 52.)* Rate of ectopic pregnancy in women with previous known PID is estimated as up to 10 times higher than in women with no previous history of PID **(answers a, b, d, and e)**.

Urinary System

Questions

255. Acetazolamide, a member of the sulfonamide family of antibacterial drugs, blocks carbonic anhydrase activity. Which of the following would most likely occur after treatment with acetazolamide?

a. Metabolic alkalosis
b. Increased excretion of hydrogen ions from the kidney
c. Decreased bicarbonate in the pancreatic juice
d. Increased bone resorption
e. Increased acid production by parietal cells
f. Inhibition of diuresis

256. A 39-year-old man reports that his urine is light tea-colored and is becoming progressively darker. It was "Coca-Cola" color during a recent upper respiratory infection. His blood pressure has increased steadily over the course of his annual physical examinations and serum IgA is now elevated. Renal biopsy shows IgA deposits in the region delineated with the asterisk in the accompanying transmission electron micrograph. What is the function of this cell?

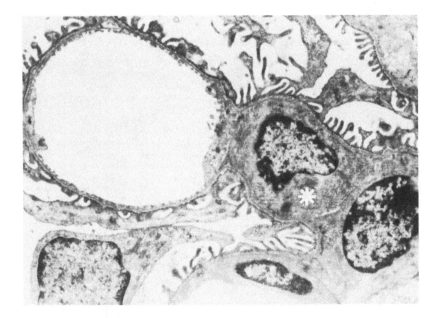

a. Synthesizes extracellular matrix for support of the capillary wall
b. Exerts an antithrombogenic effect
c. Forms the visceral layer of Bowman capsule
d. Separates the urinary space and the blood in the capillaries
e. Forms the filtration slits through the interdigitations of the pedicels

257. A 15-year-old adolescent presents with hematuria, hearing loss, lens dislocation, and cataracts. Genetic analysis shows a mutation of the *COL4A5* gene. A renal biopsy is performed. In which area labeled A to E on the accompanying electron micrograph would you expect to see the primary site of damage?

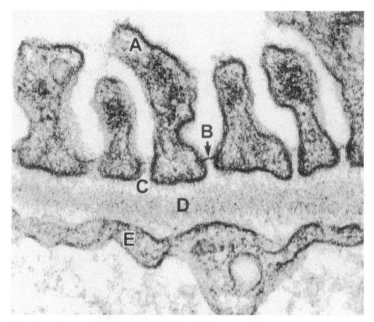

(Electron micrograph courtesy of Dr. Dale R. Abrahamson.)

a. Area A
b. Area B
c. Area C
d. Area D
e. Area E

258. A 14-year-old adolescent presents in the pediatric nephrology clinic with fatigue, malaise, anorexia, abdominal pain, and fever. She reports a loss of 6 lb in the last 2 months. Serum gamma globulin as well as the immunoglobulins: IgG, IgA, and IgM are all elevated. She is diagnosed with bilateral photophobia as a result of nongranulomatous uveitis. Her serum creatinine is 1.4 mg/dL (normal 0.6-1.2 mg/dL) and urinalysis of glucose and protein are 2⁺ on dipstick test confirmed by the laboratory at 8.0 g/dL and 0.95 g/dL, respectively. A renal biopsy is prepared for light and electron microscopy. Lymphocytes, plasma cells, and eosinophils are found within infiltrates with pathological change in the tubular basement membrane. The cell most affected is shown in the accompanying transmission electron micrograph. Which one of the following is a correct statement about this cell?

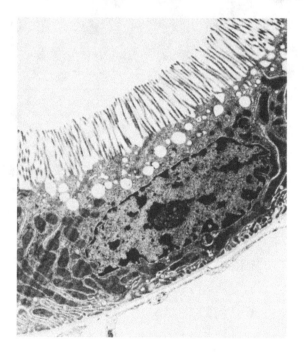

a. Impermeable to water despite the presence of ADH
b. The site of the countercurrent multiplier
c. The site of action of aldosterone
d. The source of renin
e. The primary site for the reduction of the tubular fluid volume

259. A 38-year-old African American man presents with blood pressure of 165/130 mm Hg, proteinuria, edema, and a recent weight gain of 15 lb. After a renal biopsy, he is diagnosed with nephrotic syndrome and focal segmental glomerulosclerosis. This disease is caused by a mutation in the *TRPC6* gene leading to malfunction in the cell shown between the arrows in the accompanying scanning electron microscope image. Which one of the following best describes the function of this cell?

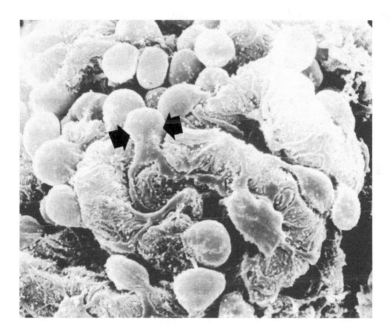

a. Regulates size selectivity and glomerular filtration rate
b. Secretes type II collagen that contributes to the glomerular basal lamina
c. Constitutes the parietal layer of Bowman capsule
d. Phagocytoses immunoglobulins trapped in the glomerular basal lamina
e. Regulates blood flow through the glomerular capillaries by contraction of the pedicels in response to Angiotensin II
f. Synthesizes the mesangial matrix
g. Lines the glomerular capillaries
h. Releases angiotensin II
i. Determines distal tubular osmolarity

260. In a patient with diabetes mellitus of 30 years' duration, complications related to kidney function may include which of the following?

a. Enhanced selectivity of the filtration barrier
b. Decreased permeability to plasma proteins
c. Increased glomerular filtration rate
d. Decreased secretion of aldosterone
e. Glycation of proteins in the basal lamina

261. A 45-year-old man presents with nephrolithiasis. The process of calcium oxalate stone formation as seen in this patient begins with Randall plaques found in the basement membrane of which one of the following structures found only in the renal medulla?

a. Proximal convoluted tubules
b. Distal convoluted tubules
c. Collecting ducts
d. Afferent arterioles
e. Thin loops of Henle

Urinary System

Answers

255. The answer is c. (*Kierszenbaum, pp 144-145, 160. Mescher, pp 264, 307.*) Carbonic anhydrase (CA) is a critical enzyme that plays an essential role in a number of cells by catalyzing the hydration of carbon dioxide and the dehydration of bicarbonate. In the pancreas, blocking CA results in a reduction in secretion of bicarbonate into the pancreatic juice by the pancreatic duct cells. Blockage of CA results in alkalinization of the urine and metabolic acidosis not alkalosis **(answer a)** because of loss of bicarbonate and the decrease in renal tubular excretion of hydrogen ions from the kidney **(answer b)**. In osteoclasts, blockage of CA would result in decreased bone resorption **(answer d)**. In parietal cells, blocking CA activity results in reduction in protons moving toward the lumen and bicarbonate toward the blood **(answer c)**. Acetazolamide is a diuretic **(answer f)**.

256. The answer is a. (*Kierszenbaum, pp 405-409. Mescher, pp 335, 339.*) The cell labeled in the transmission electron micrograph of the renal corpuscle is a mesangial cell that synthesizes extracellular matrix that supports the capillary wall. Mesangial cells are morphologically similar to pericytes found in association with other systemic blood vessels. The mesangial cells surround glomerular capillaries as illustrated in this transmission electron micrograph and function as phagocytes and regulators of glomerular blood flow. Mesangial cells synthesize cyclooxygenase-2 (COX-2 [a critical enzyme in prostaglandin synthesis]) and nitric oxide, two molecules involved in vasoactive regulation. Mesangial cell proliferation and matrix accumulation are major contributors to the development of glomerulosclerosis. Like endothelial cells, mesangial cells synthesize endothelin. Endothelial cells are anti-thrombogenic **(answer b)**. An endothelial cell within a glomerular capillary is shown below the mesangial cell. A podocyte with its processes in close association with the glomerular capillary is also observed below the mesangial cell. The podocytes form the visceral layer of the Bowman capsule **(answer c)** and possess processes that interdigitate to form the pedicels **(answer e)**. The outer layer of the Bowman capsule is formed by parietal cells, one of which is located in the lower left corner of the micrograph. The urinary space and the blood are separated by the glomerular basement membrane (**answer d**) formed from the fusion of the capillary and podocyte-produced basal laminae. The patient in the vignette has Berger disease, also known as IgA nephropathy, the most common cause of glomerulonephritis.

257. The answer is d. *(Kierszenbaum, pp 407-408. Mescher, pp 333-335, 338. Kumar, pp 931-932.)* The genetic mutation in *COL4A5* leads to a defect in the α-chains that comprise type IV collagen found in the lamina densa labeled **A** on the accompanying transmission electron micrograph of the basement membrane. The glomerular basement membrane will therefore show abnormal splitting and thinning in the lamina densa and overall thickening. The hematuria results from breakdown of the basal lamina allowing the passage of red blood cells and eventually protein (proteinuria). The patient is diagnosed with Alport syndrome resulting from a mutation of the α5 chain of type IV collagen. Remember that type IV collagen consists of three alpha chains forming a triple helix. The noncollagenous C-terminal (NC1) and the 7S N-terminal are particularly important for the cross-linking of type IV collagen. The cross-linking forms the scaffolding necessary for the normal filtration properties of the basal lamina. Proliferation of mesangial cells and increased production of mesangial matrix are typical of later stages of Alport syndrome when glomerulonephritis is a prominent feature of the disease.

The glomerular filtration barrier consists of the pedicel (**A**) of the podocyte, the basal lamina (**C** = lamina rara, **D** = lamina densa) synthesized by the podocyte, and the endothelial cell (**E**). The podocyte consists of a "cell body" of cytoplasm with long processes that encircle the glomerular basement membrane. The filtration slits are labeled **B** and are located between adjacent pedicels (foot processes of the podocytes). The remainder of the filtration barrier is formed by the glomerular basement membrane, which contains type IV collagen and heparan sulfate. As seen in the accompanying high magnification electron micrograph, there are three distinct layers within the glomerular basement membrane: (1) an electron-dense lamina densa (type IV collagen) in the center surrounded by (2) the lamina rara externa on the glomerular side and by (3) the lamina rara interna on the capillary endothelial side.

The glomerular filtration barrier is a physical and charge barrier that exhibits selectivity based on molecular size and charge. The presence of collagen type IV in the lamina densa of the basement membrane presents a physical barrier to the passage of large proteins from the blood to the urinary space. Glycosaminoglycans, particularly heparan sulfate, produce a polyanionic charge that binds cationic molecules. The foot processes are coated with a glycoprotein called podocalyxin, which is rich in sialic acid and provides mutual repulsion to maintain the structure of the filtration slits. It also possesses a large polyanionic charge for repulsion of large anionic proteins. Patients with a mutation in the gene encoding for nephrin are diagnosed with congenital nephritic syndrome characterized by proteinuria resulting in excessive edema. Nephrin is the key protein comprising the slit diaphragm; it functions to inhibit the passage of molecules through the filtration slits. It is an integral membrane protein, which is anchored by other proteins to the cytoskeleton of the pedicel of the podocyte.

258. The answer is e. (*Mescher, pp 335-338, 341, 342. Kumar, pp 938-948.*) Tubulointerstitial nephritis uveitis (TINU) is an autoimmune disease in which autoantibodies are targeted against the renal tubular cells. The transmission electron micrograph illustrates a proximal convoluted tubule cell, the primary site for reduction of the tubular fluid volume by reabsorption from the glomerular filtrate. The elaborate microvilli at the apical surface and the extensive endocytic vacuoles are "designed" for protein reabsorption and are the distinguishing features of proximal convoluted tubule cells. Numerous mitochondria, within basal folds, provide energy for transport. In the distal tubule, there are very few microvilli.

The afferent arterioles contain the juxtaglomerular cells, modified arterial smooth muscle cells that produce renin **(answer d)**, a major factor in blood pressure regulation. The thin loop of Henle is responsible for the production of the countercurrent multiplier **(answer b)**, which allows the kidneys to produce a hyperosmotic medulla. The multiplier moves Na^+ and Cl^- out of the ascending limb (which is impermeable to water) and into the medullary interstitial fluid. Subsequently, the descending limb, which is permeable to water, takes up the Na^+ and Cl^- from the interstitium. The vasa rectae adjust their osmolarity to that of the medulla.

The distal convoluted tubule (DCT) has the highest concentration of Na^+, K^+-ATPase. The DCT pumps Na^+ against a concentration gradient and is relatively impermeable to water, leading to the production of a hypotonic tubular fluid. The distal tubules empty into the connecting and collecting ducts, which are permeable to water under the regulation of ADH **(answer a)**. ADH stimulation increases collecting duct permeability to water, allowing the production of hyperosmotic urine. Without ADH, the urine leaving the kidney would be hypo-osmotic. The collecting duct principal cells are the ADH responsive cells and contain fewer mitochondria and basal infoldings than occur in the cells of the distal convoluted tubule. Aldosterone (answer c) also acts on the principal cells and secondarily on the thick ascending limb of Henle to increase reabsorption of NaCl.

259. The answer is a. *(Kierszenbaum, pp 405-408. Mescher, pp 333-334, 337, 338, 339. Ross, pp 653-660.)* The cell in the scanning electron micrograph is a podocyte (visceral epithelial cell) that, along with other factors, regulates size selectivity and the filtration rate of the glomerular basement membrane. Each podocyte has foot processes, called pedicels, that extend around the glomerular capillaries and interdigitate with pedicels from adjacent podocytes. The space between adjacent pedicels is the filtration slit and adjacent pedicels are linked by filtration slit diaphragms comprised of nephrin (answer c). Basement membrane collagen, type IV (not type II), is synthesized by podocytes and glomerular endothelial cells (answer b). Mesangial cells are involved in turnover of the glomerular basal lamina and phagocytose immunoglobulins trapped in the basal lamina (answer d). They contract in response to angiotensin II binding thus regulating blood flow through the glomerular capillaries (answer e), and synthesize the mesangial matrix (answer f). Endothelial cells line the glomerular capillaries (answer g) and possess many aquaporin water channels. Angiotensin II receptors are found on mesangial cells. Angiotensin II is formed from angiotensin I by endothelial cells, particularly in the lung (answer h).

The patient in the vignette has focal segmental glomerulosclerosis resulting from a mutation in the TRPC6 cation-channel protein, found in the pedicels. The mutation leads to impaired channel function and decreased adaptation to physiological challenges.

The macula densa is a portion of the distal tubule that is specialized for determination of distal tubular osmolarity (answer i).

260. The answer is e. *(Fauci, pp 1749, 1762-1764. Kumar, pp 934-995, 1141-1143. Kierszenbaum, pp 404-409. Mescher, pp 333-334, 338.)* In patients with long-term diabetes mellitus, glycation (nonenzymatic addition of sugar to proteins and other molecules) occurs in response to high-blood glucose levels. The critical renal changes are the thickening of the glomerular basement membrane, elimination of the separation of laminae rarae and densa, loss of anionic repulsion of sugar groups, and obliteration of the filtration slits. These renal changes are known as nephrotic syndrome and lead to loss of selectivity of the filtration barrier (answer a) and increased permeability to proteins (answer b). This causes the loss of protein from the blood to the urine (proteinuria). The liver adjusts to the proteinuria by producing more proteins (eg, albumin). After continued proteinuria, the liver is unable to produce sufficient protein, which results in hypoalbuminemia leading to an overall decrease in osmotic pressure. Edema then occurs as fluid leaves the vasculature to enter the tissues. The movement of fluid from the vasculature to the tissues results in reduced plasma volume and decreased glomerular filtration rate (GFR [answer c]). The overall effect is further edema because of compensatory release of aldosterone (answer d) coupled with reduced GFR and the already existing edema.

Glycation results in the production of advanced glycation end-products (AGE, see figure that follows), which alters the properties of the glomerular basement membrane. The cellular receptor for AGE is called RAGE and is a multiligand member of the immunoglobulin superfamily of cell surface molecules. In addition to its role in diabetes, RAGE interacts with molecular pathways that regulate homeostasis, development, and inflammation and plays a role in pathological conditions such as Alzheimer disease and diabetes mellitus. Binding of a ligand to RAGE activates key cell signaling pathways, such as p21 (ras), MAP kinases, and NF-kappa-B (NFκB), thereby reprogramming cellular characteristics. The interactions and terminology are further complicated by the presence of ENRAGE (extracellular

Dangers of Diabetic Hyperglycemia

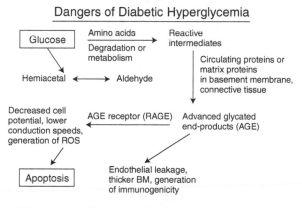

AGE = advanced glycation end-products,   RAGE = age receptor,

BM = basement membrane,   ROS = reactive oxygen species

newly identified RAGE-binding protein) that interacts with cellular RAGE on endothelial cells, macrophages, lymphocytes, and other cells to activate proinflammatory mediators. Interactions between AGE, RAGE, and ENRAGE may explain many diabetic complications including delayed wound healing. AGE derivatization is probably nonspecific and involves not only basal lamina-specific molecules, but also a vast array of extracellular and intracellular proteins (transcription factors, structural proteins, and membrane transporters). Hence, cellular coordination/communication becomes slowly, but progressively hampered in the kidney and other organs.

261. The answer is e. (*Mescher, pp 334, 335, 343.*) Only the thin loops of Henle are found exclusively in the medulla. The collecting ducts are found in both the cortex and medulla of the kidney **(answer c)**. Cortical collecting ducts are found in the medullary rays, whereas medullary collecting ducts are found in the medulla and lead into the papillary duct. The convoluted portions of the proximal and distal tubules are found exclusively in the cortex **(answers a and b)**. Afferent arterioles **(answer d)** are found adjacent to the vascular pole of the glomeruli within the cortex. Plaques, defined as sites of interstitial crystal deposition at or near the papilla tip, are found in kidneys of calcium oxalate-stone formers.

Eye and Ear

Questions

262. A 42-year-old woman underwent LASIK for myopia in both her eyes. In LASIK, the shape of the cornea is flattened. This will result in which of the following?

a. Decreased refraction of light by the cornea
b. A decreased amount of light entering through the cornea
c. Conversion of the cornea from a "stationary" to an "adjustable" form of refraction
d. Maintenance of the lens in a more flattened state
e. Focusing of light on the retina at a point other than the fovea

263. Retinal detachment most commonly results from which of the following?

a. Local swelling in specific retinal layers
b. Leakage of blood from the inner retinal capillaries
c. Fluid accumulation between the retina and the retinal pigment epithelium (RPE)
d. Impaired pumping of water toward the photoreceptors by the RPE
e. Increased phagocytosis of outer segments by the RPE cells

264. A 47-year-old woman is referred to her ophthalmologist. She reports difficulty with tasks at night or in dark places that has occurred for the past 4 to 5 years. Specifically, she has trouble walking in dim-lit rooms and the movie theater. She has given up night driving and also describes a prolonged adaptation period going from light to dark. She describes her daylight vision as "tunneled" as she frequently walks into furniture. A family history indicates that her father had a similar condition. In this disease, a single point mutation in the rhodopsin gene leads to disruption of signal transduction. Visual transduction involves which of the following?

a. Inactivation of phosphodiesterase
b. Increase in cGMP levels
c. Conversion of all-*trans*-retinal to 11-*cis*-retinal
d. Closing of a Na^+ channel
e. Depolarization of the rod cell membrane

265. The RPE is characterized by which of the following?

a. The presence of the photoreceptor (rod and cone) perikarya
b. Phagocytosis of worn-out components of photoreceptor cells
c. Origin from the inner layer of the optic cup during embryonic development
d. Presence of amacrine cells
e. Synthesis of aqueous humor

266. A 47-year-old woman, who was diagnosed with type I diabetes mellitus at age 12 experiences floaters and blurred vision. She is diagnosed with diabetic retinopathy. Which of the following occurs in this complication of diabetes?

a. Reduction in the thickness of the basal lamina of small retinal vessels
b. Microaneurysms
c. Decreased capillary permeability
d. Increased retinal blood flow
e. Loss of phagocytic ability of the pigmented epithelium

267. Which of the following statements describes the structure labeled B in the figure below?

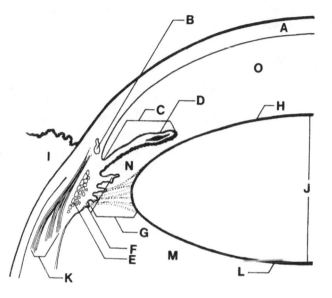

a. It is responsible for the production of aqueous humor
b. It is the location of vitreous humor outflow from the posterior chamber
c. It is a site of blockage in glaucoma
d. It is involved in the regulation of accommodation
e. It is the major corneal artery

268. Data from the photoreceptors are integrated in which of the following?

a. Outer segment of the rod
b. Inner segment of the rod
c. Ganglion cell layer
d. Inner nuclear layer of the retina
e. Outer plexiform layer of the retina

269. The direction in which vestibular hair cell stereocilia are deflected is important for which of the following reasons?

a. Differentiates between type I and type II hair cells
b. Determines whether cells are depolarized or hyperpolarized
c. Determines whether linear or angular acceleration is detected
d. Determines the direction of blood flow in the stria vascularis
e. Is determined by the frequency of the sound

270. A 3-year-old girl who has had numerous episodes of otitis media is referred to an otorhinolaryngologist. She has a hearing deficit and delayed speech milestones. Inflammation and diminished movement of the tympanic membrane with insufflation is revealed by pneumatic otoscopy. There is decreased visibility of the landmarks of the middle ear. A myringotomy is carried out and her hearing returns to normal. Which of the following is directly involved in the normal sound transduction in this patient?

a. Deflection of the tectorial membrane
b. Shearing motion of the tympanic membrane against hair cell stereocilia
c. Movement of the tectorial membrane resulting in hair cell depolarization
d. Equalization of the pressure in the middle ear and nasopharynx by the Eustachian tube
e. Vibration at the round window via the stapes

271. During a boxing match, a 23-year-old boxer sustains a direct blow to his right ear. He presents with dizziness, vertigo, imbalance, nausea, vomiting, tinnitus, and fullness in the ears. His vertigo increases with activity and is relieved by rest. He has some hearing loss. The symptoms worsen with coughing, sneezing, or blowing his nose, as well as with exertion and activity. He is diagnosed with a perilymphatic fistula. The fistula allows leakage of perilymph. In which of the following structures is perilymph normally found?

a. Utricle
b. Saccule
c. Semicircular canals
d. Scala media
e. Scala tympani

272. A 44-year-old woman is referred to an otorhinolaryngologist with attacks of vertigo that are accompanied by vomiting and nausea. She has sudden falls that occur without warning. The attacks are preceded by fullness in one ear, hearing fluctuation, and tinnitus. Her family tells her that her "eyes jump" during these attacks. Audiometry and electrocochleography detect sensorineural hearing loss and endolymphatic hydrops. She is diagnosed with Ménière disease. How is the structure labeled "D" in the accompanying diagram related to Ménière disease?

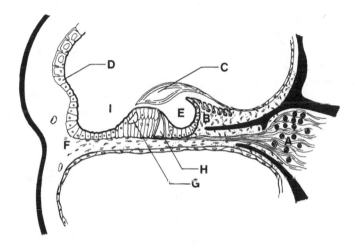

a. Transduction of the sound to a nerve impulse
b. Support of the organ of Corti
c. Overproduction of perilymph
d. Underproduction of perilymph
d. Forms the tectorial membrane
e. Overproduction of endolymph
f. Underproduction of endolymph

273. Detection of angular acceleration is accomplished by which of the following structures?

a. Maculae of the utricle and saccule
b. Hair cells of the organ of Corti
c. Cristae ampullaris of the semicircular canals
d. Interdental cells
e. Pillar cells

Eye and Ear

Answers

262. The answer is a. (*Fauci, pp 181, 1279. Riordan-Eva, p 422.*) LASIK (Laser-assisted in situ keratomileusis) has largely replaced radial, or refractive, keratotomy. Both methods can be used to decrease the refraction of light by the cornea **(answer b)**. LASIK alters corneal (not lens) anatomy to create a new shape that is more flattened in the center and higher at the periphery of the cornea **(answer d)**. This occurs because intraocular pressure will cause a reshaping of the cornea due to induced weakness produced by the laser removal of tissue. The purpose of the procedure is to reduce myopia and eliminate the need for corrective lenses. The reduction in curvature of the central portion of the cornea results in decreased refractive power of the cornea **(answers c and e)**. The removal of tissue and the degree of correction required is estimated by computer simulations. LASIK can be used to correct nearsightedness (myopia), farsightedness (hyperopia), and astigmatism, but does not correct presbyopia (an age-related progressive loss of the ability to focus at near). Most LASIK patients have myopia.

263. The answer is c. (*Riordan-Eva, pp 188, 196-198.*) Retinal detachment is the result of the accumulation of fluid between the retina and the RPE **(answers a, b, d, and e)**. In one type of detachment, rhegmatogenous retinal detachment, fluid accumulates after a break occurs in the retina. Detachments without breaks in the retina are called nonrhegmatogenous, or serous, detachments. Vitreous degeneration usually is a prerequisite for retinal detachment that results in the breaking of the retina. The breakdown of the vitreous produces traction on the retina, which may already possess an inherent area of weakness. The site of retinal detachment is the area between the inner and outer layers of the embryonic optic cup and represents a relatively weak area of adherence between the retinal and RPE layers.

264. The answer is d. (*Mescher, pp 420-421, 428. Kierszenbaum, pp 264-268.*) Visual transduction involves closing of the Na⁺ channel in rod cells in response to photons of light. Rhodopsin is the visual pigment found in the outer segments of rod cells and is composed of retinal, a vitamin A derivative, bound to opsin. When photons strike rhodopsin, 11-*cis*-retinal is isomerized to 11-*trans*-retinal (**answer c**) resulting in bleaching, which represents the dissociation of retinal from opsin. The conformationally-altered opsin then acts on transducin, a G protein that couples bleaching to cGMP through the action of a phosphodiesterase (**answer a**), the enzyme that cleaves cGMP to GMP. Breakdown of cGMP (**answer b**) results in the closing of the gated Na⁺ channels, a reduction in permeability to Na⁺, and hyperpolarization of the cell membrane. The signal spreads to the inner segment and through gap junctions to nearby photoreceptor cells. In the presence of cGMP, the Na⁺ channel remains open; in its absence, the channel closes and the cell hyperpolarizes. Therefore, the rods and cones differ from other receptors in that hyperpolarization of the cell membranes (**answer e**) occurs rather than the depolarization that occurs in other neural systems. Closing the channel slows down the release of the visual transmitter. The patient in the vignette has retinitis pigmentosa (RP), the most prevalent hereditary retinal degenerative disease. RP has been linked to over 30 different gene mutations; however, there is a final common pathway leading to death of rods. Nyctalopia (night blindness) is usually the first symptom followed by progressive loss of peripheral vision.

265. The answer is b. (*Mescher, pp 418-419, 422.*) The RPE is a single layer of cells that phagocytose old components of photoreceptor cells. It is derived from the outer layer of the optic cup (**answer c**) and is continuous from the ora serrata retinae to the optic nerve. Microvilli are prominent on the apical surfaces of the RPE and play an important role in the maintenance of the blood-retinal barrier. In addition, the RPE synthesizes melanin and stores vitamin A for the photoreceptor cells. Rod and cone perikarya and amacrine cells are found in the photosensitive retina derived from the inner layer of the optic cup (**answers a, c, and d**). Aqueous humor is synthesized by the non-pigmented epithelium of the ciliary body (**answer e**).

266. The answer is b. (*Kumar, pp 1359-1363. Fauci, p 2287. Riordan-Eva, pp 191-193. Kierszenbaum, p 564.*) Retinopathy is one of the major complications of diabetes mellitus. In diabetic retinopathy, pathologic changes usually begin with thickening of the basement membrane of small retinal vessels (**answer a**). The abnormal vessels develop microaneurysms, which leak and hemorrhage (**answer c**) with resultant ischemia (**answer d**) of the retinal tissue. New vessels proliferate in response to ischemia and production of angiogenic factors, such as vascular endothelial growth factor (VEGF). Loss of phagocytic capacity (**answer e**) of the RPE occurs in retinal dystrophy, but is not a characteristic of diabetic retinopathy. Retinopathy also occurs with prematurity when initial retinal vascularization is disturbed.

267. The answer is c. (*Mescher, pp 414, 417, 418.*) The structure labeled B is the sinus venosus sclerae (canal of Schlemm), which carries aqueous humor to the scleral veins and the systemic vasculature. Blockage of the canal of Schlemm, the trabecular meshwork, or the scleral veins results in glaucoma. The overall figure shows the region of the iridocorneal angle and other associated structures in the eye. This region is extremely important in the production and outflow of the aqueous humor and in the distribution of zonule fibers to the lens. The iris (**C**) contains both sphincter (**D**) and dilator muscles, which work in opposition to one another and are innervated by parasympathetic and sympathetic fibers, respectively. The center of the iris is a "hole," the pupil.

The ciliary body contains the ciliary muscles (**E** and **K**). The ciliary muscles stretch the choroid and relax the lens, which is essential for the process of lens accommodation. The ciliary processes (**F**) extend from the ciliary body and produce aqueous humor. They are also the origin of the zonule fibers (**G**), which anchor the lens. The zonule fibers are involved in accommodation. When the ciliary muscles contract, causing forward displacement of the ciliary body, the tension on the zonule fibers is reduced, which leads to an increase in lens thickness and maintenance of focus. The aqueous humor produced by the ciliary processes (**F**) is transported into the posterior chamber (**N**) and flows into the anterior chamber (**O**) through the pupil. Outflow from the anterior chamber occurs through the trabecular meshwork at the iridocorneal angle and flows through the canal of Schlemm.

The cornea (**A**) forms the transparent, avascular anterior portion of the eye. The outer anterior surface of the cornea is covered by an epithelium. Beneath the epithelium is Bowman membrane, the corneal stroma, Descemet membrane, and the endothelium (at the posterior surface of the cornea), which lines the anterior boundary of the anterior chamber.

The lens (**J**) is formed embryologically from a thickening of the surface ectoderm called the lens placode, which eventually forms a lens vesicle.

Lens fiber production continues throughout life. New fibers are added under the anterior epithelium (**L**), and contain nuclei and other light-scattering organelles, which disappear toward the center of the lens. The lens-specific cytoskeletal proteins that maintain lens fiber conformation and transparency are: the crystallins (members of the lenticular chaperone family) and the beaded-filament structural proteins, filensin, and phakinin ([CP49] members of the intermediate filament protein family). Interactions between these unique proteins and the cytoskeleton maintain normal lens fiber structure and are modified during normal aging, leading to decreased flexibility and onset of presbyopia. Mutations in the genes transcribing those proteins are associated with cataract formation. The lens is surrounded by a capsule (**H**).

The three compartments of the eye include the posterior and anterior chambers, which are filled with aqueous humor, and the vitreous body (**M**), which is filled with a gel consisting of hydrated hyaluronic acid and other glycosaminoglycans.

The conjunctiva is the mucosa, or lining, of the eyelid and is labeled **I** in the figure.

268. The answer is d. (*Mescher, pp 419, 424, 426.*) The inner nuclear layer is responsible for the integration of data from adjacent photoreceptors (**answers a → c and e**). The retina consists of 10 layers:

1. The RPE is derived from the outer wall of the optic cup. The RPE functions in the phagocytosis of rod disks.
2. The photoreceptor layer consisting of the rods and cones is the outer layer of the retina.
3. The outer limiting membrane is formed by the junctional complexes between Müller cells and the membranes of photoreceptor cells.
4. The outer nuclear layer contains the nuclei of rod and cone cells and the surrounding cytoplasm (perikarya).
5. The outer plexiform layer contains rod and cone synapses as well as the cell processes of bipolar, horizontal, and photoreceptor cells.
6. The inner nuclear (bipolar) layer is composed of the nuclei and perikarya of the bipolar and amacrine cells as well as the nuclei of Müller cells.
7. The inner plexiform layer consists of amacrine cells dispersed between the processes of bipolar and ganglion cells. This layer is responsible for modulation of signals from the ganglion to the photoreceptor cells.

8. The ganglion cell layer contains the ganglion cells separated by the cytoplasm of astrocyte-like glia (Müller cells).
9. The nerve fiber layer consists of axons of the ganglion cells that will form the optic nerve.
10. The internal limiting membrane is located between the vitreous body and the retina. The photoreceptors are of two types: rods and cones. The nuclei of the rods and cones are found in the outer nuclear layer and extend across the outer limiting membrane in one direction and toward the outer plexiform layer in the other direction. The outer segment is the photon-sensitive portion of the rod and cone and contains membranous disks. Rhodopsin is composed of opsin and retinal. It is responsible for transduction of light (photons) into hyperpolarization of the cell membrane. Rhodopsin is present in the disks of the outer segment of the rod. The inner segment contains numerous mitochondria, glycogen, and protein synthetic apparatus. Rods are responsible for night vision, whereas the cones are responsible for color vision, which is best resolved at the fovea. The fovea, which is the center of the macula, is composed exclusively of cones and is the site of optimal resolution.

The choroid is a highly vascular layer that consists of three parts: stroma, choriocapillaris, and Bruch membrane. Blood supply to the retina is derived from the choriocapillaris of the choroid. The sclera is a layer of relatively avascular dense connective tissue.

269. The answer is b. *(Kandel, pp 597, 614-615, 803.)* The vestibular hair cells are the sensory transduction system of the inner ear and are responsible for the conversion of mechanical energy into an electrical signal for cranial nerve VIII. These cells are called hair cells because their surface contains stereocilia. These are modified microvilli that contain a large number of actin filaments and extend from the surface of the cell. The stereocilia are different lengths and are arranged in order by size with a large kinocilium at one end. The arrangement of the stereocilia is very important because bending in one direction (ie, toward the kinocilium) depolarizes the cell and leads to excitation, whereas bending them in the other direction (ie, away from the kinocilium) results in hyperpolarization and inhibition **(answers a, c → e)**. The classification of type of hair cell (I or II) is based on the pattern of efferent and afferent innervation.

270. The answer is c. (*Mescher, pp 434-437.*) Movement of the tectorial membrane results in hair cell depolarization and the release of neurotransmitter onto afferent endings of the auditory (VIII) cranial nerve leads to initiation of an action potential **(answer b).** Sound waves are directed toward the tympanic membrane by the pinna and the external auditory canal of the external ear. The vibration of the tympanic membrane is transmitted to the oval window by way of the ossicles of the middle ear. Induction of waves in the perilymph results in the movement of the basilar and vestibular membranes toward the scala tympani and causes the round window to bulge outward **(answer e).** The movement of the hair cells is facilitated because the tectorial membrane is rigid **(answer a)** and the pillar cells form a pivot. The stabilization of the pressure between the middle ear and the nasopharynx is not directly related to the mechanism of sound transmission **(answer d).**

271. The answer is e. (*Mescher, pp 427, 431.*) The scala tympani contains perilymph. Endolymph is similar to extracellular fluid (high K^+, low Na^+). It is found in the utricle, saccule, semicircular canals, and scala media (cochlear duct), which are parts of the membranous labyrinth **(answers a, b, c, and d).** Endolymph is synthesized by the highly vascular stria vascularis in the lateral wall of the scala media. The endolymphatic sac and duct are responsible for absorption of endolymph and the endocytosis of molecules from the endolymph.

272. The answer is e. (*Young, pp 415-421, 423. Mescher, pp 427, 431, 434, 436. Fauci, pp 145, 202-203.*) The stria vascularis **(D)** is found in the lateral wall of the cochlear duct (scala media, I) and is responsible for the production of endolymph. Patients with Ménière disease present with a triad of vertigo, sensorineural hearing loss, and tinnitus resulting from overproduction of endolymph and distension of the endolymph-filled system of the cochlea. The organ of Corti is found within the cochlear duct and contains the hair cells that are responsible for transduction of the sound to a nerve impulse. It rests on the basilar membrane, which separates it from the epithelial lining of the tympanic cavity. The inner tunnel **(H)** of the organ of Corti separates the outer from the inner hair cells. The outer hair cells possess microvilli that are attached to the tectorial membrane **(C).** In contrast, the inner hair cells are unattached. Supportive cells include the phalangeal and pillar cells, which are not labeled on the figure. The spiral lamina is a bony structure that protrudes from the modiolus. The spiral limbus (**B**) is a connective tissue structure superior to the unattached edge of the spiral lamina. Along the outer wall of the canal of the organ of Corti is a thickened projection of periosteum known as the spiral ligament (**F**). The spiral ganglion is labeled **A** on the figure and contains bipolar cells. Peripheral processes of spiral ganglion cells reach the organ of Corti, whereas central processes terminate in nuclei located in the medulla. The internal spiral tunnel is labeled **E** in the figure.

273. The answer is c. (*Mescher, pp 427-429, 431-432, 434. Sadler, pp 327-330. Moore and Persaud, pp 430-434.*) The semicircular canals, which extend from the utricle, contain the cristae ampullares and detect angular acceleration. The utricle represents the dorsal portion of the otocyst-derived inner ear; the saccule represents the ventral portion. Both the utricle and saccule contain maculae that detect linear acceleration (**answer a**). The maculae of the utricle and saccule are perpendicular to one another. These maculae contain type I and type II hair cells, which differ in their innervation. The hair cells have stereocilia and a kinocilium embedded in a membrane that contains otoconia (statoconia) composed of calcium carbonate. The stereocilia and kinocilia are embedded in the cupola, which does not contain the otoconia found in the maculae. The endolymph turns right when the head turns left and vice versa. Movement stimulates the stereocilia and induces depolarization. The interdental cells (**answer d**) produce the tectorial membrane, which is essential for the development of the shearing force for sound transduction in the organ of Corti (**answer b**). It detects sound vibration and is responsive to variation in the frequency of sound waves. There are two types of pillar cells: inner and outer. The pillar cells along with the inner and outer (Deiters) phalangeal cells provide cellular mechanical coupling between the mechanosensory hair cells and the basilar membrane (**answer e**).

Head and Neck

Questions

274. When a physician examines the "corneal reflex" in a patient, she/he touches the cornea with a wisp of cotton that causes the eyelid to rapidly shut. As with most reflexes, one is testing both the afferent information that is carried back to the central nervous system and the reflex motor response. What specific cranial nerve branches are responsible for both the afferent and efferent parts of the corneal reflex?

a. Short ciliary nerve (CN III); zygomatic and temporal branches of the facial nerve (CN VII)
b. Short ciliary nerve (CN III); oculomotor nerve (CN III)
c. Long ciliary nerve (CN V^1); zygomatic branches of the facial nerve (CN VII)
d. Long ciliary nerve (CN V^1); infraorbital branch of the trigeminal nerve (CN V^2)
e. Infraorbital nerve (CN V^2); zygomatic branches of the facial nerve (CN VII)

275. A 79-year-old man is brought to a family practice office by his wife because he "keeps running into things" on his right side. His wife also reports that he seems to ignore objects on his right. Testing his vision in each eye his physician determines that the patient cannot see anything in the right visual field of either eye. The physician orders a head MRI because he suspects which one of the following?

a. A pituitary tumor compressing his optic chiasm
b. A tumor in the medial wall of the right orbit compressing the optic nerve
c. An aneurysm of the left middle cerebral artery compressing the left optic tract
d. A tumor in the middle cranial fossa compressing the right optic tract
e. An aneurysm in the arterial supply to the visual cortex

276. A 23-year-old woman presents with concern over a hyperpigmentation spot that has enlarged after her weeklong vacation in Cancun, Mexico. The woman is blond with fair skin. The pigmented spot is on her cheek, below the medial portion of her eye and lateral to the dorsal surface of the nose, but just above her labial malar (nasolabial) skin fold. The spot has grown to about 6 mm laterally and 4 mm cranially/caudally with irregular borders and two tones of brown pigmentation. What two regional lymph nodes should specifically be palpated during her physical examination?

a. Buccal and submandibular nodes
b. Buccal and submental nodes
c. Jugulodigastric and juguloomohyoid nodes
d. Parotid and mastoid nodes
e. Submental and submandibular nodes

277. The central nervous system is bathed in 135 to 150 mL of cerebrospinal fluid (CSF). In adults, this fluid is produced at the rate of 450 to 500 mL per day from the choroid plexus within the ventricular system and should have a pressure of less than 20 cm of water. Most of the absorption of cerebrospinal fluid occurs at arachnoid villi. The arachnoid villi allow cerebrospinal fluid to pass between which of the following two spaces?

a. Choroid plexus and subdural space
b. Subarachnoid space and subdural space
c. Subarachnoid space and superior sagittal sinus
d. Subdural space and cavernous sinus
e. Superior sagittal sinus and jugular vein

278. A 44-year-old attorney presents to a family practice office with a hat on her head and wearing dark sunglasses even though it is an overcast January day. Upon taking off her glasses and hat a series of vesicles are visible above her left eye continuing to her hairline. The vesicles stop at the midline of her forehead, but extend onto the dorsal surface of her nose and onto her left upper eyelid. There are no vesicles around or above her ears. She reports that she had pain in a similar pattern for a couple of days before the vesicles suddenly appeared. She can think of no change in habits or travel to account for the vesicles; she has infrequently left her home and office during the past 2 weeks since she is preparing for a case before the Cailfiornia Supreme Court. She had both chickenpox and mumps as a child. What is the working diagnosis and explanation for the unique pattern of the vesicles?

a. Herpes zoster affecting the mandibular division of the trigeminal cranial nerve
b. Herpes zoster affecting the ophthalmic division of the trigeminal cranial nerve
c. Herpes zoster affecting the zygomatic branch facial cranial nerve
d. Mumps affecting the maxillary division of the facial cranial nerve
e. Mumps affecting her parotid salivary gland

279. A 28-year-old man is treated in the emergency department (ED) for a superficial gash on his forehead. The wound is bleeding profusely, but examination reveals no fracture. While the wound is being sutured, he relates that while he was using an electric razor, he remembers becoming dizzy and then waking up on the floor with "blood everywhere." The physician suspects a hypersensitive cardiac reflex. The patient's epicranial aponeurosis (galea aponeurotica) is penetrated, resulting in severe gaping of the wound. The structure overlying the epicranial aponeurosis is which one of the following?

a. A layer containing blood vessels
b. Bone
c. The dura mater
d. The periosteum (pericranium)
e. The tendon of the epicranial muscles (occipitofrontalis)

280. A 52-year-old woman is referred to the dermatologist. Unlike many patients she is not concerned about the lines and wrinkles that are beginning to appear on her face, but she is concerned because she has been told repeatedly by friends that she looks "sad" recently. She has brought in a 10-year-old picture of herself. When examining her face you notice that the inferior corners of her mouth droop downward. Which muscle of facial expression will the dermatologist inject with botulinum toxin (Botox) to improve her smile?

a. Depressor anguli oris muscle
b. Mentalis muscle
c. Orbicularis oculi muscle
d. Orbicularis oris muscle
e. Zygomaticus major muscle

281. A 19-year-old teenager comes into the emergency department (ED) at 5:00 PM with cotton in his nose and blood running down the front of his T-shirt nearly to his belt. He was in the ED the night before. The previous night, gauze soaked in procoagulant had stopped the problem, but not now. No history of trauma was reported. Upon removing the blood soaked gauze, blood pumped from an artery in Kiesselbach area, on the nasal septum, just superior and posterior to the external nasal aperture. An ENT was called in to cauterize the boy's nose. There are four major blood vessels that normally supply blood to the Kiesselbach area. Describe how, for at least two of the arteries, a physician can have the boy apply pressure elsewhere (not directly on the pulsating artery) that may successfully cut off blood to the pulsating artery, while the ENT cauterizes the blood vessel.

a. Hold both sides of the bridge of the nose at the apex from the exterior.
b. Hold both sides of the upper lip between his fingers.
c. Hold both sides of the nose at the junction of the nasal bones with the lateral nasal cartilages.
d. Apply pressure from the oral cavity over the incisive foramen.
e. a and b
f. b and d

Questions 282 and 283

A 42-year-old Asian woman presents to her family practice physician with a bulge in the middle of her neck in front of her trachea. The growth has become bothersome when she swallows and has been noticed by family and friends. An ENT physician performs a fine-needle biopsy, taking samples from both the right and left side of the thyroid gland and sends the sample for pathological analysis. The pathology report is returned with a diagnosis of papillary thyroid cancer and the ENT recommends surgical removal of all of the thyroid gland.

282. What risk factors does the surgeon warn the patient about before reassuring the woman that he has removed hundreds of cancerous thyroid glands without such complications?

a. Creation of a tracheostomy stoma for breathing and loss of peristaltic function due to cutting of the vagus nerve
b. Creation of a tracheostomy stoma for breathing and placement of a gastric stoma to bypass loss of swallowing function
c. Loss of peristaltic function due to cutting of the vagus nerve and hypoparathyroidism due to removal of the parathyroid glands
d. Loss of voice due to creation of a tracheostomy stoma for breathing and loss of peristaltic function due to cutting of the vagus nerve
e. Loss of singing voice due to cutting the recurrent laryngeal nerve and hypoparathyroidism due to removal of the parathyroid glands

283. Which muscles must be retracted to gain access to the thyroid gland during its removal?

a. Longus coli, longus capitus, and anterior scalene muscles
b. Mylohyoid, anterior belly of the digastrics, genioglossus, and geniohyoid muscles
c. Platysma, sternohyoid, sternothyroid, and omohyoid muscles
d. Superior, middle, and inferior pharyngeal constrictors
e. Trapezius, rhomboids, and levator scapulae muscles

284. A 53-year-old woman has paralysis of the right side of her face that produces an expressionless and drooping appearance. She is unable to close her right eye, has difficulty chewing and drinking, perceives sounds as annoyingly intense in her right ear, and experiences some pain in her right external auditory meatus. Physical examination reveals loss of the blink reflex in the right eye on stimulation of either cornea and loss of taste from the anterior two-thirds of the tongue on the right. The inability to close the right eye is the result of involvement of which one of the following?

a. Zygomatic branch of the facial nerve
b. Buccal branch of the trigeminal nerve
c. Levator palpebrae superioris muscle
d. Superior tarsal muscle (of Müller)
e. Orbital portion of the orbicularis oculi muscle

285. A 62-year-old rock musician falls out of a palm tree while vacationing in Fiji. He climbed the tree and fell while trying to reach one of the coconuts. He didn't think he had broken any bones in the fall. While he felt fine the day of the fall, the next morning he awoke with a bad headache and was relatively incoherent. At the Fiji ED, both frontal and lateral skull plain films show no evidence of any fracture, but during the physical examination papilledema is noted in both eyes. He is flown to New Zealand where head CT findings are consistent with which one of the following diagnoses?

a. Epidural hematoma
b. Subdural hematoma
c. Pituitary tumor
d. Graves disease
e. Trigeminal neuralgia

286. A 1-week-old neonate is brought to the pediatric office by her first time mother. The 8 lb 3 oz baby girl is alert, but arrives at the office in the detachable car seat with her head turned to the left while tilting her head toward the right as if she is trying to touch her right ear to her chest. The muscles on the left side of her neck are slightly stretched and the baby can move her head around a little bit, but not far from the tilted and turned position. This condition was not noticed at birth, and the new mother and baby left the hospital just 24 hours after the vaginal delivery. What muscle in the baby's neck was likely torn during the vaginal delivery and what is the name for the condition?

a. Anterior scalene muscle, congenital muscular torticollis
b. Sternocleidomastoid muscle, congenital muscular torticollis
c. Sternocleidomastoid muscle, spasmodic torticollis
d. Trapezius muscle, floppy head syndrome
e. Trapezius muscle, spasmodic torticollis

287. A 37-year-old mother delivers a full-term 7 lb, 10 oz baby boy. The baby boy has a left cleft of the upper lip that extends upward toward the left nostril and left anterior cleft of the primary palate just deep to the cleft lip. The mother has two other children without clefts at home. The obstetrician explains to the mother that these defects are most likely due to a failure of which one of the following embryonic processes?

a. Mandibular process to fuse with the lateral nasal process
b. Mandibular process to fuse with the medial nasal process
c. Maxillary process to fuse with the lateral nasal process
d. Maxillary process to fuse with the medial nasal process
e. Lateral and medial nasal processes to fuse with each other

288. A 2-month-old infant is brought to a pediatric ophthalmology practice by her father. The baby girl almost always holds her head down with her chin resting on her chest. The father thinks that the baby's left eye has normal function and follows a bright and noisy rattle, however, the baby girl's right eye cannot follow any object held below the horizon of her normal gaze. When the ophthalmologist holds the baby's head gently in the normal anatomic position relative to her body and the rattle is held and shaken either medially or laterally above the girl's head both right and left eyes follow the rattle. However, the baby's right eye cannot follow the rattle when it goes below the horizon of her visual field. Which extraocular muscle does the ophthalmologist suggest be injected with botulinum toxin to potentially correct the baby's strabismus?

a. Right inferior oblique muscle
b. Right inferior rectus muscle
c. Right lateral rectus muscle
d. Right superior oblique muscle
e. Right superior rectus muscle

289. A 9-year-old girl is brought to the pediatric office by her mother because the girl has been complaining about a very sore throat. The mother notes that her daughter has started to snore loudly at night. Examination of the girl's mouth and oropharynx reveals the likely source of the problem to be extremely large palatine tonsils. Surgical removal of the tonsils is the suggested treatment, but it is explained that there is a small risk associated with the surgery, which may result in which one of the following?

a. Loss in the ability to taste salt on the anterior two-thirds of the tongue
b. Loss in the ability to protrude her tongue, thus limiting her ability to lick an ice-cream cone
c. Weakness in the ability to open her mouth fully when eating an apple due to damage to the innervation of the lateral pterygoid muscle
d. Loss in the ability to taste on the posterior one-third of the tongue and perhaps some difficulty in swallowing
e. Weakened ability to move her jaw from side-to-side because of loss in innervation of the medial pterygoid muscle

290. A 9-year-old boy is brought to the emergency department by his mother. He tripped on the carpet while playing tag with his sister in the living room and fell face-first onto the corner of a wooden coffee table. Fortunately, his eye just missed the corner of the table, however, his left cheek hit the table just below his eye forcing the lower lateral margin of the eye away from the orbit. Gentle palpation indicates that both his zygomatic bone and a lateral portion of the maxilla are broken and dislocated from the rest of his face. The boy's nose, medial portion of the maxillary bone and maxillary teeth are all intact. When the "H" test is performed, the left eye has more limited movement than the right eye and cannot look above the horizon. Which extraocular muscle is likely trapped in which facial bone?

a. Inferior rectus muscle in the ethmoid bone
b. Inferior rectus muscle in the maxillary bone
c. Medial rectus muscle in the frontal bone
d. Medial rectus muscle in the maxillary bone
e. Superior rectus muscle in the sphenoid bone

291. A 43-year-old mother of two watching her son play baseball is hit on the side of the head with a foul ball from another field. She is knocked unconscious for a few seconds and is taken to the ED of a local hospital by her husband. At the ED in addition to observing a growing "goose egg" over her right temporal region, examination of her fundi with an ophthalmoscope shows subtle papilledema. She is immediately sent for frontal and lateral skull films, which show a fracture in the frontal bone near the pterion. Head CT shows an accumulation of blood near the fracture under the frontal bone, but anterior to the coronal suture. What is the most likely working diagnosis provided to the on call neurosurgeon to bring her into the hospital on a Saturday afternoon?

a. Extracranial hematoma
b. Extracranial and epidural hematomas
c. Extracranial and subdural hematomas
d. Subarachnoid hemorrhage
e. Extracranial hematoma and subarachnoid hemorrhage

292. A 23-year-old Caucasian man boxes semiprofessionally. He was once knocked out by a right "hook" to the head, and for about a week afterwards he had frequent headaches and a very runny nose, which finally stopped running by itself. However, he still remains unable to smell with his left nostril. What is the most likely site of injury that explains the symptoms?

a. Fracture at the cribriform plate
b. Fracture of the lacrimal bones
c. Fracture of the nasal bones
d. A Le Fort II fracture
e. A Le Fort III fracture

293. A 19-year-old undergraduate student arrives at the emergency department (ED) via ambulance. He was in a bicycle accident in which he flew over his handlebars and landed on the edge of the curb, striking the right side of his mandible. The ED physician determines that the mandible is broken by holding both sides of the mandible and feeling independent movement of the right and left sides. Not only has the teenager fractured his mandible, but his maxillary incisors have cut completely through his lower lip on the right side. While suturing the lower lip laceration it is noticed that the teenager has no sensation within his lower lip on the right side, while the left side of the lower lip has normal sensation. Based on the loss of sensation within the lower lip, what is the location of the fracture?

a. Body of the mandible posterior to the mental foramen
b. Coronoid process of the mandible
c. Mandibular symphysis in the midline
d. Neck of the mandible inferior to the condyle
e. Ramus of the mandible superior to the mandibular foramen

294. A 17-year-old adolescent arrives at the ED with her jaw wide open and an apple core in her left hand. She is in obvious pain from dislocating her jaw, displacing the articular disk beyond the articular tubercle of the temporomandibular joint while eating the apple. The dislocation was the result of excessive contraction of which one of the following muscles?

a. Buccinator
b. Lateral pterygoid
c. Medial pterygoid
d. Masseter
e. Temporalis

295. A physician views the anterior neck of a 24-year-old male medical student. He has a reddish spot (in circle) that is in the center of a slightly raised area just anterior to his sternocleidomastoid muscle about one and a half inches superior to his jugular notch. This reddish raised area has existed for as long as he can remember. When the physician gently pushes on it, it feels attached to a structure that extends superiorly from this location. The patient reports that "at times it leaks a little clear fluid" after he has been heavily exercising for long periods of time. Which one of the following is the most likely congenital anomaly in this patient?

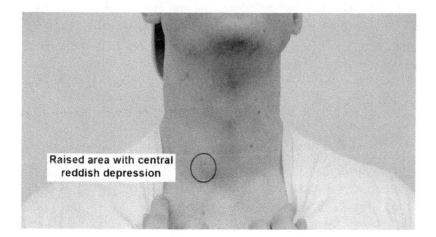

Raised area with central reddish depression

a. Glossopharyngeal fistula
b. An internal branchial sinus
c. A branchial fistula
d. A hyperactive sebaceous gland
e. Spina bifida occulta
f. Thyroglossal duct cyst

Questions 296 and 297

A 42-year-old woman is watching her son play baseball when a stray foul ball from another field unexpectedly strikes her in the back of the head and neck behind her left ear. A subcutaneous bulge rapidly appears, but she stays to watch the rest of the game and ices the bump when she arrives at home. The next day much of the swelling is diminished, but when she tries to eat an apple, or even when she swallows, it hurts deep behind her left ear. In addition, the patient reports the sensation of a foreign body in her throat and discomfort when turning her head. She travels to the urgent care clinic where the physician orders a lateral skull film that shows no fracture of her mastoid process.

296. The styloid process is fractured and displaced from the skull. To which one of the following bones is the styloid process attached?

a. Ethmoid bone
b. Mandible
c. Occipital bone
d. Sphenoid bone
e. Temporal bone

297. Which structure is most likely to cause tension on the styloid process when opening the jaw widely?

a. Stylohyoid ligament
b. Stylohyoid muscle
c. Styloglossus muscle
d. Stylomandibular ligament
e. Stylopharyngeus muscle

298. A 53-year-old banker develops paralysis on the right side of his face, which produces an expressionless and drooping appearance. He is unable to close the right eye and also has difficulty chewing and drinking. Examination shows loss of the blink reflex in the right eye to stimulation of either right or left cornea. Lacrimation appears normal on the right side, but salivation is diminished and taste is absent on the anterior right side of the tongue. There is no complaint of hyperacusis. Audition and balance appear to be normal. Where is the lesion located?

a. In the brain and involves the nucleus of the facial nerve and superior salivatory nucleus
b. Within the internal auditory meatus
c. At the geniculate ganglion
d. In the facial canal just distal to the genu of the facial nerve
e. Just proximal to the stylomastoid foramen

299. The dark structure in the midbrain indicated by the arrow in this midsagittal MRI represents a passage within the brain. What would be the consequence if this passage is obstructed?

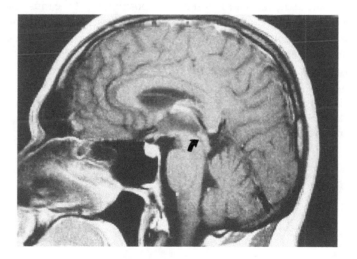

a. Venous blood would appear in the subarachnoid space.
b. Arterial blood from the basilar artery would appear in the subarachnoid space.
c. Neurons of the corticospinal tract would no longer function.
d. Cerebrospinal fluid would accumulate within the ventricles.
e. Spinothalamic (sensory) fibers would no longer function.

300. An ENT is about to remove a pair of enlarged palatine tonsils from an 11-year-old boy who had chronic tonsillitis over the past 3 years. The palatine tonsils are located between the anterior and posterior palatine (faucial) pillars. The anterior and posterior palatine pillars are formed, respectively, by which of the following muscles?

a. Levator veli palatini and tensor veli palatini
b. Palatoglossus and palatopharyngeus
c. Palatopharyngeus and salpingopharyngeus
d. Styloglossus and stylopharyngeus
e. Superior constrictor and middle constrictor

301. A 6 lb 14 oz baby girl was born to a 20-year-old mother. When the baby cried with her first few breaths the obstetrician noticed that the baby had a normal upper lip but a complete cleft of her hard and soft palate. The cleft prevents the baby from developing sufficient negative pressure for breast-feeding because of the continuity of the oral and nasal cavities. While bone and tissue can be pulled medially during surgery to repair the defect in the hard palate, separating the nose from the oral cavity, the most difficult part of the reconstruction is the repositioning of the muscles of the soft palate for proper function. Which perioral muscle aids in opening the Eustachian/auditory tube during each swallow to allow proper middle ear function and thus hearing?

a. Masseter muscle
b. Musculus uvulae muscle
c. Palatoglossus muscle
d. Palatopharyngeus muscle
e. Tensor veli palatini muscle

302. An 87-year-old man had been sitting on the toilet when suddenly he fell to the left side against an adjacent wall. Fortunately his wife heard him hit his head against the tiled wall and found him partially wedged against it. While he is conscious, he has difficulty speaking and little control of his left side, though he is capable of some movement. The paramedics arrive, lift him from his stuck position, give him oxygen during the ambulance trip, hook up ECG leads, and find normal heart rhythm and patterns. By the time he arrives in the ED, he is a little more responsive, but his speech is slurred. A head CT is immediately performed and is read as normal other than slight age-associated shrinkage of the brain. He has a bad headache and stiff neck. There is no papilledema, so a spinal tap is performed to determine whether to start tissue plasminogen activator (TPA) treatment. There is some blood found equally within all four tubes collected, so TPA is not initiated. Which one of the following is the most likely diagnosis?

a. Subarachnoid hemorrhagic stroke, which had stopped by the time the CT was performed
b. Ischemic stroke, which had opened by the time the CT was performed
c. Subdural hematoma
d. Epidural hematoma
e. Alzheimer dementia

303. A patient is observed to suffer from hypoglossal hemiplegia. There is atrophy of the tongue on the right side and deviation of the protruded tongue to the right. In addition, the patient exhibits upper motoneuron paralysis on the left side of the body. Deviation of the tongue toward the right involves which one of the following?

a. Left nucleus ambiguus
b. Left pyramidal tract caudal to the decussation
c. Right hypoglossal nerve
d. Right nucleus ambiguus
e. Right pyramidal tract rostral to the decussation

304. A woman is found to have internal (medially directed) strabismus of the left eye, paralysis of the muscles of facial expression on the left side, hyperacusis of the left ear, and loss of taste from the anterior two-thirds of her tongue on the left. Her mouth is somewhat drier than normal. In addition, there is a lack of tearing in her left eye, and a blink reflex cannot be elicited from the stimulation of either the right or the left cornea. She has upper motor neuron paralysis of the right side of her body. Internal strabismus results from paralysis of which one of the following cranial nerves?

a. Cranial nerve II
b. Cranial nerve III
c. Cranial nerve IV
d. Cranial nerve V
e. Cranial nerve VI

305. During a neck dissection, the styloid process is used as a landmark. Which one of the following statements correctly pertains to one of the five structures that attach to the styloid process?

a. The stylohyoid muscle attaches to the lesser horn of the hyoid bone.
b. The styloglossus muscle acts to protrude the tongue.
c. The stylohyoid ligament attaches to the lingula of the mandible.
d. Distally the stylopharyngeus muscle is split by the digastric muscle.
e. The stylomandibular ligament attaches to the lingula of the mandible.

306. A very concerned mother brings her teenager into their family practice office. The teenager awoke in the morning with a large swollen mass that filled part of his upper eyelid and medial forehead just above his left eye. His eyelid is so swollen he can barely keep it open. His history reveals indoor allergies and a persistent head cold. During the physical examination it is noted that purulent nasal discharge is present along with extreme tenderness to percussion over his paranasal sinuses. The large swollen mass in his eyelid and forehead is pliable. The physician prescribes intravenous antibiotics and provides which one of the following explanations to the very concerned mother and teenager?

a. He suffers from trigeminal neuralgia that affects the ophthalmic portion of cranial nerve V.
b. He suffers from tic douloureux that affects the ophthalmic portion of cranial nerve V.
c. He suffers from sinusitis, which has eroded through the wall of the frontal sinus, and since the frontalis muscle is not attached to bone, allowed pus to leak into the upper eyelid.
d. He has Bell palsy, which is generally caused by herpes simplex virus infection of the facial nerve within the facial canal that caused the loss of ability to raise the upper eyelid and thus allow fluid to accumulate within it.
e. He suffers from a sty, which is an inflammation of meibomian or tarsal glands, which lie on the inner surface of the eyelid.

307. During a prenatal ultrasound, images suggest that the fetus has a defective lower thoracic spinal cord. α-fetoprotein levels are two standard deviations above normal. It is suggested to the mother that the child be delivered via a Cesarean section to reduce the chances of damaging any protruding spinal cord and meninges. After birth, an ultrasound study determines that the covering of the spinal cord, along with the intact spinal cord, forms a saclike projection through a dorsal defect in the vertebral column. What is the proper term for this congenital condition?

a. Rachischisis
b. Anencephaly
c. Meningocele
d. Meningomyelocele
e. Hydrocephaly

308. A teenage baseball player is hit in the base of the skull by a thrown bat. He is hoarse and complains of difficulty swallowing. The cranial x-ray indicates a basal skull fracture that passes through the jugular foramen. The examining physician notes a large hematoma behind the ear on the injured side. If the nerves passing through the jugular foramen are severed as a result of the cranial fracture, which one of the following muscles will remain functional?

a. Palatoglossus muscle
b. Sternocleidomastoid muscle
c. Styloglossus muscle
d. Stylopharyngeus muscle
e. Trapezius muscle

309. A tall, skinny, 14-year-old teenage boy is brought into the family practice office by his mother. She noticed that he snores loudly at night. When questioned, the teenager admits to having a sore throat ever since the family's new golden retriever started sleeping in his room several months ago. The boy failed to tell his mother about the sore throat because he always wanted a pet. When the physician examines the teenager, she notices enlarged submandibular lymph nodes. When the teenager opens his mouth, the potential cause of the problem is visible superior and lateral to the posterior of his tongue. What is the most likely cause of nighttime snoring in this teenager?

a. A short uvula
b. Eruption of wisdom teeth prematurely
c. Enlarged lingual tonsils
d. Enlarged palatine tonsils
e. Mandibular tori
f. The tongue stud he had gotten without his mother's noticing

310. Muscle relaxants are used routinely during anesthesia with resultant closure of the vocal folds. Laryngeal intubation by the anesthesiologist is necessary because which one of the following muscle(s) is/are unable to keep the glottis open?

a. Cricothyroid muscles
b. Lateral cricoarytenoid muscles
c. Posterior cricoarytenoid muscles
d. Thyroarytenoid muscle
e. Transverse arytenoid muscles

311. A 55-year-old husband is brought to his internist by his wife of 27 years. She claims that his head is getting bigger. The husband admits that his ears and nose are getting bigger, but claims that he still wears the same hat he has worn for decades. Within the midsagittal MRI below, which structure would one suspect of enlargement if the wife's claim is correct?

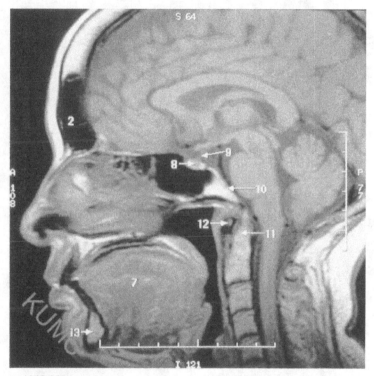

(Image 1302-003, used with permission from the Radiological Anatomy web site, University of Kansas, School of Medicine, http://classes.kumc.edu/som/radanatomy/.)

a. 2
b. 7
c. 8
d. 9
e. 10
f. 11
g. 12

312. A 42-year-old man is involved in a motor vehicle accident which causes a fracture to the base of his skull with compression of the structure that passes through foramen 42. Which one of the following actions would most likely be lost or weakened?

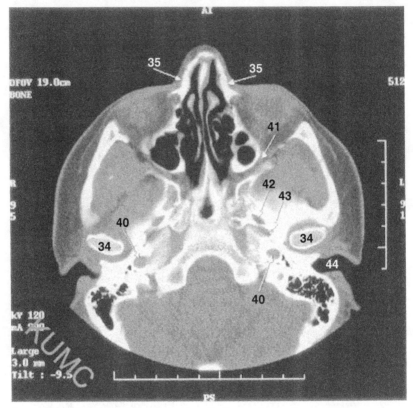

(Image 1205-028, used with permission from the Radiological Anatomy web site, University of Kansas, School of Medicine, http://classes.kumc.edu/som/radanatomy/.)

a. Facial expression on the left side
b. Ability to chew on the left side
c. Ability to turn head
d. Quality and strength of voice
e. Ability to shrug shoulders

313. A 32-year-old woman was brought into the ED from a car accident. She was conscious, but had been knocked unconscious for a couple of minutes by the force of a car that had run a stop sign, broad-siding her vehicle. She has a hematoma over the parietal bone on the left side of her head. She complains of a stiff neck and tilts her head slightly to the right. While performing a cranial nerve examination, it is noted that her left eye has difficulty moving inferiorly from a fully adducted horizontal position, when she looks down at her feet. A head CT is ordered with specific imaging of which one of the following cranial nerves?

a. Right cranial nerve III
b. Left cranial nerve III
c. Right cranial nerve IV
d. Left cranial nerve IV
e. Left cranial nerve VI

314. A 58-year-old man presents to the ENT clinic with complaints of headaches and nasal drainage. He has seasonal allergies, but this year he complains of headaches along with his allergies. The headache often feels as if it is between his eyes or "on top of his head." Upon examination of his nose and mouth, a large nasal polyp is seen on the medial aspect of the superior turbinate of his left nostril. A CT confirms a large nasal polyp in the left sphenoethmoid recess and sinusitis within an adjacent sinus. The sinusitis is most likely causing the headaches within which one of the following locations?

a. Anterior ethmoid sinuses
b. Frontal sinus
c. Middle ethmoid sinuses
d. Maxillary sinus
e. Sphenoid sinus

315. The parents of a 3-year-old are upset because he has had six middle ear infections, forcing them to miss many days of work in order to stay home with the boy rather than send him to daycare. Most likely the boy's Eustachian (auditory) tube is not functioning correctly. In order to treat recurrent middle-ear infections, pressure-equalization (PE) tubes (or tympanostomy tubes) may be placed at what location within the tympanic membrane?

a. At the umbo of the tympanic membrane
b. At the attachment of the manubrium with the tympanic membrane
c. At the pars flaccida of the tympanic membrane where the fibrous layer is missing
d. In the inferior half of the tympanic membrane
e. In the eustachian tube to keep it open, because that is often the cause of the initial problem

316. A 72-year-old grandmother is watching her grandson play baseball on one field, when a foul ball from another baseball diamond strikes the right side of her face, knocking her unconscious. She regains consciousness in the ambulance on the way to the hospital. Skull films reveal fractures of both her right zygomatic arch and the coronoid process on the right side of the mandible. Which two of the following muscles either originate from or insert onto the fractured structures, thus weakening the woman's ability to chew?

a. Medial and lateral pterygoid
b. Masseter and lateral pterygoid
c. Masseter and medial pterygoid
d. Stylohyoid and posterior belly of the digastric
e. Temporalis and masseter

317. A 63-year-old man is on the hospital service for workup of a stiff neck, the "worst headache" of his life, and general malaise. Two days earlier, he had a spinal tap, which was bloodless and consistent with viral meningitis. This morning the patient needs to turn his whole head when he looks at the nurse as she enters his hospital room. While his headache is improving, both his eyes have reduced ability to move laterally; rather he tends to turn his head. Ophthalmoscopic visualization of his fundi shows no evidence of papilledema. The site of his spinal tap is oozing some fluid. The rest of the cranial nerve examination is normal. Which one of the following is the most likely cause of his reduced eye movement?

a. Viral meningitis
b. Stretching of cranial nerve VI
c. Excess cerebral spinal fluid that is stretching just cranial nerves III
d. Bilateral tumors at the superior orbital fissures
e. Normal stiffening process following hospitalization for couple of days

318. An 87-year-old man is having difficulty swallowing and often chokes on his food. You check his gag reflex by touching the posterior one-third of his tongue and palatine tonsil area. Which one of the following cranial nerves provides the afferent limb of the gag reflex?

a. Cranial nerve I
b. Cranial nerve II
c. Cranial nerve III
d. Cranial nerve IV
e. Cranial nerve V
f. Cranial nerve VI
g. Cranial nerve VII
h. Cranial nerve VIII
i. Cranial nerve IX
j. Cranial nerve X
k. Cranial nerve XI
l. Cranial nerve XII

319. A 93-year-old nursing home patient is seen during morning rounds. She is quite upset because she awoke with double vision and an inability to open her left eye completely. Her physician performs a complete cranial nerve examination. Her left eye, under her drooping eyelid, is dilated and rotated down and outward. It lacks the normal pupillary reflex. There is no evidence of papilledema in either eye. The rest of the cranial nerve examination is normal. Which one of the following is the most likely explanation for this condition?

a. An aneurysm of the left posterior cerebral artery compressing cranial nerve III
b. An aneurysm of the right anterior cerebral artery compressing cranial nerve III
c. A tumor at the left optic canal
d. Glaucoma
e. A left parotid gland tumor compressing cranial nerve VII

320. A 73-year-old man presents because of repeated biting of his tongue and cheek, and difficulty chewing. The left side of his tongue is somewhat swollen and he has two different cuts on it. His left cheek is slightly less full over the angle of the mandible compared to the right side. He has very little sensation over his left mandible, along the side of his head, and on the left side of his tongue. He has weakened ability to elevate his mandible on the left side. Taste sensation on his tongue is normal. He also complains of slight dryness on the left side of his mouth. The rest of his cranial nerve examination is normal. A head CT is ordered because his physician suspects which one of the following?

a. A tumor at the left superior orbital fissure
b. A tumor blocking the left foramen rotundum
c. A tumor blocking left foramen ovale
d. A tumor blocking the left internal acoustic meatus
e. A tumor blocking the right internal acoustic meatus

321. A 43-year-old man presents with left-sided maxillary tooth pain of one week's duration. Because he thought it might have been one of his maxillary fillings (the newer plastic polymers) he visited his dentist first, but his dentist was unable to identify any dental problems. His physician taps on his maxillae and elicits sharp pain when she taps on the left, but not right side of his face. While he does not think he has any allergies, he admits that his girlfriend has recently bought a cat that lives inside. A sinus series is ordered because his physician suspects which one of the following?

a. Sphenoid sinusitis
b. Anterior ethmoidal sinusitis
c. Posterior ethmoidal sinusitis
d. Maxillary sinusitis
e. Frontal sinusitis

322. Access to the heart is typically obtained by placing venous catheters. While at times the cephalic vein is used, other times a location closer to the heart is desired. It is essential to access a low-pressure central vein, rather than a high-pressure central artery. When performing a cardiac catheterization of the right heart chambers it is important for the cardiologist to remember that the carotid sheath contains which of the following?

a. Internal carotid artery (lateral), internal jugular vein (medial), and sympathetic chain
b. Internal carotid artery (medial), external jugular vein (lateral), and sympathetic chain
c. Internal carotid artery (medial), external jugular vein (lateral), and phrenic nerve
d. Internal carotid artery (lateral), internal jugular vein (medial), and phrenic nerve
e. Internal carotid artery (medial), internal jugular vein (lateral), and the vagus nerve

323. A physician witnesses a choking incident in a restaurant. The Heimlich maneuver is unsuccessful at removing the food from the pharynx. The victim is having extreme difficulty breathing and starts to pass out. Where is the best location to produce an emergency airway?

a. In the midline just superior to the hyoid bone
b. In the midline just inferior to the hyoid bone
c. At the laryngeal notch
d. At the junction between the thyroid cartilage and cricoid cartilage
e. At tracheal ring 2 to 3 below the cricoid cartilage

324. Recent examination of human cadavers indicates that only about two-thirds of the human population have the risorius muscles. In about one-third of individuals this muscle fails to develop. From which structure of the embryonic branchial apparatus illustrated below would the risorius muscle develop?

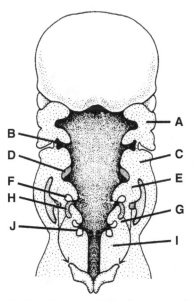

(Reproduced, with permission, from Sweeney L. Basic Concepts in Embryology: A Student's Survival Guide. New York, NY: McGraw-Hill; 1998.)

a. A
b. B
c. C
d. D
e. E
f. F
g. G
h. H
i. I
j. J

325. A 68-year-old woman presents to the ENT clinic because of a small lump on the right side of her face just anterior to her ear. At first it is thought to be an enlarged lymph node, but careful examination of her ear and scalp fails to confirm the diagnosis. The small lump appears to be within the superficial portion of the parotid salivary gland, anterior to the external ear and posterior to the masseter muscle. A needle biopsy of the lump is performed and sent for pathological assessment. The diagnosis is a pleomorphic adenoma of the parotid gland. The tumor needs to be surgically removed. Which one of the following is a serious potential risk of the surgical resection procedure?

a. Loss of her ability to taste on the right side of her tongue
b. Loss of her ability to chew on the right side of her mouth
c. Right-sided facial muscle paralysis
d. Loss of her ability to move the right side of her tongue
e. Increased sensitivity to sounds on the right side

326. A 53-year-old woman presents with hearing loss and ringing in her left ear. About a month ago she experienced dizziness and felt sick, but that seemed to pass. She describes recent and numerous headaches, always on the left side. A complete cranial nerve examination is completed. Everything is normal except for the hearing loss and weakness in her left facial muscles. A head MRI is ordered because of concerns about which one of the following?

a. Conductive hearing loss
b. Ménière disease
c. Acoustic neuroma
d. Tic douloureux
e. Parotid gland tumor

327. A 13-month-old baby boy is brought into the pediatric office by his concerned mother. The boy is just beginning to talk and seems to have difficulty speaking some sounds. The mother also notes that his tongue seems "sort of stuck in his mouth" compared to her two older children. Examination of the baby, including his mouth, confirms that his tongue seems to be stuck in the floor of his mouth. Which one of the following is the correct explanation of this part of tongue development?

a. The hypoglossal nerves that control the tongue failed to develop
b. The problem could likely be corrected by cutting the lingual frenulum
c. The problem could likely be corrected by shortening the posterior belly of the digastric muscle
d. The problem could likely be corrected by cutting the pterygomandibular raphe
e. The problem is not correctable and speech therapy is the best option

328. A 19-year-old man presents in extreme pain holding a handkerchief over his right eye. He explains that he was accidentally struck in the eye with a pool cue and the he can't see anything other than a milky white cloud in his right eye. On examination of his right eye, there appears to be a scratch on the cornea, the anterior chamber of the eye is partially filled with blood, but the eye has not ruptured. Intraocular pressure as measured with a tonometer is normal. The patient is told that it is important to avoid any other blows to the head since the retina is at increased risk for detachment and to return to the office the next day to determine if the intraocular pressure has risen. There are abnormal red blood cells in the aqueous humor that may plug the normal site of drainage, leading to excessive intraocular pressure if left untreated. Where in the anterior chamber of the eye does aqueous humor normally drain?

a. Trabecular meshwork that leads to the scleral venous sinus (canal of Schlemm)
b. Ciliary muscle which has zonular fibers (suspensory ligament of the lens) attached to it
c. Ciliary process
d. Lens
e. Retina

Head and Neck

Answers

274. The answer is c. (*Moore, pp 903-905, 912.*) During the corneal reflex the long ciliary (CN V^1) nerve carries pain information from the eye, which causes the eye to close due to firing of the muscle of facial expression innervated by the zygomatic branch of the facial nerve (CN VII). Short ciliary nerves (**answers a and b**), by definition, have traveled through the ciliary ganglia (some have synapsed) and, therefore, are postganglionic parasympathetic fibers, which will innervate the intraocular eye muscles for accommodation of the iris and pupil. The infraorbital branch of CN V^2 (**answers d and e**), while sensory, does not innervate the eye, but does innervate the skin and lower eyelid.

275. The answer is c. (*Moore, pp 1061-1063, 1080. Fauci, pp 184-185.*) Information from the nasal retinal field crosses the midline at the optic chiasm; thus images from the right visual fields strike the left retinal fields of both eyes and from the right eye cross at the optic chiasm (see High-Yield Facts, Figure 18, p 77).

The images that strike the left temporal retina (from the right visual field) of the left eye stay on the left and join the nasal retinal field of the right eye in the left optic tract. An aneurysm in the left middle cerebral artery, if large enough, would likely impinge on the left optic tract. A pituitary tumor (**answer a**) would likely compress the optic chiasm leading to a loss of the temporal visual fields in both eyes (bilateral tunnel vision or bitemporal hemianopsia). A tumor in the right orbit that compresses the right optic nerve (**answer b**) would lead to loss of vision in only the right eye. Compromise of the right optic tract (**answer d**) would lead to loss of left visual fields in both eyes. An aneurysm affecting the arterial supply to the occipital visual cortex (**answer e**) would be very unlikely to produce the symptoms described.

276. The answer is a. (*Moore, pp 858-859.*) The buccal and submandibular nodes should be specifically palpated. The hyperpigmentation lesion could be malignant melanoma, which can spread to regional lymph nodes. The spot is just above the nasolabial skin fold so it should drain first into buccal (or facial) lymph nodes, which then drain into submandibular lymph nodes. Submental nodes (answers b and e) receive lymph from the lower lip and chin area. Jugulodigastric and juguloomohyoid nodes (answer c) are named members of deep neck lymph nodes and would not be the first nodes to receive metastatic cells. The parotid and mastoid nodes (answer d) are just in front of and behind the ear, respectively and receive most of their lymph from the pinna of the ear or areas superior to this region.

277. The answer is c. (*Moore, pp 866, 878-882.*) Cerebrospinal fluid (CSF) formed in the choroid plexus circulates in the subarachnoid space and is absorbed by the venous sinuses through the arachnoid villi, some of which project into the superior sagittal sinus and its lateral lacunae. Lateral lacunae are areas of expansion of the superior sagittal sinus. CSF protects the nervous system during impact and against mechanical injuries and is important for metabolism. It circulates slowly through the ventricles of the brain, out of the fourth ventricle, and through the meshes of the subarachnoid space.

278. The answer is b. (*Moore, pp 96-97, 849-853.*) The attorney is diagnosed with herpes zoster affecting the ophthalmic division of the trigeminal cranial nerve. Herpes zoster is the reemergence of varicella-zoster virus after it has lay dormant within the sensory ganglia (the trigeminal ganglia in this case). Herpes zoster produces pain and vesicles (shingles) along a dermatomal pattern. Her vesicle pattern matches the left ophthalmic division of the trigeminal cranial nerve. The trigeminal ganglia contain nerve cell bodies, which receive and transmit sensory information into the brain stem from the face. The mandibular division of the trigeminal cranial nerve (answer a) runs along the mandible and anterior to her ear along the side of her head. The zygomatic branch of the facial nerve (answer c) is a motor nerve, and these are not usually affected by varicella-zoster virus. Mumps is caused by the mumps virus and often causes painful swelling of the parotid salivary gland (answer d and e), which is unaffected in this woman. (Also see Question and Answer 137.)

279. The answer is a. (*Moore, pp 843-844, 860.*) A mnemonic device for remembering the order in which the soft tissues overlie the cranium is SCALP: skin, connective tissue, aponeurosis, loose connective tissue, and periosteum (answer d). The scalp proper is composed of the outer three layers, of which the connective tissue contains one of the richest cutaneous blood supplies of the body. The occipitofrontal muscle complex inserts into the epicranial aponeurosis, which forms the intermediate tendon of the digastric muscle (**answer e**). This structure, along with the underlying layer of loose connective tissue, accounts for the high degree of mobility of the scalp over the pericranium. If the aponeurosis is lacerated transversely, traction from the muscle bellies will cause considerable gaping of the wound. Secondary to trauma or infection, blood or pus may accumulate subjacent to the epicranial aponeurosis. Bone (**answer b**) is too deep, as is the dura mater (**answer c**).

280. The answer is a. (*Moore, pp 844-849.*) Botulinum toxin injection inhibits acetylcholine release at the neuromuscular junction, leading to flaccid (sagging) paralysis of muscle. If injected into the depressor anguli oris muscles at each corner of the mouth, the levator anguli oris and zygomaticus major muscles, which are unaffected, will better be able to lift the corners of her mouth, giving her a more youthful smile. The mentalis muscle (**answer b**) is more medial in location than the corner of the mouth and tends to pull the lower lips inferiorly and medially. The orbicularis oculi muscle (**answer c**) surrounds the eye and closes the eyes (producing "crow's feet" at the lateral canthus of the eye). The orbicularis oris muscle (**answer d**) surrounds the lips and allows them to close tightly as when kissing. The zygomaticus major muscle (**answer e**) tends to raise the corner of the mouth and upper lips and is needed for smiling, so it should not be injected.

281. The answer is f. (*Moore, pp 959-960,964.*) Nosebleed blood flow to Kiesselbach area may be reduced by holding both sides of the upper lip and also pressing on the incisive foramen. Kiesselbach area on the nasal septum is just superior and posterior to the external nasal aperture. Many nosebleeds (or epistaxis) occur in this area since it is exposed to most of the incoming air. There are four blood vessels that supply blood to this area: (1) anterior ethmoid artery (a branch off the ophthalmic artery); (2) sphenopalatine artery (a branch off the maxillary artery that exits the sphenopalatine foramen); (3) greater palatine artery (a branch also off the maxillary artery, but traverses both the greater foramen and the incisive foramen to reach the nose); and (4) septal branch artery (a branch off the superior labial artery which is derived from the facial artery). While the lay press often suggests holding the bridge of the nose **(answers a and e)**, that would only block blood within the infratrochlear artery, which mainly serves the exterior dorsal surface of the nose. Holding **(answer c)** both sides of the nose at the junction of the nasal bones with the lateral nasal cartilages would tend to block blood flow within the external branch of the anterior ethmoid. This might actually increase the blood coming from an artery in Kiesselbach area. Thus **(answer b)** holding both sides of the upper lip between his fingers will cut off blood to the septal branch of the superior labial artery, and applying pressure from the oral cavity over the incisive foramen **(answer d)** would cut off blood coming from the greater palatine arteries. Note that it is difficult to stop blood within either the sphenoid palatine artery or anterior ethmoid arteries by applying any external pressure.

282. The answer is e. (*Moore, pp 1043-1046.*) During removal of the thyroid gland the surgeon must be careful not to cut the recurrent laryngeal nerve and cause hypoparathyroidism by incidental removal of the parathyroid glands. The thyroid gland often wraps itself around the trachea within pretracheal fascia, and the recurrent laryngeal nerve runs alongside the trachea in between the trachea and the esophagus, so those nerves that control the larynx are at risk. The parathyroid glands normally lie on the deep surface of the thyroid gland and typically receive their blood supply from the inferior thyroid arteries. If all four of the parathyroid glands are removed then parathyroid hormone (PTH) would not be produced. PTH is essential for maintaining proper calcium levels and hypocalcemia and eventual tetany would result. Removal of the thyroid gland often decompresses the trachea, so creation of the tracheostomy **(answers a and b)** would rarely, if ever, be needed. The vagal nerves run as a plexus upon the esophagus, which is posterior to the trachea, so, rarely would a vagus nerve **(answer c and d)** or peristaltic function be at risk.

283. The answer is c. (*Moore, pp 999-1001.*) The platysma, and the strap muscles: sternohyoid, sternothyroid, and omohyoid would be retracted during thyroid gland removal. The thyroid gland lies in pretracheal fascia, which is deep to those four muscles. The sternocleidomastoid, and trapezius are within the investing fascia of the neck, which is superficial to both the thyroid gland (in pretracheal fascia) and in the infrahyoid strap muscles. The sternocleidomastoid muscle might also need to be retracted. The longus coli, longus capitus muscle, and anterior scalene muscles **(answer a)** are all anterior to the vertebral column surrounded by prevertebral fascia and are posterior to the thyroid gland. The mylohyoid, anterior belly of the digastrics, genioglossus, and geniohyoid muscles **(answer b)** are all superior to the hyoid bone and, therefore, superior to the thyroid gland. The superior, middle, and inferior pharyngeal constrictors **(answer d)** are all posterior or superior to the thyroid gland and thus would not be retracted. The trapezius, rhomboids, and levator scapula muscles **(answer e)** are all posterior to the neck and back and would not need to be retracted to gain access to the thyroid gland.

284. The answer is a. *(Moore, pp 853-854.)* The woman in the scenario has symptoms of Bell palsy. Palpebral portion of the orbicularis oculi muscle (innervated by the zygomatic branch of the facial nerve) produces the blink, whereas the orbital portion **(answer e)** is involved in "scrunching" the eye shut. In some individuals the temporal branch of the facial cranial nerve also innervates the upper portion of the orbicularis oculi muscle. The buccal branch of the facial nerve innervates muscles of facial expression (including the buccinator muscle and upper portion of orbicularis oris muscle) between the eye and the mouth, whereas the buccal branch of the trigeminal nerve **(answer b)** is sensory. The levator palpebrae superioris muscle **(answer c)**, which elevates the upper eyelid, is innervated by the oculomotor nerve, whereas the involuntary superior tarsal muscle **(answer d)** is supplied by sympathetic nerves.

285. The answer is b. *(Moore, pp 876-877, 908.)* The head CT findings were consistent with subdural hematoma. This is the most likely finding. Falls in older adults (while 62 many not be old for those young at heart) that do not produce skull fracture may still provide enough force to cause the brain to move in relationship to the meningeal layers causing bleeding inside the skull. (Older brains tend to shrink due to slow neuronal loss leaving more space for movement within the skull.) Subdural hematomas are often due to a tearing of cerebral veins as they enter the superior sagittal sinus. As the vein tears, it often bleeds into a potential space inside the dura mater, but outside the fluid-impervious outer layer of the arachnoid mater. Those are veins that bleed into this potential space, so bleeding is often slow to develop. Subdural hematomas are usually treated by drilling a small hole in the skull over the center of the hematoma and removing the blood clot. Normally the initial tear of the vein repairs itself with time.

Epidural hematomas (**answer a**) are rare if there are no skull fractures. A pituitary tumor (**answer c**) might affect vision, but normally does not cause papilledema. Graves disease (**answer d**) may produce exophthalmus and would be present before the fall. Trigeminal neuralgias (**answer e**) are rarely produced by falls.

286. The answer is b. (*Moore, pp 1007, 1008.*) The sternocleidomastoid muscle most likely became overstretched during the birthing process. As the muscle fibers start the process of repair, the remaining muscle fibers contract to limit head movement, a process called guarding. Generally physical therapy involving gently stretching the sternocleidomastoid muscle is effective at slowly reversing the condition. A modified cervical collar, called a tubular orthosis for torticollis is effective in aiding proper head positioning if the condition persists beyond 4 months of age. Spasmodic torticollis (**answer c**) is a sudden contraction of the sternocleidomastoid muscle and usually presents in adulthood. The anterior scalene muscle (**answer a**) connects from transverse cervical processes down to the superior surface of the first rib and would simply cause the neck to tilt to one side, with little or no head rotation. Tearing of the trapezius muscle (**answers d and e**) during birth is very rare and would cause the baby's head to tilt upward and to one side. Floppy (or dropped) head syndrome (**answer d**) is a condition that occurs in adults and may be associated with a variety of neuromuscular diseases including amyotrophic lateral sclerosis (ALS) also known as Lou Gehrig disease, Parkinson disease, myasthenia gravis, polymyositis, and genetic myopathies.

287. The answer is d. (*Moore, pp 946, 949. Sadler, pp 284-285.*) The lateral nasal process forms the alar region of the nose. Normally the maxillary process grows medially and fuses with the medial nasal process at the philtrum on both sides of the upper lip. The fact that the cleft involves both the lip and bony primary palate suggests failure of the maxillary process to fuse with the medial nasal process. The mandibular process (**answers a and b**) does not normally fuse with either the lateral or medial nasal processes (**answer c**). This would reduce the size of the mouth. The lateral and medial nasal processes (**answer e**) fuse to form a nostril separate from the oral cavity.

288. The answer is e. (*Moore, pp 898-903.*) The baby's right eye is unable to be depressed below the horizon of normal gaze because of tonic contraction of the superior rectus muscle. Normally both the inferior rectus and superior oblique muscles help depress the eye and allow downward gaze. Botulinum toxin (Botox) inhibits acetylcholine release at the neuromuscular junction thus causing a flaccid paralysis of the muscle that is injected. The other extraocular muscles may then be able to function and permit downward gaze. If the right inferior oblique muscle **(answer a)** is injected, the eye would tend to migrate downward, but outward. If the right inferior rectus muscle **(answer b)** is injected with Botox, then the eye would tend to migrate further upward and medially. If the right lateral rectus muscle **(answer c)** is injected and becomes flaccid, then the eye would tend to gaze only medially. If the right superior oblique muscle **(answer d)** is injected with Botox, then the eye would tend to migrate upward and laterally.

289. The answer is d. (*Moore, p 1047.*) The palatine tonsil sits in the lateral wall of the oropharynx in the palatine arch posterior to the palatoglossus muscle and anterior to the palatopharyngeus muscle. The glossopharyngeal CN (IX) traverses the bed of the palatine tonsil and carries afferent information to the brain regarding both general sensation and the special sense of taste from the posterior one-third of the tongue. The glossopharyngeal nerve is at risk for being cut during tonsillectomy. The ability to detect taste from the anterior two-thirds of the tongue **(answer a)** is not at risk because that information is carried by the lingual nerve, below the tongue. The ability to protrude the tongue **(answer b)** is provided by innervation from the hypoglossal nerve, which innervates all the intrinsic tongue muscles and lies below the tongue and is not a risk. The mandibular division of the trigeminal CN V (V^3) does not course near the palatine arch and would not be at risk. It aids in the opening of the mouth **(answer c)** and movement of the mandible from side-to-side **(answer e)**.

290. The answer is b. (*Moore, p 909.*) Inferior rectus muscle was trapped in the maxillary bone. The breaking and dislocation of the zygomatic bone and part of the maxillary bone would be a modified type II Le Fort fracture, typical of a so-called "blowout" fracture. Since the left eye could not gaze above the horizon, the inferior rectus muscle was most likely trapped in the inferior orbital fissure, a site of weakness of the maxillary bone. The ethmoid bone **(answer a)** forms part of the medial wall of the orbit adjacent to the medial rectus muscle **(answers c and d)**, both of which are uninvolved in this injury. The superior rectus muscle **(answer e)** elevates the eye allowing superior gaze. It runs along the frontal bone and is not affected in this scenario.

291. The answer is b. (*Moore, pp 876-877.*) The most likely diagnosis is extracranial and epidural hematomas. The extracranial hematoma is the growing "goose egg" that was developing on the outside of her head. This condition is not life threatening. The physical findings of papilledema, frontal bone skull fracture, and accumulating blood inside the cranial bones anterior to the cranial suture are all consistent with epidural hematoma. Most likely the frontal bone fractured, lacerating the frontal branch of the middle meningeal artery and veins which run in grooves near the pterion. The temporal region of the skull is particularly thin in this region and more prone to compression fractures. Subdural hematomas **(answer c)** rarely present in a limited area, rather they occupy one complete cerebral hemisphere as the arachnoid mater separates from the dura mater. It is unlikely that a spinal tap, if performed would contain blood (indication of subarachnoid hemorrhage [**answers d and e**]).

292. The answer is a. (*Moore, pp 1054-1058, 1078.*) A fracture through the cribriform plate would likely cause both a leaking of cerebrospinal fluid (CSF) out of the nose (rhinorrhea) and headaches. It would likely shear off the olfactory nerves that pass through the cribriform plate of the ethmoid bone, resulting in left-sided anosmia (inability to smell). The lacrimal bone **(answer b)** surrounds the nasal lacrimal duct and if fractured might lead to a runny nose, but this would not explain the anosmia. The nasal bone **(answer c)** forms the root of the nose and is often broken in boxers, but such a fracture would not necessarily lead to a runny nose or continued headaches. Le Fort fractures **(answers d and e)** are fractures of the face involving the displacement of the maxillary and nasal region (type II) including displacement of the maxilla and zygomatic arch, thus displacing the maxillary teeth, nose, and zygomatic arch (type III). Neither of the Le Fort fractures would fit with the symptoms.

293. The answer is a. (*Moore, p 927.*) The mandible is fractured posterior to the mental foramen, since the mental nerve is cut. The inferior alveolar nerve enters the ramus of the mandible at the mandibular foramen, then supplies all the mandibular teeth, but gives off the mental nerve that exits the mental foramen and innervates the lower lip. Thus, a fracture across the body of the mandible anterior to the angle and posterior to the mental foramen would likely sever the inferior alveolar nerve, resulting in the loss of sensation within the lower lip. A fracture at the coronoid process of the mandible (**answer b**) would only detach the temporalis muscle from its insertion onto the mandible. A fracture at the mandibular symphysis (**answer c**) would not affect lower lip sensation since there are no nerves that cross the midline. A fracture at the neck of the mandible (**answer d**) would only compromise blood supply to the head of the mandible, which usually does not undergo necrosis as a consequence of its small size. A fracture at the ramus of the mandible superior to the mandibular foramen (**answer e**) would not affect the inferior alveolar nerve.

294. The answer is b. (*Moore, pp 921-922, 927.*) The temporalis, masseter, and medial and lateral pterygoid muscles are the muscles of mastication that attach to the mandible. The buccinator muscle (**answer a**), which controls the contents of the mouth during mastication, is innervated by the facial CN VII. The lateral pterygoid muscles, acting bilaterally, protract the jaw and, acting unilaterally, rotate the jaw during chewing. Because the fibers of the superior head of the lateral pterygoid muscle insert onto the anterior aspect of the articular disk of the temporomandibular joint as well as onto the head of the mandible, spasm of this muscle, such as in a yawn, can result in dislocation of the mandible by pulling the disk anterior to the articular tubercle. Reduction is accomplished by pushing the mandible downward and backward, so that the head of the mandible reenters the mandibular fossa. The temporalis (**answer e**), medial pterygoid (**answer c**), and masseter (**answer d**) muscles primarily elevate the jaw in molar occlusion.

295. The answer is c. (*Moore, p 1048-1049.*) This congenital anomaly is a branchial fistula. When the pharyngeal pouches persist, they may form connections to the exterior of the neck immediately anterior to the boundary of the sternocleidomastoid muscle. Since this weeps fluid it is most likely a fistula or external cyst (not one of the options). An internal branchial sinus (**answer b**) would be a blind pouch off the pharynx and have no external connections. The internal opening for this fistula would most likely be within the bed of the palatine fossa (from the second pharyngeal pouch) or further inferiorly within the pharynx if it is from the third or lower pharyngeal pouches. Persistent glossopharyngeal fistula (**answer a**) (opening of the embryonic glossopharyngeal duct) more rarely makes a connection to the surface ectoderm and like a thyroglossal duct cyst (**answer f**) would be a midline structure. A hyperactive sebaceous gland (answer d) would not secrete a clear fluid. Spina bifida occulta (answer e) is associated with a tuft of hairy skin over a defect in the posterior arch of the spinal cord.

296. The answer is e. (*Moore, pp 826, 831.*) The styloid process is attached to the temporal bone. The temporal bone has five major parts: the squamous, zygomatic, petrous, mastoid, and tympanic, in addition to the styloid process. The styloid process is not present in newborns, but grows as a bony projection from the temporal bone to serve as the site of attachment for two ligaments and three muscles. The ethmoid bone (answer a) lies superior to the nose. The occipital bone (answer c) forms the base of the skull around the foramen magnum and the caudal, posterior part of the skull. The sphenoid bone (answer d) constitutes a large part of the base of the skull more anteriorly and medially than the temporal bone.

297. The answer is d. (*Moore, pp 919, 922, 923.*) The stylomandibular ligament connects the styloid process to the inferior angle of the mandible along the posterior edge of the ramus. When the jaw is opened wide, especially when biting an apple or yawning, stress is placed on the ligament, causing pain. The stylohyoid ligament connects the styloid process to the lesser horn of the hyoid bone and generally limits the extent to which the hyoid bone and the larynx moves inferiorly. The larynx rises during swallowing, resulting in shortening of the stylohyoid ligament (answer a). Therefore, this is the least likely source of pain. The stylohyoid muscle (answer b) raises the hyoid bone and larynx during swallowing, but not when yawning. During yawning the larynx tends to move inferiorly, not superiorly. The styloglossus muscle (answer c) raises and retracts the base of the tongue during swallowing, but is not likely to be active during yawning. The stylopharyngeus muscle (answer e) helps raise the pharynx during swallowing, but is unlikely to specifically contract during yawning.

298. The answer is d. (*Moore, pp 861, 1081.*) The patient has facial paralysis, which indicates injury to the facial nerve. A problem in the internal auditory meatus (answer b) usually affects hearing and balance. That the superior salivatory nucleus (answer a) is normal is indicated by normal lacrimation. Hence, the lesion must be distal to the origin of the greater superficial nerve at the genu of the facial nerve (answer c). However, absence of hyperacusis (inability to tolerate everyday sounds) indicates that the branch to the stapedius muscle is functioning normally, and suggests that the lesion is close to the stylomastoid foramen. Loss of taste and diminished salivation place the lesion proximal to the origin of the chorda tympani nerve. If the lesion were proximal to the stylomastoid foramen (**answer e**), taste and salivation would have been normal, with facial paralysis as the only sign.

299. The answer is d. (*Moore, pp 923-926.*) The passage in the brain indicated by the arrow is the cerebral aqueduct (of Sylvius), which is the narrow canal connecting the third and fourth ventricles. The cerebrospinal fluid produced in the lateral and third ventricles must reach the fourth ventricle to escape into the subarachnoid space through the foramina or lateral apertures (of Luschka) and median aperture (of Magendie). If either the cerebral aqueduct or apertures of the fourth ventricle become blocked then this condition is called "obstructive" (older term "internal") hydrocephalus. Venous blood (**answer a**) would also appear dark on this MRI but would appear along the superior sagittal sinus. The basilar artery (**answer b**) would be located just anteriorly, along the clivus. Neuronal tracts (**answers c and e**) do not appear dark in an MRI.

300. The answer is b. (*Moore, pp 936-938.*) The anterior palatoglossal arch, or anterior faucial pillar, is formed by the mucosa overlying the palatoglossal muscle. The posterior faucial pillar, or palatopharyngeal arch, likewise is formed by the palatopharyngeus muscle. The palatoglossus and palatopharyngeus muscles insert into the tongue and pharynx, respectively, and both are innervated by the pharyngeal branch of the vagus nerve (CN X). The tensor veli palatini and levator veli palatini, which arise from opposite sides of the auditory tube and base of the skull, insert into the soft palate. They are innervated, respectively, by the trigeminal nerve and the pharyngeal branch of the vagus nerve. The salpingopharyngeus muscle (**answer c**), also innervated by the pharyngeal branch of the vagus nerve, arises from the torus tubarius at the opening of the auditory tube and inserts into the pharyngeal musculature. The superior and middle pharyngeal constrictors (**answer e**) are innervated by the pharyngeal branch of the vagus nerve. The stylopharyngeus and styloglossus muscles (**answer d**) originate from the styloid process and insert onto the lesser horn of the hyoid and into the tongue, respectively. They are innervated by the glossopharyngeal and hypoglossal nerves, respectively. Levator veli palatini and tensor veli palatini muscles (**answer a**) are above the soft palate.

301. The answer is e. (*Moore, p 970.*) The tensor veli palatini muscle has two functions: one to elevate the soft palate and second to open the Eustachian tube during each swallow (or yawn) to allow air to pass from the nasopharynx into the middle ear. The masseter (**answer a**) is a muscle of mastication that lies outside the oral cavity and raises the mandible during chewing and has nothing to do with soft palate function. The musculus uvulae muscle (**answer b**) raises the uvula. The palatoglossus muscle (**answer c**) forms the anterior edge of the palatine arch and helps lower the soft palate. The palatopharyngeus muscle (**answer d**) forms the posterior edge of the palatine arch and helps lower the soft palate and raises the pharynx during swallowing.

302. The answer is a. (*Moore, pp 887-888.*) The most likely diagnosis is a subarachnoid hemorrhagic stroke, which had stopped by the time the CT was performed. While most strokes present with sudden onset of neurological symptoms, the majority of strokes (~80%) are ischemic (**answer b**) in nature due to cerebral blood clots. This man probably had a hemorrhagic stroke as a consequence of increased blood pressure due to straining, to relieve his constipation. This is consistent with his developing headache, stiff neck, and blood within the CSF collected by spinal tap. One would not want to give TPA to a patient with a hemorrhagic stroke because it would probably make conditions worse. The CT was normal because the blood vessel had spontaneously stopped bleeding and the amount of blood was too small to detect radiographically. Subdural hematoma (**answer c**), while common in the elderly, would not result in a bloody spinal tap. Epidural hematoma (**answer d**) would not result in a bloody spinal tap. Alzheimer dementia (**answer e**) is not relevant to this case.

303. The answer is c. (*Moore, p 1082.*) Atrophy of the intrinsic musculature of the tongue on one side is due to a lesion of the ipsilateral hypoglossal nerve. Deviation of the tongue to the right on protrusion results from the unopposed action of the left genioglossus muscle, which is innervated by the left hypoglossal nerve. The hypoglossal nerve also innervates numerous other tongue muscles involved in deglutition. The question only asks about the cause of the tongue deviation so the other answers (**answers a, b, d, and e**) are not involved in controlling the tongue, rather CN X or limb functions.

304. The answer is e. *(Moore, pp 913, 1081.)* The abducent nerve (CN VI) innervates the lateral rectus muscle. Remember, the "formula" LR₆SO₄. Lateral rectus is innervated by CN VI, superior oblique by CN IV, and the remainder of the extrinsic eye muscles by CN III. Loss of innervation to the lateral rectus results in unopposed tension by the medial rectus, which produces internal strabismus. The oculomotor nerve (CN III) innervates the medial, superior, and inferior recti, the inferior oblique, and the levator palpebrae superioris muscles. Paralysis of this nerve **(answer b)** would result in lateral deviation of the eye (external strabismus) accompanied by ptosis (drooping eyelid). In addition, mydriasis (dilated pupil) results from loss of function of the parasympathetic component of the oculomotor nerve. Damage to the trochlear nerve (CN IV) results in paralysis of the superior oblique muscle with impaired ability to direct the eye downward and outward **(answer c)**. The optic nerve **(answer a)** is responsible for receiving the special sense of sight. The trigeminal cranial nerve **(answer d)** carries pain information from the eye.

305. The answer is a. *(Moore, pp 984, 1002.)* The stylohyoid muscle inserts onto the lesser horn of the hyoid bone (both derivatives of the second branchial arch) and raises that bone during swallowing. The distal tendon of the stylohyoid muscle is split by the digastric muscle **(answer d)** passing through its trochlea attached to the lesser horn. The styloglossus muscle acts to retract the tongue **(answer b)**. The sphenomandibular ligament inserts onto the lingula of the mandibular foramen **(answer c)**; the stylohyoid ligament inserts onto the lesser horn of the hyoid bone. The stylopharyngeus muscle inserts into the middle pharyngeal constrictor. The stylomandibular ligament **(answer e)** attaches to the posterior edge of the ramus of the mandible not to the lingula of the mandible.

306. The answer is c. *(Moore, pp 964-965.)* He suffers from sinusitis, which has eroded through the wall of the frontal sinus, and since the frontalis muscle is not attached to bone, allows pus to leak into the upper eyelid. Inflammation of the mucous membrane that lines the sinuses may sometimes lead to a buildup of pus that can block the normal drainage pathways. If pressure builds, erosion of the bony wall of the sinus can occur. In this instance, the anterior wall of the frontal sinus was compromised and pus escaped into the forehead and into the upper eyelid, since the frontalis muscle, a normal barrier, attaches only into skin of the forehead. In order to allow movement, the skin of the eyelid is only attached to underlying structures by loose areolar connective tissue, through which infections easily spread. Intravenous antibiotics were initiated. The swelling spontaneously reduced after the first week of treatment and no visible defects were noted 1 month later. Trigeminal neuralgia or tic douloureux (**answers a and b**) is characterized by sudden sharp pains over the distribution of one or more branches of the trigeminal nerve. Although pain is perceived within the ophthalmic division, the teenager would not suffer from sudden sharp twinges of pain, rather a dull constant pain from swollen tissue. Bell palsy (**answer d**) is generally caused by a herpes simplex virus infection of the facial nerve within the facial canal. The resulting unilateral facial paralysis limits one's ability to close the upper eyelid, not raise it. A sty (**answer e**) is an inflammation of the sebaceous gland, associated with each eyelash or cilia. A chalazion is an inflammation of a meibomian or tarsal gland, which lies on the inner surface of the eyelid. This could cause a bulge in the upper eyelid, but does not fit with the other clinical findings.

307. The answer is d. (*Moore, p 463. Sadler, pp 302-303.*) In the family of conditions known as spina bifida, failure of the dorsal portions of the developing vertebrae may expose a portion of the spinal cord and its covering. This usually occurs near the caudal end of the neural tube, often in the lumbar region. If there is no projection of the spinal cord or its covering through the bony defect, the condition is "hidden" (spina bifida occulta). However, the term spina bifida cystica is used when the spinal meninges are displaced from the spinal canal and into the defect. In a meningocele (**answer c**), there is a saclike projection formed only by the meninges. If the projection contains neural material, it is a meningomyelocele, which is the case for this newborn. Most newborns with lumbar meningomyelocele have loss of function of lower extremities and may also have bowel and bladder dysfunction because the spinal cord does not make proper neural connections as a result of its growing outside the normal spinal canal. Rachischisis, also known as myeloschisis (**answer a**), is an extreme example of spina bifida cystica in which the neural folds underlying the vertebral defect fail to fuse, leaving an exposed neural plate. Anencephaly (**answer b**) occurs when the cranial neural tube fails to fuse, thus resulting in lack of formation of forebrain structures and a portion of the enclosing cranium. Hydrocephaly (**answer e**) results from blockage of the narrow passageways between the ventricles or between the ventricles and the subarachnoid space. Resultant swelling of the ventricles compresses the brain against the cranial vault and may cause serious mental deficits.

308. The answer is c. (*Moore, pp 1009, 1082.*) Cranial nerves IX, X, and XI pass out of the skull at the jugular foramen. The styloglossus muscle is innervated by the hypoglossal nerve, which leaves the posterior cranial fossa by way of the anterior condylar canal. In addition to the internal jugular vein, the jugular foramen contains the glossopharyngeal nerve (innervating the stylopharyngeus muscle [**answer d**]), the vagus nerve (innervating palatal [**answer a**], pharyngeal, and laryngeal musculature), and the spinal accessory nerve innervating the sternocleidomastoid (**answer b**) and trapezius muscles (**answer e**).

309. The answer is c. (*Moore, p 949. Fauci, p 1666.*) Removal of enlarged palatine tonsils will often reduce snoring especially in children and teenagers, though less frequently than in adults. The enlarged pharyngeal tonsils or adenoids may also cause snoring, but they are located in the posterior of the nasopharynx. Obesity is a leading cause of snoring in adults, but this teenager was described as skinny. An enlarged or infected uvula may cause snoring, so a short uvula (**answer a**) is very unlikely to cause snoring. Premature eruption of the wisdom teeth (**answer b**) rarely causes snoring, but may cause impaction or crowding of existing teeth. Lingual tonsils (**answer c**) are found in the tongue and do not cause snoring. Mandibular tori are benign bony protrusions of the mandible toward the oral cavity that are covered with oral mucosa. Unless the mandibular tori (**answer e**) grow extremely large, they are unlikely to cause snoring. While the piercing of the tongue in order to place the tongue stud (**answer f**) produces swelling of the tongue that normally goes away by 7 to 10 days, a tongue stud is unlikely to cause snoring. In most states a minor would need parental permission for getting his tongue pierced.

310. The answer is c. (*Moore, pp 1045-1046.*) The posterior cricoarytenoid muscles rotate the arytenoids laterally, which swings the vocal process of that cartilage outward to abduct the vocal cords and open the glottis. These are the sole abductors of the vocal folds. The lateral cricoarytenoid muscles (**answer b**) and the unpaired transverse arytenoid muscle (**answer e**) adduct the vocal folds. The thyroarytenoid muscle (**answer d**) and its innermost portion, the vocalis muscle, act to tense the cords. The cricothyroid muscle (**answer a**) lengthens the vocal cords.

311. The answer is c. (*Moore, p 961. Fauci, pp 2209-2210.*) Structure 8 is the pituitary gland. The anterior pituitary produces growth hormone from somatotropes. Growth hormone secreting tumors often cause an enlargement of the skull and the pituitary gland. The pituitary gland sits in the sella turcica which is surrounded by the large sphenoid air sinus (black region) just inferior to the pituitary gland. Cancers of the pituitary gland are often removed by operating through the nose and the sphenoid air sinus, leaving the brain relatively undisturbed. Other labeled structures are as follows: 2 **(answer a)**, frontal sinus (this might undergo some enlargement if a growth hormone secreting pituitary tumor were present); 7 **(answer b)**, tongue genioglossus; 8 **(answer c)**, pituitary gland; 9 **(answer d)**, infundibular stalk; 10 **(answer e)**, clivus portion of the occipital bone; 11 **(answer f)**, odontoid process of axis (C2); 12 **(answer g)**, anterior arch of atlas (C1); and 13, mandible.

312. The answer is b. *(Moore, p 833, 1078-1079.)* Structure 42 is the foramen ovale. It transmits the mandibular division of the trigeminal cranial nerve (CN V^3), responsible for innervating the muscles of mastication. The patient would also show loss of sensation along the mandible due to interruption of transmission of sensory information within the mandibular division of cranial nerve V. Weakened muscles of facial expression **(answer a)** would result from compromising the stylomastoid foramen, which transmits part of the facial cranial nerve (CN VII; not on this image). Weakened ability to turn one's head **(answer c)** and shrug **(answer e)** would be the result of damage to the accessory cranial nerve (CN XI), which exits the skull through the jugular foramen (not numbered on this image). The vagus **(answer d)** cranial nerve (CN X) exits through the jugular foramen along with CN IX and XI. Structure 40 is the carotid canal. Other labeled structures are as follows: 34, condyle of the mandible; 35, frontal process of the maxilla; 41, inferior orbital fissure; 43, foramen spinosum; and 44, external auditory canal.

313. The answer is d. *(Moore, pp 902, 1080-1081.)* Cranial nerve IV has a long intracranial course, so it has an increased chance of injury. The nerve originates from the trochlear nucleus in the midbrain and is the only cranial nerve to exit the brain on the dorsal rather than ventral surface. It exits the middle cranial fossa by exiting the superior orbital fissure (along with CN III, V^1, and VI). The nerve also does not pass through the common tendinous ring to reach the superior oblique muscle; CN IV is the only extraocular muscle to pass through a pulley, the trochlea. A patient with a cut CN IV tends to tilt her/his head toward the unaffected side (in this case to the right, thus not [answer c]). A physician examines individual extraoc-ular muscle function by performing the "H" test (see High Yield Facts, Figure 17). To test the function of the superior oblique muscle (innervated by the trochlear nerve) the patient first looks medially (adduction) and then inferiorly (toward the nose). Cranial nerve III (answers a and b) is involved with the bulk of the other extraocular eye movements and is normal. Cranial nerve VI (answer e) innervates the lateral rectus muscle, which is responsible for abducting each eye, and is normal in this patient.

314. The answer is e. (*Moore, 956-958.*) A nasal polyp within the sphenoethmoid recess is very likely to inhibit proper drainage of the sphenoid sinus increasing the likelihood of sphenoid sinusitis. While pain from sphenoid sinusitis can be described as behind or between the eyes, classically it refers pain to the vertex of the head. Sinusitis is a common cause of headaches. Pain for sinusitis within the anterior ethmoid sinuses (answer a) generally occurs between the eyes and the anterior ethmoid sinuses drain under the middle turbinate. Pain from sinusitis within the frontal sinus (answer b) presents as pain directly superficial to the frontal bone between the eyes within the glabellar regions. The frontal sinus drains inferior to the middle turbinate. Pain from sinusitis within the middle ethmoid sinuses (answer c) normally presents as pain between the eyes. The middle ethmoid sinuses drain inferior to the middle turbinate. Pain from sinusitis within the maxillary sinus (answer d) presents as pain within or cranial to the maxillary teeth. The maxillary sinus drains inferior to the middle turbinate.

315. The answer is d. (*Moore, pp 978-979.*) PE or tympanostomy tubes that look like little plastic bobbins are typically positioned by cutting the inferior posterior portion of the tympanic membrane in a radial fashion. The umbo (answer a) is where the tip of the manubrium of the malleus is attached to the tympanic membrane (answer b) and would not be a site of insertion of a PE tube; thus both answers a and b are wrong. The pars flaccida (answer c) of the tympanic membrane is near the course of the chorda tympani nerve which is therefore a dangerous location for incisions to place tubes. It would be difficult to place a tube within the Eustachian tube (answer e), even though that is the site of the malfunction. PE tubes typically are pushed out of the tympanic membrane as the stratified squamous epithelium continually sloughs off cells at its surface, pushing on the external flang, and thus naturally popping the bobbin-like tube out of the membrane months later.

316. The answer is e. (*Moore, pp 921-923.*) The temporalis muscle elevates the mandible by inserting onto the coronoid process of the ramus of the mandible. The masseter muscle elevates the mandible by originating from the zygomatic arch and inserting on the outer angle of the mandible. The medial and lateral pterygoid muscles (**answer a, b, and c**) originate from the medial and lateral pterygoid plates which lie medial to the ramus and angle of the mandible and are not fractured in this vignette. The stylohyoid and posterior belly of the digastric (**answer d**) originate from the styloid process and mastoid process, respectively, and neither of those bones are fractured. Contraction of the temporalis, masseter, and medial pterygoid muscles helps elevate the mandible. The lateral pterygoid, stylohyoid, and posterior belly of the digastric muscles help lower or open the mandible.

317. The answer is b. (*Moore, pp 505-506, 1081.*) A head CT is ordered with specific imaging of cranial nerve VI. One of the possible consequences of a spinal tap is continued leakage of cerebral spinal fluid (cerebrospinal fluid, CSF) at the site of the tap since the meninges have been compromised. If CSF continues to leak then autologous blood is injected at the site of the spinal tap to stimulate closing of the hole in the meninges. Sliding of the brain toward the foramen magnum occurs as a rare consequence of spinal taps. Since cranial nerve VI exits the brain at the junction of the medulla and the pons and then enters the Dorello dural cave along the clivus, it cannot slide down with the brain and thus would be subject to stretching. Stretching of the abducent nerve would likely lead to bilateral compromised ability to look laterally since no other cranial nerves can cause abduction of the eyes. Viral meningitis (**answer a**) would not cause a selective loss of both abducent cranial nerves. Excess CSF causes CN VI palsy, but generally not CN III palsy (**answer c**). Bilateral tumors at the superior orbital fissures (**answer d**) are unlikely, and also would compromise other cranial nerves as well. Loss of the ability to look laterally is not part of a normal course of hospitalization (**answer e**).

318. The answer is i. (*Moore, pp 949, 1082.*) The cranial nerve that provides the afferent limb of the gag reflex is the glossopharyngeal, IX cranial nerve (**answers a→h and j→l**). Cranial nerve IX provides general sensation from the posterior one-third of the tongue and palatine tonsil area. The response to touching this area is to contract the soft palate and pharynx in a protective manor or gag reflex. The motor aspects of this reflex are mainly mediated by the vagus, cranial nerve X.

319. The answer is a. (*Moore, pp 913, 1080.*) This condition is most likely due to an aneurysm of the left posterior cerebral artery compressing cranial nerve III. The woman's symptoms, ptosis of the upper eyelid, an eye that is rotated downward (because superior oblique muscle, innervated by CN IV is still functioning functional) and outward (because the lateral rectus muscle, innervated by CN VI is still functioning) with a dilated pupil (because sympathetics, which innervate the dilator pupil muscles are still functional) are all consistent with loss of function of cranial nerve III. An aneurysm in either the posterior cerebral or superior cerebellar artery often compresses cranial nerve III as it exits the midbrain. An aneurysm of the right anterior cerebral artery **(answer b)** would be very unlikely to cause a problem for the left third cranial nerve. A tumor within the left optic canal **(answer c)** would affect the left optic nerve which passes through it. Cranial nerve III passes into the orbit through the superior orbital fissure along with CN IV, V^1, and VI. Neither glaucoma **(answer d)** nor a parotid gland tumor **(answer e)** would present with those symptoms.

320. Answer is c. (*Moore, pp 1065-1067.*) It is suspected that a tumor is blocking the left foramen ovale. The mandibular division of the trigeminal cranial nerve exits the skull through the foramen ovale. This division provides general sensation to the tongue (via the lingual nerve) and mandibular teeth (via the inferior alveolar nerve) and area over the mandible (via the buccal nerve). In addition, the mandibular division of the trigeminal also innervates eight muscles (the four muscles of mastication [temporalis, masseter, medial, and lateral pterygoid muscles], two associated with the floor of the mouth [the mylohyoid and anterior belly of the digastric muscles], and two tensors [tensor tympani in the middle ear and tensor veli palatini in the soft palate]). In addition, preganglionic nerves from cranial nerve IX (via the lesser petrosal nerve) also pass through the foramen ovale on their way to stimulate the parotid salivary gland. A tumor at the superior orbital fissure **(answer a)** would affect eye movements and forehead sensation. A tumor at the foramen rotundum **(answer b)** would affect sensation under the eye on the face and maxillary teeth pain. A tumor at the internal acoustic meatus **(answers d and e)** would affect the facial nerve, hearing, and balance.

321. The answer is d. (*Moore, p 964.*) A sinus series is ordered because his physician suspects that he has maxillary sinusitis. The maxillary sinus is the most frequent site of sinusitis. This is likely due to the fact that its ostium is high on the medial wall of the sinus, thus requiring ciliary action to drain the sinus when in the anatomical position. Lying on his right side may help this patient drain his left maxillary sinus. The maxillary sinus ostium is generally large enough that a cannula can be threaded into the sinus and vacuum applied to help drain it. Sphenoid sinus pain (**answer a**) is generally referred to the top of the skull near the vertex. Anterior (**answer b**) and posterior (**answer c**) ethmoidal sinus pain refers to areas around the eyes (either medial or lateral). Frontal sinusitis pain (**answer e**) presents over the frontal sinus and tapping on the forehead there will elicit pain.

322. The answer is e. (*Moore, pp 999-1000, 1011.*) The correct answer is the internal carotid artery (medial), internal jugular vein (lateral), and the vagus nerve. **Answers a and b** are not correct because the carotid sheath contains the vagus, not the sympathetic chain, nor the phrenic nerve (**answers c and d**). The internal carotid artery (which has a palpable pulse) is medial and the internal jugular vein, into which the cardiac catheter is inserted, has a lateral location within the carotid sheath.

323. The answer is d. (*Moore, pp 1044-1045.*) The food is most likely stuck in the laryngeal pharynx, so you must produce an alternative airway (called a tracheostomy) below the glottis, which reflexly closes. Locations around the hyoid bone (**answers a and b**) and above the laryngeal notch (**answer c**) are above the blockage and would not get air into the lungs. The isthmus of the thyroid gland generally lies in front of the second and third tracheal ring (**answer e**), and because it is so highly vascular, it is not an ideal location for an emergency airway. An additional alternative location for an emergency airway would be the jugular notch, but is not preferred because of the occurrence of a thyroid ima artery below the isthmus, in a small percentage of the population.

324. The answers is c. (*Sadler, pp 268-269.*) The muscles of facial expression are derived from the second pharyngeal/branchial arch. A, C, E, G, and I denote the first, second, third, fourth, and sixth branchial arches, respectively. B, D, F, H, and J denote the first, second, dorsal third, ventral third, and fourth branchial pouches, respectively. B will become the auditory tube; D will become the palatine tonsillar fossa; F will become the inferior parathyroid glands; H will become the thymus; the dorsal part of J will form the superior parathyroids and the ventral portion of J will form the ultimobranchial body (C cells of the thyroid). (See High-Yield Facts, Figure 1, Tables 2 and 3).

325. The answer is c. *(Moore, pp 926, 1081.)* One of the risks of the surgical resection is that she may develop right-sided facial muscle paralysis. About 80% of salivary gland tumors originate from within the parotid salivary gland. The facial nerve sends out motoneurons from the stylomastoid foramen. That nerve then branches into 5 to 7 major branches that innervate the muscles of facial expression (derived from the second branchial arch). The branches divide while passing through the substance of the parotid salivary gland. The branches are named for the anatomic regions that they serve: temporal; zygomatic; buccal; mandibular; cervical; and posterior auricular branches. While it is unlikely that all of those branches would be cut while removing the parotid tumor, they all are potentially at risk. The tumor is described as superficial within the parotid gland and since the facial nerve normally passes through the middle of the gland, the facial nerve might be spared. The patient in the vignette is very unlikely to lose the sense of taste **(answer a)**. That information is carried in the lingual and chorda tympani nerves, which are much deeper and unlikely to be at risk. The mandibular division of the mandible innervates the muscles of mastication and exits the skull at the foramen ovale deep to the parotid and protected by the lateral pterygoid muscles, so losing the ability to chew on the right side is unlikely **(answer b)**. The hypoglossal nerve innervates tongue muscle **(answer d)** from below the tongue, so is not in jeopardy of being cut. The tensor tympani receives innervation from the mandibular division of the trigeminal nerve as it exits the foramen ovale which is deep to the surgical area, thus not in danger **(answer e)**.

326. The answer is c. *(Moore, p 1082.)* An acoustic neuroma is a benign tumor of the Schwann cells that myelinate the vestibular portion of the VIII cranial nerve. Even though the tumor arises on the vestibular portion of the VIII cranial nerve, hearing loss **(answer a)** is usually the first reported symptom. Tinnitus or ringing in the ear and headaches are also frequently reported. While the vestibular system may be disrupted (this patient complained of dizziness) the vestibular system on the right side is functioning normally and provides enough information once the individual becomes accustomed to the loss. In this case the tumor has started to affect the VII cranial nerve which controls the muscles of facial expression. Her symptoms go beyond conductive hearing loss (she is also young [53] to be suffering from conductive hearing loss). Ménière disease (answer b) is an excess accumulation of endolymph, which is usually associated with hearing loss, tinnitus, and vertigo (all reported in this woman), but would not be associated with any facial paralysis. Tic douloureux (or trigeminal neuralgia; answer d) is characterized by sudden pain along the distribution of the trigeminal nerve and is not a presenting problem. A parotid gland tumor (answer e) could result in the loss of control of the muscles of facial expression, but hearing and balance would generally be unaffected.

327. The answer is b. (Moore, p 950.) The pediatrician explains that the problem could be corrected by cutting the lingual frenulum. The boy is currently "tongue-tied." The frenulum of the tongue limits its ability to protrude from the mouth. The inferior aspect of the genioglossus and the geniohyoid muscles contract in order to pull the hyoid bone forward allowing one to stick their tongue out of their mouth. All the intrinsic and three quarters of the extrinsic muscles of the tongue are innervated by the hypoglossal nerve (XII CN). It is very unlikely that the XII cranial nerve never developed (answer a), since the child would then have no tongue movement and the tongue would atrophy. Shortening the posterior belly of the digastric (answer c) would worsen the problem by pulling the tongue up and back within the mouth. Cutting the pterygomandibular raphe (answer d) would serve no function. Speech therapy (answer e) would be the second best answer in that it might stretch the frenulum over time.

328. The answers is a. (Moore, pp 907, 912.) Aqueous humor is produced by the ciliary processes which project from the ciliary body (answer c), in the posterior chamber. Aqueous humor flows through the pupil into the anterior chamber, where it normally drains through the trabecular meshwork that leads to the scleral venous sinus (canal of Schlemm, see Question 267 and feedback). This trabecular meshwork can become plugged with red blood cells, especially if some blood clotting occurs. If the trabecular meshwork is blocked, then intraocular pressure builds up in the eye, which if excessive, can lead to blindness. This is the reason for daily intraocular pressure monitoring until the blood clears. When intraocular pressure increases suddenly (hours) it is very painful, and the pressure must be relieved by inserting a small needle at the corner of the cornea and applying pressure elsewhere, thus releasing fluid in a procedure called "burping the eye." As the intraocular pressure is normalized, the eye pain subsides. Gradual increases in intraocular pressure, however, may go undetected because they are not always painful (such as in the case of glaucoma). The ciliary muscle which has zonular fibers (suspensory ligament of the lens) attached to it **(answer b)** controls the shape of the lens, but does not drain aqueous humor. It also lies in the posterior not the anterior chamber of the eye. The lens **(answer d)** is not the site of drainage of aqueous humor and is located in the posterior chamber of the eye. The retina **(answer e)** is not the site of drainage of aqueous humor and is located in the posterior four-fifths of the eye surrounding the vitreous body (humor) of the eye (Also see Question 267 and feedback).

Thorax

Questions

329. A new mother brings her 6-month-old infant to the pediatric clinic. She reports that the new day care provider thinks that the baby boy is a slow bottle feeder, breathes heavily, and turns bluish while feeding. He is much less active than the other boys and is small for his age. A systolic murmur (continuously between S1 and S2 heart sounds) loudest at the left sternal border at about the third intercostal space is detected. The sound of the murmur is significantly reduced in the back. All heart valve sounds are normal. The lungs sound congested. The baby boy is sent for an echocardiogram. Which one of the following is the most likely congenital cardiac anomaly in the child in this vignette?

a. Aortic valve stenosis
b. Transposition of the great arteries
c. Persistent ligamentum arteriosum
d. Pulmonary valve stenosis
e. Ventricular septal defect (VSD)

330. A mother brings her 11-month-old girl to her pediatric office for her annual physical. The baby girl has normal height and weight for her age. The baby's heart has a split S2 heart sound, which does not vary with the baby's breathing patterns, even as she starts to cry a little. The sound is easily heard at the left upper sternal border. All other heart valve sounds are normal. The lungs sound normal. What congenital cardiac anomaly is likely present?

a. Aortic valve stenosis
b. Atrial septal defect (ASD)
c. Coarctation of the aorta
d. Transposition of the great arteries
e. Ventricular septal defect

331. A mammogram of a woman, age 48, reveals macrocalcification within the right upper, lateral quadrant of the breast, indicating the need for a biopsy. The surgeon closely examines the nipple for indications of ductal carcinoma. At surgery for the biopsy, a locator needle is inserted into the region of macrocalcification and the position confirmed by mammography. The surgeon incises the skin and dissects a block of tissue. The pathology report indicates ductal carcinoma with microinvasion necessitating surgery. Both patient and surgeon agree that a modified radical mastectomy offers the best prognosis in her case. At surgery for mastectomy, the surgeon carries the dissection along the major pathway of lymphatic drainage from the mammary gland. The major lymphatic channels parallel which one of the following?

a. Subcutaneous venous networks to the contralateral breast and abdominal wall
b. Tributaries of the axillary vessels to the axillary nodes
c. Tributaries of the intercostal vessels to the parasternal nodes
d. Tributaries of the internal thoracic (mammary) vessels to the parasternal nodes
e. Tributaries of the thoracoacromial vessels to the apical (subscapular) nodes

332. A 48-year-old woman undergoes a complete mastectomy, including removing several axillary lymph nodes. The lymph nodes are all negative for evidence of metastasis. However, the patient is found to have winging of the scapula when her flexed arm is pressed against a fixed object. This indicates injury to which one of the following nerves?

a. Axillary
b. Long thoracic
c. Lower subscapular
d. Supraclavicular
e. Thoracodorsal

333. A mother of three older children brings her 1-month-old infant to her pediatrician's office. The baby was born 1 month prematurely, breathes rapidly, especially when trying to feed, and she is not gaining weight. Her heart beat is rapid with a "machinelike" murmur that masks the S2 heart sound and is loudest at the left upper chest. The baby's peripheral pulse is bounding with a sudden drop-off in systolic pressure. An echocardiogram is ordered because which one of the following congential heart anomalies is suspected?

a. Aortic valve stenosis
b. Atrial septal defect
c. Coarctation of the aorta
d. Patent ductus arteriosus
e. Ventricular septal defect

334. A mother brings her 4-year-old boy into the pediatric clinic. He is normal for height and weight for his age, but he has just joined a soccer team to become socialized prior to kindergarten, since he is the only child of a stay-at-home mother. The mother notes that her son needs to stop and rest in the middle of the field after running hard. All heart sounds are normal with the exception of a murmur at the second intercostal space along the left sternal border. Which one of the following is the most likely cardiac problem in this boy?

a. Aortic valve stenosis
b. Atrial septal defect
c. Coarctation of the aorta
d. Patent ductus arteriosus
e. Pulmonary valve stenosis

335. When examining an anteroposterior (AP) chest film of a 57-year-old man with a systolic ejection-type cardiac murmur, the radiologist notices that the arch of the aorta forms a typical aortic knob on the left of the mediastinal border, but also appears as a bulge on the right upper mediastinal border, suggesting an enlarged ascending aorta. In addition, the left ventricular heart border appears prominent. There is no evidence of pulmonary hypertension in this patient. An echocardiogram is ordered because it is suspected that this patient has which one of the following conditions?

a. Tetralogy of Fallot
b. Pulmonary valve stenosis
c. Atherosclerosis
d. Aortic valve stenosis
e. Defective tricuspid valve

336. A 38-year-old woman with a body mass index (BMI) of 31 presents with pain to the right side of the neck, extending laterally to the right clavicle for an hour or two after meals. A careful physical examination of her neck and shoulder region suggests that the pain may be referred pain, since manipulation of the right shoulder and neck does not reproduce the vague pain. Which one of the following nerves is responsible for referred pain in this woman?

a. Cervical cardiac accelerator nerves
b. Posterior vagal trunk
c. Right intercostal nerves
d. Right phrenic nerve
e. Right recurrent laryngeal nerve

337. An 82-year-old woman visits the hospital emergency department with the recent onset of grotesque swelling of the right arm, with slight swelling of her right neck, and face. Her right jugular vein is visibly engorged and her right brachial pulse is diminished. On the basis of these signs, her chest x-rays might show which one of the following?

a. A left cervical rib
b. A mass in the upper lobe of the right lung
c. Aneurysm of the aortic arch
d. Right pneumothorax
e. Thoracic duct blockage in the posterior mediastinum

338. A frantic young mother brings her 3-year-old boy to the emergency department. The child is suspected of aspirating a small (0.6 cm in diameter), cloth-covered metal button since one is missing from his teddy bear and when asked where it went, he said he ate it. Although the child does not complain of pain, he has a persistent and frequent coughing. Diminished breath sounds in this patient are most likely to be heard in which one of the following?

a. In both lungs
b. In the lingula of the left inferior lobe
c. In the right inferior lobe
d. In the left superior lobe
e. In the right superior lobe

339. A 36-year-old woman delivers a 7 lb 2 oz, 20.5 inch baby girl at 39 weeks. This is her fourth child. About 2 hours after delivery, the mother calls the nursing staff because the baby has taken on a slightly bluish-gray color. The child is breathing fairly rapidly, but without much effort or strain. The baby's heart and lung sounds are normal, other than a mild systolic murmur. The baby is placed on supplemental oxygen hoping that she will "pink up," but the baby's color and rapid breathing does not change. An echocardiogram is ordered because of the suspicion that the baby has what life threatening congenital heart anomaly?

a. Aortic valve stenosis
b. Atrial septal defect
c. Coarctation of the aorta
d. Patent ductus arteriosus
e. Transposition of the great arteries

340. An otherwise healthy married 25-year-old female medical student is referred to the cardiology clinic by her primary care physician for consultation and evaluation. She has told her primary care physician that she is thinking of starting a family. She has an artrial septal defect (ASD), diagnosed at age 5, but it was not repaired because of parental concerns about their healthy daughter undergoing open-heart surgery. Why should her cardiologist recommend that she at least consider getting her ASD surgically repaired prior to her planned pregnancy?

a. The pregnancy adds significant additional resistance to the peripheral venous system because of the size of the placenta. This will cause a left to right atrial shunt, leading to hypertrophy of the left ventricle. In addition, there are clamshell devices that may be inserted intravenously to repair the ASD that do not require open-heart surgery.

b. The pregnancy adds significant additional resistance to the peripheral venous system because of the size of the fetal circulatory system. This will cause a right to left shunt, leading to hypertrophy of the left atrium. In addition, there are clamshell devices that may be inserted intravenously to repair the ASD that do not require open-heart surgery.

c. No treatment is recommended because living with an ASD carries no risk if you have lived with it for 25 years.

d. Pregnancy increases the chances of venous emboli, which may lead to stroke because emboli can bypass the lung by traversing the ASD. In addition, there are clamshell devices that may be inserted intravenously to repair the ASD that do not require open-heart surgery.

e. The pregnancy adds significant additional resistance to the peripheral venous system because of the size of the fetal circulatory system. This will cause a left to right shunt, leading to hypertrophy of the right atrium. In addition, now that she is older the risks of open-heart surgery are significantly reduced compared to surgery as a child because the heart is much larger.

341. Failure of which developmental process is common to the following congenital heart defects: pulmonary stenosis; tetralogy of Fallot; and transposition of the great arteries?

a. Failure of the conotruncal ridges to spiral and meet each other as they separate the truncus arteriosus into an aorta and pulmonary trunk

b. Failure of the superior and inferior endocardial cushions to meet in the middle allowing separation of the truncus arteriosus into an aorta and pulmonary trunk

c. Failure of the septum primum to fuse with the septum secundum thus allowing the separation of the truncus arteriosus into an aorta and pulmonary trunk

d. Failure of neural crest cells to migrate into the septum primum to fuse with the septum secundum thus allowing the separation of the truncus arteriosus into an aorta and pulmonary trunk

e. Failure of the muscular septum to meet the membranous septum thus allowing the separation of the truncus arteriosus into an aorta and pulmonary trunk

342. A 28-year-old woman comes into the emergency department exhibiting dyspnea and mild cyanosis, but no signs of trauma. Her chest x-ray is shown below. The most obvious abnormal finding in the inspiratory posteroanterior (PA) chest x-ray of this patient (performed in the anatomic position) is a left pneumothorax (collapsed lung) as indicated by the dark appearance of the left lung and the shifting of the heart to the right. Which one of the following structures is indicated by the arrow?

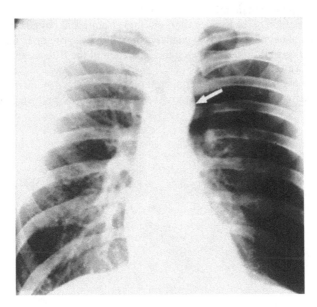

a. Left atrium
b. Grossly enlarged heart
c. Aortic arch
d. Pulmonary trunk
e. Left ventricle

343. A 23-year-old, semiconscious man is brought to the emergency department following an automobile accident. He is tachypneic and cyanotic. The right lower anterolateral thoracic wall reveals a small laceration and flailing. Air does not appear to move into or out of the wound, and it is assumed that the pleura have not been penetrated. After the patient is placed on immediate positive pressure endotracheal respiration, his cyanosis clears and the abnormal movement of the chest wall disappears. Radiographic examination confirms fractures of the fourth through eighth ribs in the right anterior axillary line and of the fourth through sixth ribs at the right costochondral junction. There is no evidence that bony fragments have penetrated the lungs or of pneumothorax (collapsed lung). Several hours later, the cyanosis returns. The right side of the thorax is found to be more expanded than the left, yet moves less during respiration. Upright chest x-rays are shown below.

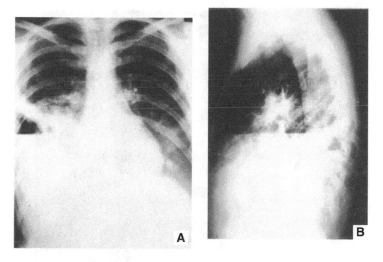

Which of the following is the most obvious abnormal finding in the inspiratory PA and lateral chest x-ray of this patient (viewed in the anatomic position)?

a. Flail chest
b. Right hemothorax
c. Right pneumothorax
d. Paralysis of the right hemidiaphragm
e. Left hemothorax

344. A 37-year-old man was pinned against the wall of a loading dock when a forklift backed into him, breaking two ribs and causing a hemothorax. A negative pressure drain (chest tube) must be inserted into the pleural space in order to remove blood from his pleural cavity. What would be a typical location for placement of the chest tube?

a. At the apex of the pleural space between the clavicle and first rib
b. Costomediastinal recess on the left, adjacent to the xiphoid process
c. Right fourth intercostal space in the midclavicular line
d. Right sixth intercostal space in the midaxillary line
e. Right eighth intercostal space in the midaxillary line

345. A 47-year-old woman presents to her internist with a persistent cough that has lasted 6 weeks. A PA chest film was taken. Within which one of the five lung lobes is the presumed pneumonia the worst?

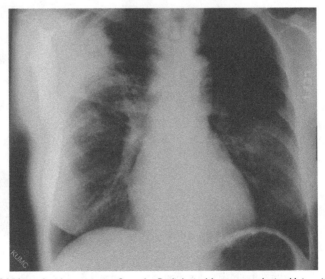

(Image 3151 used with permission from the Radiological Anatomy web site, University of Kansas, School of Medicine, http://classes.kumc.edu/som/radanatomy/.)

a. Right upper lobe
b. Right middle lobe
c. Right lower lobe
d. Left upper lobe
e. Left lower lobe

346. The miscarriage rate in humans is estimated to be as high as 15% of all pregnancies. These most often occur very early in pregnancy due to major defects in vital organs. Failure of the sixth aortic arch arteries to form would lead to loss of blood supply to which one of the following essential organs?

a. Right side of the heart
b. Face
c. Thyroid gland
d. Lungs
e. Upper digestive tract

347. Coronary arteries supply blood to the myocardium and pacemaker centers of the heart from branches that come off either the right or left coronary arteries. While some regions of the myocardium may receive blood from two different coronary arteries, the pacemaker centers of the heart normally only receive blood from a single coronary artery, but the pattern varies in the human population. The blood supply to the sinoatrial (SA) and atrioventricular (AV) nodes is derived from which coronary artery(ies)?

a. Both the SA and AV nodes receive blood from the right coronary artery or its branches.
b. Both the SA and AV nodes receive blood from the left coronary artery or its branches.
c. In 60% of the population, the SA node receives its blood from the right coronary artery. In 85% of the population, the AV node receives its blood from the right coronary artery via the posterior interventricular artery.
d. In 15% of the population, the SA node receives its blood supply from the right coronary artery. In 15% of the population, the AV node receives its blood supply from the right coronary artery via the posterior interventricular artery.
e. In 60% of the population, the SA node receives its blood supply from the left coronary artery. In 85% of the population, the AV node receives its blood supply from the left coronary artery via the posterior interventricular artery.

348. The mother of a 4-year-old girl is talking with the pediatric cardiologist. She has just come from her daughter's echocardiogram appointment. Several days earlier at the pediatrician's office, the pediatrician heard a split S2 heart sound at the upper left edge of the child's sternum and recommended the cardiac echo study. The patient has a 1.5 cm ASD and judging from the superior location in the atrial septum it maybe due to an abnormally large ostium secundum. The mother asks the cardiologist to explain an ostium secundum. What will the cardiologist most likely say?

a. An ostium secundum is the second hole in the first septum that forms to separate the left from the right atrium and is usually located cranially on the interatrial wall.

b. An ostium secundum is the second hole in the second septum that forms to separate the left from the right atrium and is usually located cranially on the interatrial wall.

c. An ostium secundum is the second hole in the first septum that forms to separate the left from the right atrium and is usually located caudally on the interatrial wall.

d. An ostium secundum is the second hole in the membranous septum that forms to separate the left from the right atrium and usually located caudally on the interatrial wall.

e. An ostium secundum is an alternative name for the foramen ovale that forms to separate the left from the right atrium and it is usually located caudally on the interatrial wall.

349. A 36-year-old male bartender is brought by ambulance to the emergency department because a patron jumped over the bar, grabbed an ice pick, and stabbed him in the chest rather than pay his bar tab at the end of the night. The ice pick entered the chest about 2 cm to the left of the sternum in between the fourth and fifth rib. Upon examining the bartender, there is very little blood coming from the puncture wound and normal lung sounds can be heard from both the right and left lung. However, his heart is beating rapidly at 100 beats per minute, his external jugular veins are bulging, and his heart sounds are becoming difficult to hear. A stat ultrasound is ordered because which one of the following conditions is likely present?

a. Hemothorax
b. Pneumothorax
c. Cardiac tamponade
d. Aortic valve stenosis
e. Deep venous thrombosis

350. During a bar fight a 23-year-old man's chest is punctured to the left of his sternum with an ice pick. He is brought to the emergency department because he is feeling faint and unable to walk due to weakness. He is placed on oxygen as he is evaluated. All his heart sounds are distant and muffled and his blood pressure is low despite a very rapid pulse. His lungs sound normal. His jugular veins are becoming more and more distended. How would one use a 3 inch, 19 gauge needle to help the bar fight victim?

a. Insert it just under the left tip of the xiphoid process in an effort to remove blood from the pericardial cavity.

b. Insert it at the second intercostal space on the left side of the sternum in an effort to inject nitroglycerine to increase the strength of cardiac contractions.

c. Insert it at the ninth intercostal space at the left midclavicular line in an effort to remove blood from the pleural cavity.

d. Insert it at the fourth intercostal space on the right side in an effort to remove blood from the right pulmonary artery.

e. Insert it just under the left clavicle in an effort to remove blood from the right cephalic vein.

351. A patient reports that he spent two weeks on a desert island as part of a television survival show. It rained and was cool the last 5 days, and he developed a cough. He is now in the emergency department with a productive cough that produces rusty and bloodstained sputum. He complains of significant pain that appears to be pleural in origin. Pneumococcal lobar pneumonia is suspected. From the accompanying CT scan at the T4 level, which one of the following lung lobes (indicated by the asterisk) is involved with the pneumonia?

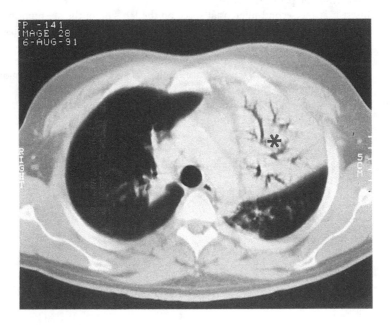

a. Right upper lobe
b. Right middle lobe
c. Right lower lobe
d. Left upper lobe
e. Left lower lobe

352. A 62-year-old man is brought by ambulance to the emergency department. He collapsed with severe tearing chest pain while trying to carry two bags of groceries in from his car. He is given oxygen and electrocardiogram (ECG) leads are applied in the ambulance. The ECG appears relatively normal. In the emergency department, he is alert, but breathing rapidly and has severe chest pain that radiates to his back. The pain does not radiate to his left arm. The heart sounds are all normal, but his lung sounds are diminished on the left side. A CT is ordered immediately because of fear that he may have which one of the following conditions?

a. Development of a patent foramen ovale
b. Dissection of the thoracic aorta
c. Rib fracture on the left side
d. Blockage of the left anterior descending artery
e. A diaphragmatic hernia on the left side

353. A 7 lb 10 oz, 21 inch baby boy is born to a mother who already has 2 children at home. After the baby is cleaned by the nurse, he is returned to the mother who attempts to breast-feed the boy. While the baby boy roots and finds the nipple, he immediately starts to cough and choke. The baby is immediately taken for a sonogram that confirms the boy has a tracheoesophageal fistula. What is the most frequent type of tracheoesophageal fistula?

a. A blind upper segment of the trachea and an esophagus that connects to both the proximal part of the trachea and the stomach
b. A continuous esophagus containing the trachea that extends anteriorly just superior to the stomach
c. An upper segment of the esophagus that connects to the trachea below the larynx and a lower segment of the esophagus that also connects to the trachea
d. An upper segment of the esophagus that connects to the trachea inferiorly to the larynx and a lower segment that ends cranially as a blind pouch
e. An upper segment of the esophagus that ends in a blind pouch and the lower segment connects to the bifurcation of an otherwise intact trachea

354. A 6-year-old girl is brought to her pediatrician's office by her mother. The girl has just joined a recreational soccer team for the first time and she is not as fast as most of the girls her age. Both of her legs hurt "all over" during and after soccer practices. The nurse checks her blood pressure which is 150/90 mm Hg. Upon physical examination, the pediatrician reconfirms the hypertension in both arms and feels a weak femoral pulse just below her inguinal ligament. Her leg blood pressure is 85/55 mm Hg. This freestanding pediatric office does not have sonography equipment nor a CT scanner so a PA chest film is ordered because of suspicion of which one of the following anomalies?

a. A patent ductus arteriosus
b. Tetralogy of Fallot
c. Transposition of the great arteries
d. Grooving of the inferior surface of the ribs
e. An enlarged right heart border

355. A 2-month-old infant from a small rural town is brought to a regional pediatric center by her mother. Her heart's apical beat is heard on the right side of her chest. What is the name for this condition and what other congenital condition might one suspect to find associated with this finding?

a. Dextracardia and DiGeorge syndrome
b. Dextracardia and Down syndrome
c. Dextracardia and situs inversus
d. Situs inversus and anencephaly
e. Situs inversus and clubfoot

356. A family physician delivers a 6 lb 6 oz full-term baby girl. Her breathing rate is slightly elevated, and when she cries her lips turn blue. Her toes are also bluish. A pediatric cardiology consult is requested "STAT." The cardiologist orders an echocardiogram. The sonographer, who performs the echo study, is convinced that the baby girl has transposition of her great vessels. Which one of the following is the most likely additional heart anomaly that is present in this newborn girl?

a. Overriding aorta
b. Ventricular septal defect
c. Ligamentum arteriosum
d. Coarctation of the aorta
e. Aortic aneurysm

357. An ambulance brings a 52-year-old man to the ED. He was who shoveling snow off his driveway when he felt both chest pain and pain radiating down the medial aspect of his left arm, so his wife called 911. The electrocardiogram (ECG) looks fairly normal in the ambulance. After receiving oxygen in the ambulance, the pain disappeared. On arrival in the ED, creatine kinase and troponin-1 levels are normal. A second ECG appears normal, with and indication of slight hypertrophy of the left ventricle. In most hearts which three arteries and two veins drain the left ventricle?

a. Left anterior descending artery, left marginal artery, posterior interventricular artery; anterior cardiac vein and middle cardiac vein
b. Left anterior descending artery, left marginal artery, posterior interventricular artery; great cardiac vein and middle cardiac vein
c. Left anterior descending artery, left marginal artery, posterior interventricular artery; great cardiac vein and small cardiac vein
d. Left anterior interventricular artery, left anterior descending artery, posterior interventricular artery; great cardiac vein and small cardiac vein
e. Left anterior interventricular artery, left anterior descending artery, posterior interventricular artery; anterior cardiac vein and middle cardiac vein

358. When choosing vessels for bypass surgery for occluded coronary arteries, sections of the internal thoracic artery have been preferred in recent years over lower leg veins, since they seem to last longer. In coronary bypass surgery, the transplanted blood vessel is placed in which of the following positions?

a. The proximal end of the artery is anastomosed to the pulmonary trunk.
b. The distal end of the artery is anastomosed to the great cardiac vein.
c. The proximal end is attached to the ascending aorta and the distal end is attached distal to the occluded coronary artery.
d. The distal end of the artery is anastomosed to the great cardiac vein and the proximal end is attached distal to the occluded coronary artery.
e. The proximal end of the artery is anastomosed to a pulmonary vein

359. A recently married, 37-year-old woman needs a physical examination before taking out a life insurance policy for the first time. She is 5 ft 7 in tall and weights 140 lb and has been reasonably active all her life. She is often anxious and she has occasional migraine headaches. Her heart sounds at the left fifth intercostal space at about the midclavicular line are abnormal; there is an extra high pitched systolic sound. What is the most likely diagnosis?

a. Aortic valve regurgitation or insufficiency
b. Aortic valve stenosis
c. Mitral valve prolapse
d. Pulmonic valve prolapse
e. Tricuspid valve prolapse

360. A 62-year-old professor underwent his second coronary bypass surgery. During his first bypass surgery 15 years ago, the cardiothoracic surgeon bypassed a blockage in the left anterior descending artery. This time the surgeon harvested the radial artery from his left arm (he is right handed) and bypassed a blockage within his posterior interventricular artery. About 8 hours after the surgery, the surgeon returned to see the patient. He listens to the professor's heart, and is concerned about the general dampening of the heart sounds. He then orders a transesophageal echocardiogram to specifically look for leakage of blood into what space?

a. Aortic adventitia
b. Between the myocardium and epicardium
c. Left pleural cavity
d. Oblique pericardial sinus
e. Transverse pericardial sinus

361. A 3-month-old infant is seen for the first time by a physician in the local free clinic. Her mother reports that she is OK, but she "quits" physical activity after short bursts of effort, and likes to be held a lot. The girl recently appears bluish when feeding or trying to crawl. When the physician listens to her chest there is an extra sound or murmur, especially during systole. A PA chest film shows a general increased density of both lungs and the right inferior heart margin appears enlarged. There is no enlargement of the aortic knob, but the left inferior border of the heart margin also appears slightly enlarged. The girl is scheduled for an echocardiogram because the physician suspects which one of the following?

a. Tetralogy of Fallot
b. Coarctation of the aorta
c. Transposition of the great vessels
d. Aortic stenosis
e. Ventricular septal defect

362. When removing blood from the left pleural space, a chest tube is placed into the pleural space sometimes below the normal extent of the lung. The chest tubes are most conveniently placed at the midaxillary line through intercostal muscles midway between the ribs to avoid damaging subcostal nerve arteries and veins and their collateral branches. At the midaxillary line, to which rib does the left lung normally extend?

a. Fourth
b. Sixth
c. Eighth
d. Tenth
e. Twelfth

363. In the sagittal MRI of the thorax below, which one of the following is structure 8?

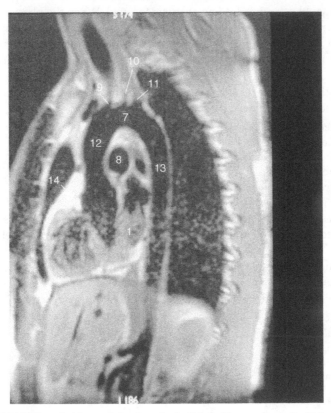

(Image 3304-007 used with permission from the Radiological Anatomy web site, University of Kansas, School of Medicine, http://classes.kumc.edu/som/radanatomy/.)

a. Left subclavian artery
b. Pulmonary trunk (bifurcated)
c. Left atrium
d. Right atrium
e. Brachiocephalic artery

364. A baby girl is born at 36 weeks of gestation weighing 6 lb 9 oz and is 19 inches long. The baby is grayish in color and an echocardiogram reveals a larger than normal ductus arteriosus, which may shut more slowly than typical and minor oxygen supplementation is initiated. Normally what are the two embryonic structures that allow blood to bypass the nonfunctional fetal lungs and what mechanism is responsible for closing those two structures after birth?

a. The ductus arteriosus and the ductus venosus both close due to decreased prostaglandin E2 levels.
b. The ductus arteriosus closes due to decreased blood flow from cutting of the umbilical cord. The ductus venosus closes due to decreased prostaglandin E2 levels.
c. The ductus arteriosus closes due to decreased prostaglandin E2 levels and the foramen ovale closes due to increased pressure within the left atrium.
d. The septum primum and septum secundum fuse due to increased pressure within the left atrium.
e. Both the septum primum and the septum secundum fuse closing off blood flow through the foramen ovale into the ostium secundum.

365. A 48-year-old man is brought to the emergency department by ambulance due to sudden shortness of breath and left-sided chest and back pain. ECG and blood work suggest normal cardiac function and no evidence of a heart attack. He has diminished lung sounds on the left side and extreme tenderness in the mid-back on the left side about 6 cm off the midline. History reveals that he was kneed in the back during a game one week ago while playing goalie. He is 5 ft 10 in and 165 lb. His urine is normal in color, smell, and volume. An AP chest film suggests fluid in the left pleural space at the costophrenic recess. CTs of the thorax and abdomen are ordered to look for which one of the following?

a. Enlarged right ventricle consistent with pulmonary hypertension
b. A cracked rib
c. Cardiac tamponade
d. Appendicitis
e. Inflamed gallbladder

366. Coronary artery disease is a frequent cause of myocardial infarction in the United States. If an echocardiogram suggests reduced posterior ventricular wall movement, there will be reduced blood flow within which of the following coronary arteries and veins?

a. Circumflex branch of the left artery; great cardiac vein
b. Anterior interventricular artery; great cardiac vein
c. Anterior interventricular artery; middle cardiac vein
d. Right marginal branch of the right artery; small cardiac vein
e. Posterior interventricular artery; middle cardiac vein

367. A 58-year-old woman underwent open-heart surgery for a mitral valve replacement. About 3 days after the surgery, her breathing became more labored just before she was about to be discharged. The surgical resident listened to the heart and lungs and noted a decrease in breath sounds in the inferior half of the left chest. When they placed a chest tube into her pleural cavity a milky white fluid was collected. What is the likely source of the fluid and what is the normal course of the structure damaged?

a. The right lymph duct, which normally crosses the midline and carries lymph to the junction of the left subclavian vein and the internal jugular vein
b. The thoracic duct, which normally carries lymph from the cisterna chyli to the junction of the left subclavian vein with the internal jugular vein in the neck
c. The thoracic duct, which normally carries lymph from the junction of the left subclavian vein with the internal jugular vein in the neck down to the cisterna chyli in the abdomen for absorption
d. Pleural lymph from damage to the intrinsic lymphatic channels of both the right and left lungs that drain toward the bifurcation of the trachea
e. Pleural lymph from damage to the intrinsic lymph channels of the left lung as they move toward the hilar region

368. A mother brings her 1-month-old infant to the office of their family physician for his first physical since leaving the hospital. The boy is normal in height and weight for his age. The baby boy has a split S2 heart sound at the left upper sternal border. All other heart valve sounds are normal. A pediatric cardiologist is consulted and reports that the baby has a patent ostium primum. What likely failed to occur during the development of this boy's heart?

a. Failure of the conotruncal ridges to spiral as they meet each other separating the truncus arteriosus into an aorta and pulmonary trunk
b. Failure of the superior and inferior endocardial cushions to meet in the middle of the heart chambers
c. Failure of the septum primum to fuse with the septum secundum thus allowing the separation of the truncus arteriosus into an aorta and pulmonary trunk
d. Failure of neural crest cells to migrate into the conotruncal ridges
e. Failure of the muscular septum to meet the membranous septum

Thorax

Answers

329. The answer is e. (*Moore, p 152. Fauci, pp 1460-1461.*) VSDs are the most common isolated congenital heart defects, slightly more common than ASDs. A VSD occurs most frequently as a defect in the membranous portion of the interventricular septum cranial to the more muscular portion of the septum, which lies more inferiorly and toward the cardiac apex. The shunt may not be detected at birth as the vascular resistance of the lungs continues to decrease for several days following birth. More blood moves through the VSD with time as the right-sided pressure drops and the pressure difference from the higher left-sided pressure increases. Since blood is flowing through the VSD during systole, from the left ventricle into the right ventricle, in an anterior direction, the murmur is best heard at the left of the sternum near the third intercostal space. The lungs sound congested due to increased blood flow. Aortic valve stenosis (**answer a**) produces a murmur loudest at the right upper sternal border. Transposition of the great arteries (**answer b**) would have been detected within hours after birth due to cyanosis, and not in a 6-month-old infant. Persistent ligamentum arteriosum (**answer c**) is not a congenital anomaly, but a normal process. Pulmonary (pulmonic) valve stenosis (**answer d**) would best be heard on the left side of the upper sternal border.

330. The answer is b. (*Moore, p 152. Fauci, p 1460.*) Many children with ASD have no symptoms. If the defect is small, then relatively little blood flows from the slightly higher pressure left atrium into the lower pressure right atrium. If the ASD is large, then oxygenated blood is mixed with poorly oxygenated blood and returned to the lungs. The characteristic initial presentation of an ASD is a so called "fixed split S2 sound" when the closure of the pulmonic valve is delayed compared to the closure of the aortic valve. Normally the closure of the pulmonary and aortic valves occur at the same time and form the S2 heart sound. In most individuals there is a splitting of S2 upon deep inspiration, which causes the right side of the heart to fill with more blood thus increasing pulmonic arterial flow closing the valve. Aortic valve stenosis (**answer a**) would cause a murmur to the right of the cranial end of the sternum. Coarctation of the aorta **(answer c)** causes higher blood pressure in the arms than in the legs. A mid-systolic murmur that is best heard between the scapulae on the back is also normally present. Transposition of the great arteries **(answer d)** is life threatening, and the child would not live to the age of 11 months without intervention. VSDs **(answer e)** produce murmurs more inferiorly, and occur continuously during systole. VSDs, typically present with more severe symptoms than ASDs.

331. The answer is b. (*Moore, pp 99-101.*) The lymphatic drainage of the mammary gland, which follows the path of its blood supply, generally parallels the tributaries of the axillary, internal thoracic (mammary), thoracoacromial, and intercostal vessels. Because about 75% of the breast lies lateral to the nipple, the more significant lateral and inferior portions of the breast drain toward the axillary nodes. The smaller medial portion drains to the parasternal lymphatic chain paralleling the internal thoracic vessels **(answers c and d)**, whereas the very small superior portion drains toward the nodes associated with the thoracoacromial trunk and the supraclavicular nodes. Lymph rarely crosses the midline **(answer a)**. Lymph reaches subscapular (apical axillary) nodes after passing through axillary nodes **(answer e)**.

332. The answer is b. (*Moore, pp 709-710.*) The serratus anterior muscle (protractor and stabilizer of the scapula) is innervated by the long thoracic nerve (of Bell), which arises from roots C5 to C7 of the brachial plexus. (Remember: SALT, serratus anterior innervated by long thoracic.) During modified radical mastectomy, this nerve is usually spared to maintain shoulder function. However, its location places it in jeopardy during the lymphatic resection. The suprascapular nerves **(answer d)** are sensory branches of the cervical plexus. The axillary nerve **(answer a)**, deep in the brachial portion of the axilla, innervates the deltoid muscle. The thoracodorsal nerve **(answer e)**, which arises from the posterior cord of the brachial plexus, innervates the latissimus dorsi. The lower subscapular nerve **(answer c)** innervates the teres major muscle and a portion of the subscapularis muscle.

333. The answer is d. (*Fauci, p 1461.*) Patent ductus arteriosus is fairly common in premature infants. The "machinelike" murmur is best heard in the left upper chest. The female-to-male ratio for patent ductus arteriosus is 2:1. Aortic valve stenosis (**answer a**) would cause a murmur at the right upper sternal border. ASDs (**answer b**) produce a fixed split S2 sound. Coarctation of the aorta (**answer c**) causes higher blood pressure in the arms than in the legs and a mid-systolic murmur that is best heard between the scapulae. VSDs (**answer e**) produce murmurs between the S1 and S2 heart sounds that are best heard more inferiorly along the sternum than the machinelike murmur of a patent ductus arteriosus.

334. The answer is e. (*Moore, p 154. Fauci, p 1463.*) Isolated pulmonary valve stenosis is rare and often occurs in conjunction with tetralogy of Fallot. If the stenosis of the pulmonary valve is mild, there are often few symptoms and the defect may go undetected for years. Pulmonic valve stenosis in mild cases may be treated by balloon dilation or in more severe cases by surgical replacement. Aortic valve stenosis (**answer a**) would cause a murmur at the right upper sternal border. ASD (**answer b**) produces a fixed split S2 sound. Coarctation of the aorta (**answer c**) causes higher blood pressure in the arms than the legs and a mid-systolic murmur that is best heard between the scapulae. Patent ductus arteriosus (**answer d**) presents with a "machinelike" murmur.

335. The answer is d. (*Moore, p 154. Fauci, pp 1474-1475. Kumar, pp 544-545.*) The presence of a systolic ejection-type murmur suggests that blood is becoming turbulent during contraction of the ventricles, consistent with aortic valve stenosis. Aortic stenosis (often discovered in adults due to a congenital bicuspid aortic valve) produces a jet of blood, which in turn causes the subsequent dilation of the ascending aorta. Secondarily, the left ventricle hypertrophies in size due to the increased resistance of forcing blood through a small valve. Tetralogy of Fallot (**answer a**) would generally be diagnosed in cyanotic newborns. Pulmonary valve stenosis (**answer b**) is unlikely since the pulmonary trunk on the patient in this vignette is normal. Atherosclerosis (**answer c**) is not relevant to the physical exam and radiological findings. A tricuspid valve defect (**answer e**) would probably not produce a systolic murmur.

336. The answer is d. (*Moore, pp 125, 287, 317.*) The phrenic nerve, which arises from cervical nerves C3 through C5, mediates sensation from the diaphragmatic pleura and peritoneum, as well as from the pericardium;

in addition, it carries motor fibers to the diaphragm. Therefore, pain from the diaphragmatic pleura or peritoneum, as well as from the parietal pericardium, may be referred to dermatomes between C3 and C5, inclusive. In this case the pain following meals would be consistent with an inflamed gallbladder causing diaphragmatic irritation. The C3, C4, and C5 dermatomes correspond to the clavicular region and the anterior and lateral neck, as well as to the anterior, lateral, and posterior aspects of the shoulder. (Remember: C3, C4, and C5 keep the diaphragm alive.) Cervical cardiac accelerator nerves (**answer a**) would be sympathetic, generally from T1-T5. The vagus (**answer b**) which is a cranial nerve does not carry referred pain back to the brain. The right intercostal nerve (**answer c**) may carry referred pain from the parietal pleura to the chest wall. The right recurrent laryngeal nerve (**answer e**) is a branch of the vagus and does not carry referred pain to the brain.

337. The answer is b. (*Moore, pp 169-171. Hansen and Lambert, p 321.*) A Pancoast tumor in the apex of the right lung may compress the right brachiocephalic vein with resultant venous engorgement of the right arm and right side of the face and neck. In addition, there may be compression of the brachial artery, the sympathetic chain, and recurrent laryngeal nerve with attendant deficits. The left cervical rib (**answer a**) is on the wrong side. An aneurysm of the aortic arch (**answer c**) could reduce pulse pressures as the great vessels are occluded, but it could not explain the venous congestion. A right pneumothorax (**answer d**) would not affect blood flow within the right arm. Thoracic duct blockage in the posterior mediastinum (**answer e**) would be unlikely to affect only the right arm.

338. The answer is c. (*Moore, p 123.*) Large aspirated objects tend to lodge at the carina (both lungs affected; **answer a**). Smaller objects (less than 0.8 cm) usually lodge in the right inferior lobar bronchus (not superior [**answer e**]) because the right mainstem (primary) bronchus is generally more vertical in its course than the left (**answers b and d**) and of greater diameter. In addition, the takeoff angle of the right lower lobe bronchus is less acute than that of the right middle lobe, thereby continuing in the general direction of both the right mainstem bronchus and trachea. Blockage of the airway will produce absence of breath sounds within the lobe and eventual atelectasis and collapse. Since the button is metal it would be visible on chest films.

339. The answer is e. (*Fauci, pp 1459, 1464. Sadler, pp 183-185.*) With transposition of the great arteries the pulmonary trunk is connected to the left ventricle and the aorta is connected to the right ventricle, just the opposite of the normal configuration. Thus, the right atria and ventricle receive blood from the body and pump blood back to the body. The left side of the heart receives highly oxygenated blood from the lungs, but pumps that blood back to the lungs. The baby is kept alive because of connections between the two closed circulatory systems via a patent ductus arteriosus, and an open foramen ovale. If transposition of the great arteries is suspected, then a continuous infusion of prostaglandins is initiated to keep the ductus arteriosus open allowing oxygenated blood to cross between the two closed sides of the heart. In addition, a balloon catheter may be passed into the right atrium to form a temporary stent to allow a second connection through the foramen ovale. Ultimately, the transposition of the great arteries must be corrected by surgery after the child is stable. Correction of transposition of the great arteries is normally done in the first week of life and also requires reconnection of the coronary arteries to the new ascending aorta. Aortic valve stenosis (**answer a**) would cause a murmur at the right upper sternal border and generally is not life threatening. ASD (**answer b**) produces a fixed split S2 sound and would rarely be so large as to be life threatening. Coarctation of the aorta (**answer c**) causes higher blood pressure in the arms than in the legs and a mid-systolic murmur that is best heard between the scapulae. Patent ductus arteriosus (**answer d**) presents with a "machinelike" murmur. In the case of the boy in this vignette, it is life saving although generally a patent ductus arteriosus is not life threatening.

340. The answer is d. (*Moore, pp 152-153. Fauci, pp 1459-1560, 2517.*) Pregnancy increases the chances of venous emboli, which may lead to stroke because emboli can bypass the lung by traversing the ASD. In addition, there are clamshell devices that may be inserted intravenously to repair the ASD that do not require open-heart surgery. Normally, emboli that form in the blood develop within the venous circulatory system, especially with stasis of blood flow. During pregnancy, the weight of the fetus on the inferior vena cava tends to increase the chances of forming emboli. In a normal circulatory system those venous emboli become trapped in the first capillary bed, in the lungs, where they form small pulmonary emboli. In most young, healthy people those are a minor health risk. When an ASD is present, systemic venous emboli may pass from the right to the left atria, thus bypassing the lung capillary network and move into the brain capillaries, where even small emboli can cause strokes. There are now "clamshell" devices that can be introduced via catheterization that can be inserted to fill the ASD, thus eliminating the need for open-heart surgery. While pregnancy does add significant resistance to the peripheral venous system (**answer a**) this is only true toward the end of pregnancy and is not the reason for an ASD repair. Pregnancy would not cause a right to left shunt through an ASD (**answer b**). ASD carries risk of stroke, especially for pregnant women (**answer c**). The risk associated with open-heart surgery is generally similar whether the patient is a child or an adult (**answer e**).

341. The answer is a. (*Sadler, pp 180-182, 183-185.*) Failure of the conotruncal ridges to spiral and meet each other as they separate the truncus arteriosus into an aorta and pulmonary trunk is responsible for pulmonary stenosis, tetralogy of Fallot, and transposition of the great arteries. The outflow tract of the heart must be separated approximately equally to form both an ascending aorta and the pulmonary trunk. This is normally accomplished by the spiral growth of conotruncal ridges that grow together and meet in the midline. They spiral as they grow, so the aorta connects to the left ventricle and the pulmonary trunk connects to the right ventricle. If the spiraling fails, then transposition of the great arteries occurs. If the ascending aorta is larger than the pulmonary trunk, then pulmonary stenosis occurs. In tetralogy of Fallot, there is pulmonary stenosis in conjunction with an enlarged, overriding aorta and a VSD that causes enlargement of the right ventricle. If the endocardial cushions fail to meet (**answer b**), then the separation of the atria from the ventricles fails to occur properly. Septum primum and septum secundum (**answers c and d**) are formed in the atria to separate the right from the left atrium and have nothing to do with conotruncal ridges, nor the outflow tracts of the heart. The muscular septum meets the membranous septum (**answer e**) within the ventricles to form the interventricular septum, not the outflow tract of the heart. Neural crest cells are required for proper formation of the conotruncal ridges.

342. The answer is c. (*Moore, pp 121-186.*) The patient has a left pneumothorax. The lucidity of the left pleural cavity with the lack of pulmonary vessels indicates that the left lung has collapsed into a small, dense mass adjacent to the mediastinum. Such a nontraumatic pneumothorax may result from the rupture of a pulmonary bleb, especially in a young person. The right lung is normal. The plain film does not show a pleural fluid level indicative of hemothorax, and the near symmetry of the domes of the two hemidiaphragms on inspiration indicates normal function of the phrenic nerves. The left atrium is a posterior heart structure and is not visible in an AP chest film **(answer a)**. The heart, measuring less than one-half of the chest diameter, is of normal size **(answer b)**, but is shifted to the right. Both the pulmonary trunk **(answer d)** and the left ventricle **(answer e)** are inferior to the arrow on the left heart border.

343. The answer is b. *(Moore, pp 120-121.)* The fluid level in the right pleural cavity is indicative of hemothorax caused by bleeding into the pleural space. As blood collects, lung tissue is displaced and cannot expand fully, thereby impairing ventilation. However, perfusion continues so that the ventilation-perfusion ratio is altered. There would be no fluid line if it were a pneumothorax **(answer c)**. A puncture wound often produces a flailing chest (**[answer a]** moving inward as the rest of the thoracic cage expands during inspiration). Paralysis of the right hemidiaphragm **(answer d)** would result in the diaphragm becoming stationary near its normal expiration height. The hemothorax is on the right side, not the left side **(answer e)**.

344. The answer is d. *(Moore, pp 121-122.)* The usual location of choice for a chest tube drain is in the midaxillary or posterior axillary line, that is, the vertical line commencing at the middle or posterior axillary fold, at the approximate level of the fifth or sixth intercostal space. The midaxillary line is typically used to keep the tube out of the way since the patient would normally be bedridden. Since the lung is collapsed toward the hilum the exact level tends not to be so important since the lung has pull cranially and medially. The needle is usually inserted just below the level at which percussive dullness occurs (if hemothorax). The apex of the lung **(answer a)** is close to the brachial plexus and subclavian vessels and farthest away from accumulating blood, and therefore is not used. The costomediastinal recess on the left, adjacent to the xiphoid process **(answer b)** is used for pericardiocentesis. The midclavicular line **(answers c)** is not used because tubes placed this far anteriorly tend to be in the way of the patient and would more likely damage the lung as it collapses toward the hilar region. The eighth intercostal space in the midaxillary line **(answer e)** would not be used since this is so low that one would be in danger of piercing the diaphragm and entering the peritoneal cavity during placement of the tube.

345. The answer is a. (*Moore, pp 111-113.*) The presumed pneumonia is worst in the right upper lobe, above the horizontal fissure which is visible as a line angling upwards across the right lung. Both upper lobes of the right and left lungs are anterior/superior lobes and separated by a diagonal fissure from the lower lobes which are inferior/posterior lobes. In the right lung there is a second horizontal fissure, which separates the upper lobe from the middle lobe. The horizontal fissure is clearly present in the PA chest film as fluid accumulates above it in the upper right lobe where the pneumonia is worse. While there is some increased density in nearly all lung lobes (**answers b, c, d, and e**), the least density is seen within the left upper lung lobe.

346. The answer is d. (*Sadler, pp 186-189.*) Branches of the arteries of the sixth aortic arches form the pulmonary arteries. In addition, the left sixth arch artery forms the ductus arteriosus. The blood supply to the right side of the heart (**answer a**) is primarily derived from the right and left coronary arteries derived from the truncus arteriosus. The face (**answer b**) and thyroid gland (**answer c**) receive blood primarily from the facial and superior thyroid arteries, respectively. Those are branches of the common and external carotid arteries which, are primarily derivatives of the third aortic arch. The upper digestive tract (**answer e**) is supplied by the celiac and superior mesenteric arteries, derivatives of the vitelline arteries.

347. The answer is c. (*Moore, pp 144-147, 157-158.*) In 60% of the population, the SA node receives its blood supply from the right coronary artery. In 85% of the population, the AV node receives its blood supply from the right coronary artery via the posterior interventricular artery (**a, b, d, and e**). This is why complete occlusion of the right coronary artery is more likely to destroy the pacemaker centers of the heart, the SA and AV nodes.

348. The answer is a. (*Sadler, pp 173-175.*) The ostium secundum is the second hole in the first septum that forms to separate the left from the right atrium and it is most likely located cranially on the interatrial wall. The ostium primum is the first hole that forms as the first septum grows from cranial to caudal toward the endocardial cushions. The ostium secundum forms cranially in the first atrial septum by apoptosis just before the growing first septum grows to close the first hole. Subsequently, the second septum grows cranially to caudally on the right side of the first septum leaving the foramen ovale. Normally blood flows from the right atrium into the left atrium during embryonic development by passing first through the foramen ovale and then through the ostium secundum. There is no second hole in the second septum (**answer b**). The foramen ovale is located caudally on the atrial septal wall. The ostium secundum is high, not caudal (**answer c**) on the first septum. The membranous septum (**answer d**) is found within the ventricles, not the atrial chambers. The ostium secundum and foramen ovale are not the same structures (**answer e**) though both allow a right to left shunt that spontaneously closes when left atrial pressure exceeds right atrial pressure.

349. The answer is c. (*Moore, pp 133-134.*) The ice pick likely penetrated the left ventricle of the heart, causing blood to leak into the pericardial sac. The rapid filling of the pericardial space does not allow the heart to fully expand between contractions leading to increased venous hypertension. The result is filling of the external jugular veins. Since the heart can only pump small quantities of the blood with each beat, it speeds up (tachycardia). The heart sounds and apical heartbeat soften because the blood surrounding the heart absorbs the sounds. A hemothorax (**answer a**) and pneumothorax (**answer b**) are unlikely since both right and left lung sounds are normal and because of the location of the ice pick injury. Aortic valve stenosis (**answer d**) would not result from a puncture wound. Deep venous thrombosis (**answer e**) generally occurs in the lower extremity and results in leg pain and is not caused by a puncture wound.

350. The answer is a. (*Moore, pp 133-134.*) Draining blood from the pericardial cavity is performed by inserting a needle just under the left tip of the xiphoid process in an effort to remove blood from the pericardial cavity. This procedure is called pericardiocentesis. Blood within the pericardial sac will cause heart failure as the fluid prevents the heart chambers from expanding properly and filling with blood. Thus, the ability of the heart to pump blood is diminished. Most of the other answers (**answers b, c, d, and e**) are all too cranial and would not allow access to the pericardial space. In most emergency departments this procedure would be performed with ultrasound guidance.

351. The answer is d. *(Moore, pp 125-127.)* The lobe indicated by the asterisk is the left upper (or superior) lobe. The general orientation when viewing CTs is that the observer is looking up from the patient's feet. Therefore, the patient's left is on your right, thus it cannot be a part of the right lung **(answers a, b, and c).** On the left, the inferior (lower) lobe **(answer e)** begins relatively high in the thoracic cavity and is posterior to the upper lobe.

352. The answer is b. *(Fauci, pp 88, 1563-1564.)* Aortic dissection occurs most frequently between the ages of 50 and 70 and in men twice as often as women. Pain in the back suggests a dissection of the descending thoracic aorta. Fifty percent of patients die before reaching the hospital. A patent foramen ovale **(answer a)** would not produce severe back pain. Fractured ribs **(answer c)** are unlikely without a history of trauma. Suffering blockage of the left anterior descending artery **(answer d)** would generally produce cardiac pain and altered ECG findings. Suffering a diaphragmatic hernia on the left side **(answer e)** would generally not produce severe back pain.

353. The answer is e. *(Sadler, p 202.)* An upper segment of the esophagus that ends in a blind pouch and the lower segment that connects to the bifurcation of the trachea that is otherwise intact. About 90% to 95% of tracheoesophageal fistulas (occur about 1 per 3,000 U.S. births) have an upper esophageal segment that ends as a blind pouch that connects just inferior to the larynx. (Note: This type of tracheoesophageal fistula is also called esophageal atresia with distal tracheoesophageal fistula.) The lower segment attached to the stomach is connected cranially to the membranous portion of the trachea just superior to the bifurcation of the trachea into right and left main bronchi. This means that the baby could still swallow amniotic fluid and have it flow into the GI tract, so the normal production and circulation of amniotic fluid is unimpeded. Once the baby starts to breathe air rather than amniotic fluid, then swallowed fluids will pass into the lungs, causing pneumonia. Babies that have tracheoesophageal fistulas are much more likely to have other congenital defects as well including Down syndrome, duodenal atresia, and cardiovascular defects. Tracheoesophageal fistulas are part of the VACTERL association: vertebral anomalies, anal atresia, cardiac defects, tracheoesophageal fistula, esophageal atresia, renal anomalies and limb defects. All the other forms of esophageal/tracheal defects and fistula **(answers a, b, c, and d)** are much less frequent.

354. The answer is d. (*Moore, p 175.*) Coarctation of the aorta often causes grooving of the undersurface of the ribs. Coarctation of the aorta is a constriction of the aorta, often occurring near the attachment of the ductus arteriosus. Constriction of the aorta leads to a decrease in blood pressure in the lower limbs. Blood flows into the internal thoracic (mammary) arteries then inferiorly to the anterior portion of the intercostal arteries that subsequently carry blood posteriorly to the thoracic aorta, distal to the coarctation. The increased blood flow from anterior to posterior leads to grooving on the inferior surface of the ribs, which can be seen on a PA chest film. The constriction of the aorta may not be evident on plain films. Echocardiogram or CT of the chest should be used to confirm the diagnosis. Coarctation of the aorta is often seen in conjunction with other heart defects (bicuspid aortic valve, or VSD) and is common in Turner syndrome. A patent ductus arteriosus (**answer a**) would not cause the difference in arm and leg blood pressures. Most people with tetralogy of Fallot (**answer b**) require surgery prior to age 6. Transposition of the great arteries (**answer c**) requires immediate surgery after birth. An enlarged right heart border (**answer e**) would not occur in this girl.

355. The answer is c. (*Sadler, p 170.*) Dextracardia is defined as developmental reversal of the heart loops to the right, rather than to the left, which is typical. Isolated dextracardia occurs 1 in 12,000 births. The complete reversal of both thoracic and abdominal organs is called situs inversus or situs inversus totalis occurs more frequently (1 in 7000 births). DiGeorge syndrome (**answer a**) is due to failure of the formation of the third and fourth branchial pouches and is not associated with dextracardia. Down syndrome (**answer b**) is due to trisomy 21 and is not associated with dextracardia. Anencephalic newborns (**answer d**) do not survive postnatally. Clubfoot (**answer e**) is not associated with dextracardia.

356. The answer is b. (*Moore, p 152. Sadler, p 183.*) The additional heart anomaly present in this newborn girl is a VSD. Babies born with transposition of the great vessels normally present with symptoms of cyanosis as the ductus arteriosus closes within the first day of birth. In this anomaly, the aorta is located on top of the right ventricle and the pulmonary trunk receives blood from the left ventricle, therefore, blood is being pumped mainly to the body by the right side and mainly to the lungs by the left side. The only way oxygenated blood is traveling to the body is if the two sides are connected, often by a patent ductus arteriosus. Babies with this anomaly immediately receive oxygen, and prostaglandins are also given to help keep the ductus arteriosus open longer than normal. About 25% of the time that transposition of the great vessels is present, there is also a VSD, which aids in the intermixing of blood from the two sides of the heart. This condition must be treated surgically. Anomalies of the aortic arch are normally not present. The presence of a ligamentum arteriosum (**answer c**) would worsen the problem. Coarctation of the aorta (**answer d**) would make the problem worse. An overriding aorta (**answer a**) is the second best answer. An aortic aneurysm (**answer e**) is unlikely to be present in a newborn.

357. The answer is b. (*Moore, pp 145-148.*) The left ventricle is generally supplied with blood from three arteries. Two come off the left coronary artery (left anterior descending artery [also called the left anterior interventricular artery] and left marginal artery) and one off the right coronary artery (the posterior interventricular). In about 70% of the population the posterior interventricular artery arises from the right coronary artery, 10% of the time from the left coronary artery and 20% of the time from both right and left coronary arteries. The circumflex branch of the left coronary artery will also often supply some blood to the left ventricle. Some hearts also have a left diagonal branch off the anterior interventricular artery as well. Normally, just two veins drain blood that has served the myocardium of the left ventricle: the great cardiac vein, which starts on the anterior surface of the heart in between the two ventricles that runs in the atrioventricular sulcus to drain into the coronary sinus. The middle cardiac vein normally drains blood from the top of the posterior interventricular sulcus. None of the other answers (**a, c, d, and e**) is correct.

358. The answer is c. (*Moore, pp 156-157.*) In a coronary bypass procedure, a blood vessel is added to allow blood to flow distal to the occluded coronary artery. This is done by removing the distal end of the internal thoracic artery from the anterior intercostal arteries, threading it through the pericardial sac, and attaching its distal end distal to the occluded artery. If the left anterior descending artery is being bypassed with the internal thoracic artery, often its proximal end is left attached to its origin off the subclavian artery. If a posterior coronary artery needs bypassing, the proximal end of the internal thoracic artery is typically cut and reattached to the ascending aorta. Remember that the internal thoracic artery supplies blood to each intercostal artery, which also receives blood from the thoracic aorta. If veins such as the great saphenous vein are used for bypasses, care must be used to be sure that valves are not present or are placed in a direction that will not limit blood flow. All of the other answers **(answers b, d, and e)** involve attaching the blood vessel to a venous structure or in the case of the pulmonary trunk **(answer a)** attaching to relatively poorly oxygenated blood, which is not done.

359. The answer is c. *(Moore, pp 154, 173.)* Mitral valve prolapse is a very common condition with up to 5% of the population having some degree of prolapse. The mitral valve closes shortly after the ventricle undergoes contraction. Mitral valve prolapse generally adds a mid-systolic click. The left ventricle produces the most force of any heart chamber, thus the mitral valve is much more prone to prolapse than the lower pressure tricuspid valve. If the prolapse is severe, it can lead to regurgitation of blood from the ventricle into the left atrium. Aortic valve regurgitation, insufficiency **(answer a)**, or stenosis **(answer b)** are best heard just to the right of the sternum at the second intercostal space. Murmurs caused by defects in the pulmonic valve **(answer d)** can best be heard to the left of the sternum at the second intercostal space. Murmurs caused by defects in the tricuspid valve **(answer e)** can best be heard just to the left of the sternum at the fourth or fifth intercostal space.

360. The answer is d. *(Moore, pp 128-133.)* The pericardial sac is normally only filled with about 20 mL of serous fluid that allows lubrication between the beating heart and other mediastinal structures. When one is bedridden, such as after open-heart surgery, any bleeding into the pericardial cavity will tend to accumulate posterior to the heart in the oblique pericardial sinus. Blood is unlikely to be retained by the aortic adventitia **(answer a)**, or the epicardium **(answer b)**. Blood within the left pleural cavity **(answer c)** would not be expected since that cavity would generally not be entered during bypass surgery. The transverse pericardial sinus **(answer e)** lies superiorly within the pericardial sac and thus would be an unlikely location for blood accumulation.

361. The answer is a. *(Sadler, p 183. Fauci, pp 1463-1464. Kumar, pp 542-543.)* The girl is diagnosed with tetralogy of Fallot. Since the girl is 3 months old it is very unlikely that she would have survived transposition of the great vessels **(answer c)** without surgical intervention. Tetralogy of Fallot consists of three congenital conditions and a fourth acquired condition as a consequence of the first three. Tetralogy of Fallot consists of an overriding aorta that receives blood from both ventricles, pulmonary stenosis that tends to keep blood out of the lungs, and a VSD (otherwise the aorta could not "override"). As a consequence of the three conditions, the right ventricle tends to hypertrophy since it has to pump blood not only into the lungs, but also through the aorta to the rest of the body. Since the girl has normal blood pressure in her upper and lower limbs, coarctation of the aorta **(answer b)** is unlikely. In addition, simple aortic stenosis **(answer d)** is unlikely to produce hypertrophy of the right ventricle. A ventricular septal defect **(answer e)** is just part of the problem.

362. The answer is c. *(Moore, pp 109, 119.)* Normally the pleural space extends inferiorly about two additional ribs inferior to the lung at each location, thus at the midaxillary line the caudal portion of the lung normally lies at about the eight intercostal space and the pleural space would extend down to about rib 10. The fourth **(answer a)** and sixth **(answer b)** intercostal spaces are too cranial and tenth **(answer d)** and twelfth **(answer e)** intercostal spaces are too caudal.

363. The answer is b. *(Moore, pp 116, 137-138.)* The pulmonary trunk (8) has just bifurcated and will form the left and right pulmonary artery just inferior to the arch of the aorta. Other labeled structures are: 1, left ventricle; 7, aortic arch; 8, bifurcated pulmonary trunk (most likely left pulmonary artery in this image); 9, brachiocephalic artery; 10, left common carotid artery; 11, left subclavian artery; 12, ascending aorta; 13, descending aorta; and 14, right coronary artery (difficult to see).

364. The answer is c. *(Moore, pp 151-152. Sadler, pp 196-199.)* The ductus arteriosus closes due to decreasing prostaglandin E2 levels and the foramen ovale closes due to increased pressure within the left atrium. The ductus venosus normally closes spontaneously **(answer a and b)** due to the fact that umbilical cord blood no longer flows as the cord is clamped and cut from the placenta. Since the septum primum is thinner than the septum secundum, the foramen ovale and the ostium secundum act as a one-way valve allowing blood to flow from the right atrium to the left atrium, bypassing the lungs. As the baby takes its first few breaths after birth and blood resistance within the lungs drops rapidly, more blood passes through the lungs. The increased blood volume returning to the left atrium raises the pressure within the left atrium above the right atrium, forces the septum primum against the septum secundum, closing the atrial shunt. While **answer d and e** are correct statements, they do not relate to the closing of the ductus arteriosus.

365. The answer is b. (*Moore, pp 121-122.*) One would expect a cracked rib that allows blood from the intercostal vessels to bleed into the pleural cavity, partially collapsing the left lung, causing the shortness of breath. Blood in the pleural cavity is an irritant and causes generalized chest pain. The left-sided, mid-back pain is from the cracked eleventh rib. Because only one lung appears to have fluid accumulation and he is young and exercises regularly; pulmonary hypertension (**answer a**) is unlikely, especially given his physical findings and history and sudden onset of symptoms. Cardiac tamponade (**answer c**), which is blood within the pericardial sac, is unexpected. Neither gallbladder pain (**answer e**), nor an inflamed appendix (**answer d**) would typically cause chest pain. Note: The CT of the abdomen is required to rule out damage to the kidneys and spleen.

366. The answer is e. (*Moore, pp 144-148.*) A sonogram of the heart (or echocardiogram) that suggests decreased posterior wall movement is most likely due to local infarction or fibrosis of that portion of the heart. Infarcted or fibrotic tissue would reduce blood flow. The major blood supply to the posterior ventricular wall in most hearts is the posterior interventricular artery (or posterior descending), normally (70% of the time) a branch off the right coronary artery. If there is blockage (generally described as a percent of normal) in a coronary artery, then there should be a concomitant decrease in the blood within the vein that serves that region. The middle cardiac vein runs with the posterior interventricular artery in the sulcus of the same name. The circumflex branch of the left coronary artery runs with the great cardiac vein (**answer a**) within the atrial ventricular sulcus for a short distance, but blood flow reduction in those vessels does not fit with the echocardiographic results. The right marginal branch of the right coronary artery runs with the small cardiac vein (**answer d**), but they serve the right ventricle. The anterior interventricular artery runs with the great cardiac vein (**answer b**), not the middle cardiac vein (**answer c**), but on the anterior aspect of the heart.

367. The answer is b. (*Moore, pp 43-46, 175-176.*) The thoracic duct, which normally carries lymph from the cisterna chyli to the junction of the left subclavian vein with the internal jugular vein in the neck. About 2 to 3 liters of lymph are returned to the venous circulatory system in the neck, not to the abdomen (**answer c**) each day. The thoracic duct is injured in about 0.5% to 1% of thoracic surgeries (iatrogenic injury). The right lymph duct (**answer a**) drains lymph from the right arm, right chest, and head and neck into the junction of the right subclavian vein with the internal jugular vein. Normally lymphatic channels do not cross the midline (**answer a and d**). Pleural lymph channels drain toward the hilar region (**answer e**) but in just 3 days would not produce enough lymph to accumulate within the pleural cavity.

368. The answer is b. (*Moore, p 152. Fauci, p 1460.*) Failure of the superior and inferior endocardial cushions to meet in the middle of the heart chambers. If the superior and inferior endocardial cushions fail to meet in the middle of the heart chambers then the septum primum has nothing to meet when it grows down from the superior atrial wall, thus causing a patent ostium primum. Many children with ASD have no symptoms. If the defect is small, then relatively little blood from the slightly higher pressure left atrium flows into the lower pressure right atrium. If the defect is large, then oxygenated blood is mixed with poorly oxygenated blood and sent back to the lungs. The failure of the conotruncal ridges to spiral (**answer a**), as they separate the truncus arteriosus into an aorta and pulmonary trunk, is not directly related to the development of ASDs. Failure of the septum primum to fuse with the septum secundum (**answer c**) is not related to the separation of the truncus arteriosus. Neural crest cells are essential for proper endocardial cushion formation, but **answer d** refers to neural crest cell migration into the conotruncal ridges. Failure of the muscular septum to meet the membranous septum (**answer e**) is the most common cause of VSDs.

Abdomen

Questions

369. A 33-year-old woman (gravida 2, para 2) delivers a term 6 lb 15 oz baby girl who has an unusually formed umbilical attachment. The anterior abdominal wall is pulled inwards about a centimeter around her umbilicus. What portion of the gastrointestinal tract is most likely to be attached to the inner surface of the umbilical region via a vitelline ligament?

a. Anal canal
b. Appendix
c. Cecum
d. Ileum
e. Stomach

370. A 46-year-old woman is admitted to a hospital in acute distress. She has experienced severe abdominal pain and vomiting for 2 days. The pain, which is sharp and constant, began in the epigastric region and radiated bilaterally around the chest to just below the scapulae. Subsequently, the pain became localized in the right hypochondrium. The patient, who has a history of similar but milder attacks after hearty meals, is moderately overweight. Palpation reveals marked tenderness in the right hypochondriac region and some rigidity of the abdominal musculature. An x-ray without contrast medium shows numerous calcified stones in the region of the gallbladder. The patient shows no sign of jaundice (icterus). Diffuse pain referred to the epigastric region and radiating circumferentially around the chest is the result of afferent fibers that travel via which of the following nerves?

a. Greater splanchnic
b. Intercostal
c. Phrenic
d. Vagus
e. Pelvic splanchnic

371. Gallbladder pain often presents as epigastric pain that subsequently migrates toward the patient's right side and can even wrap around to the posterior. The somatic location of the referred pain is not the site of the problem. Anatomically where is the gallbladder located?

a. Between the left and caudate lobes of the liver
b. Between the right and quadrate lobes of the liver
c. In the falciform ligament
d. In the lesser omentum
e. In the right anterior leaf of the coronary ligament

372. A woman presents with gallstones and no jaundice. She is prepared for exploratory surgery. The lesser omentum is incised close to its free edge, and the biliary tree is identified and freed by blunt dissection. The liquid contents of the gallbladder are aspirated with a syringe, the fundus incised, and the stones are removed. The entire duct system is carefully probed for stones, one of which is found to be obstructing a duct. In view of her symptoms, where is the most probable location of the obstruction?

a. The bile duct
b. The common hepatic duct
c. The cystic duct
d. Within the duodenal papilla proximal to the juncture with the pancreatic duct
e. Within the duodenal papilla distal to the juncture with the pancreatic duct

373. A full-term 8 lb baby boy was delivered vaginally to a 36-year-old mother. At delivery he had a large scrotum. The delivering obstetrician (OB) palpated the enlarged scrotum and determined that both testicles were present. When the OB pressed gently on the newborn's abdomen the scrotum swelled even more. What congenital condition did the OB note in the chart?

a. Abdominal hernia
b. Cryptorchid (maldescended) testes
c. Varicocele
d. Hydrocele
e. Femoral hernia

374. Many Cesarean sections are performed by making a horizontal skin incision that is slightly curved (about 15 cm) on the anterior abdominal wall just superior to the pubic hairline (bikini or Pfannenstiel incision). However, this incision is often only made through the skin down to the perimysium of the rectus abdominis muscle. Which one of the following cutaneous nerves are at greatest risk with this type of incision?

a. Thoracoabdominal (intercostal) nerve (T10)
b. Thoracoabdominal (intercostal) nerve (T11)
c. Iliohypogastric nerve (L1)
d. Ilioinguinal nerve (L1)
e. Lateral (femoral) cutaneous nerve of the thigh (L2-L3)

375. A 13-year-old adolescent was vacationing with his parents in Mexico on spring break. He developed nausea and vomiting 4 days into the trip despite caution about what he ate and drank. He switched to a clear liquid diet. None of the others on the trip were sick. On his flight back to the United States, he developed a fever and increased abdominal pain, especially in the paraumbilical region. His parents took him to their pediatrician the next day as he was feeling worse and could barely move. During the physical examination the pediatrician noted tenderness around the umbilicus and rebound tenderness over McBurney point. The patient was sent for an abdominal CT. Where is McBurney point and what is the likely diagnosis?

a. At the right costal margin at the mid-clavicular line; ruptured gallbladder
b. On a line drawn between the anterior superior iliac spine and umbilicus on the right; appendicitis
c. On a line drawn between the anterior superior iliac spine and umbilicus on the left; appendicitis
d. On a line drawn between the anterior superior iliac spine and the pubic tubercle on the right; kidney stone
e. On a line drawn between the anterior superior iliac spine and the pubic tubercle on the left; kidney stone

376. A 65-year-old man presents with jaundice of 2 to 3 weeks duration, fatigue and increasing epigastric pain. He has no history of peptic ulcers and says the pain does not relate to eating in anyway. His epigastric pain is midline and he reports recent back pain. He has pale stools, dark urine, and elevated urinary and serum conjugated bilirubin. Helical CT reveals a suspicious mass in the head of the pancreas adjacent to the descending duodenum. The gallbladder is significantly enlarged. Which of the following is the likely cause of the elevated bilirubin?

a. Viral hepatitis
b. Blocked cystic duct
c. Portal hypertension
d. Blocked duodenal papilla
e. Gilbert syndrome

377. A 75-year-old woman presents to her geriatrician with increasing epigastric pain, sometimes referred to her back. The pain is not associated with eating or any particular time of day. Once she vomited bile and stomach contents. An abdominal CT with both intravenous (IV) contrast and swallowed barium is ordered to determine the cause of her pain. The results are shown in the accompanying radiological image. Which structure is the descending portion of her duodenum?

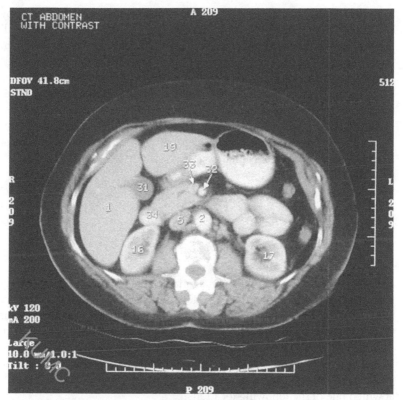

(Image 4203-013 used with permission from the Radiological Anatomy web site, University of Kansas, School of Medicine, http://classes.kumc.edu/som/radanatomy/.)

a. 1
b. 2
c. 5
d. 16
e. 17
f. 19
g. 31
h. 32
i. 33
j. 34

378. A 32-year-old mother delivers her second child, an 8 lb 1 oz baby boy. After 36 hours and several breast-feeding sessions, the baby boy still has not passed meconium. During the next 12 hours the boy's abdomen grows noticeably larger, he gains weight, and wets his diaper, but still has not had his first stool. Upon physical examination, the boy has active bowel sounds in the upper half of his abdomen, but markedly fewer sounds in the lower portion. The baby boy has a functional anus as a finger in the anus came back with meconium. The newborn vomits soon after the physician examines the boy. Which one of the following is the most likely diagnosis of the congenital condition seen in this newborn?

a. Crohn disease
b. Ulcerative colitis
c. Hirschsprung disease
d. Imperforate anus
e. Pyloric stenosis
f. Omphalocele

379. A 65-year-old man with pancreatic adenocarcinoma in the head of pancreas was taken to surgery. A PET-CT suggested metastases to both liver and multiple posterior lymph nodes. It was explained to the patient and his family that the surgery would likely not be curative, but rather palliative in that the cancer was already too far advanced for removal. Ablation of the autonomic innervation, which carries pain in this region, is performed to provide pain relief. The surgeon will inject 50% ethanol to kill nerve cells at which one of the following locations?

a. At each intercostal nerve under ribs 6 to 8
b. Around the celiac trunk
c. Around each lateral epigastric fold
d. Around the coronary ligament
e. Around the lateral arcuate ligament

380. An 11-year-old girl is brought into her pediatrician's office by her mother. She recently learned to do back flips on the balance beam, when her foot slipped off and she landed with her perineum striking the beam. She developed a massive subcutaneous hematoma filling her perineum that posteriorly formed a straight horizontal line just anterior to her anus. It extended anteriorly onto the anterior abdominal wall about half way to her umbilicus and above the inguinal ligament. No blood entered her thighs. She could still urinate and there was no blood in her urine. The hematoma was contained by what space?

a. Ischioanal fossa
b. Superficial perineal space
c. Deep perineal space
d. Femoral sheath
e. Inguinal canal

381. A 46-year-old man presents with a fever of 101°F and a 15-year history of diabetes. He has had vague lower abdominal pain for three days, but has just spiked a fever in the last 24 hours. The abdominal pain is so intense that the man can barely walk and lies curled up in a fetal position on the examining table. Gentle straightening of his left leg produces pain, while straightening his right leg does not bother him as much. He also has vague pain on the anterior surface of his left upper thigh. You order an abdominal CT because you suspect which one of the following conditions?

a. Aortic aneurysm
b. Appendicitis
c. Cirrhosis of the liver
d. Diverticulosis
e. Psoas abscess

382. The first-born baby girl of a 27-year-old mother was born vaginally at 7 lbs 11oz. An ultrasound at 39 weeks suggested polyhydramnios. However, since the woman's water broke at home, the obstetrician was unable to confirm polyhydramnios. The baby girl breast-fed about 3 hours after delivery, but the nurses reported that the baby regurgitated the milk an hour later. There is no bile present. A nasogastric tube is used to introduce barium into the baby's stomach and 55 minutes later an upper GI film (see below) was taken. What is the diagnosis?

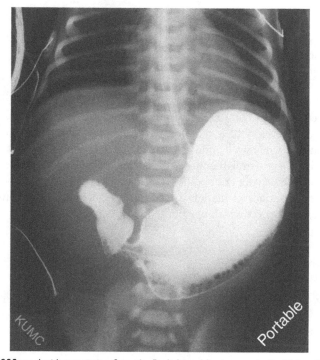

(Image 4922 used with permission from the Radiological Anatomy web site, University of Kansas, School of Medicine, http://classes.kumc.edu/som/radanatomy/.)

a. Duodenal atresia
b. Esophageal atresia
c. Pyloric stenosis
d. Iliac volvulus
e. Jejunal volvulus

383. A 19-year-old teenager is brought to the emergency department after a single car accident just 20 minutes earlier in which she lost control of her car on black ice and hit a retaining column of an overpass at about 45 miles per hour. She was wearing a seat belt but looks pale, has tachycardia and positional hypotension, is extremely nauseated, and is lying in the fetal position due to increasingly severe abdominal pain. She has no fractures and a cranial nerve test is normal. You order an abdominal CT because you suspect which one of the following?

a. Lacerated kidney
b. Ruptured spleen
c. Ruptured gallbladder
d. Diverticulitis
e. Hemorrhoids

384. A first time mother would like to deliver her first baby at home because she thinks that will be better for the baby. The obstetrician advises the mother to have a hospital delivery, but concedes that if α-fetoprotein levels are normal and an ultrasound examination of the baby at 36 weeks is normal, then she can try a home delivery. The α-fetoprotein levels are normal, but the ultrasound comes back suggesting that there is polyhydramnios. The mother says, maybe she has just been drinking too many fluids and not urinating enough so that fluid has accumulated as amniotic fluid. The obstetrician strongly encourages the mother to deliver the baby in the hospital because polyhydramnios suggests the baby may have which of the following congenital defects?

a. Lung hypoplasia
b. Anal atresia, duodenal atresia, esophageal atresia, and renal anomalies
c. Limb, vertebral, and cardiac defects
d. Renal defects, inguinal hernia, femoral hernia, hypospadia, and exstrophy of the bladder
e. Vertebral anomalies and limb defects

385. A 55-year-old woman arrives at the emergency department the day after St. Patrick's Day coughing up bright red blood. History includes excessive alcohol consumption. Using abdominal percussion it is determined that her liver extends 5 cm below the right costal margin at the mid-clavicular line. A gastroenterology consult is ordered because of suspicion that the bright red blood is most likely the result of which one of the following?

a. Hemorrhoids
b. Colon cancer
c. Duodenal ulcer
d. Gastric ulcer
e. Esophageal varices

386. An 88-year-old woman is brought by ambulance to the emergency department (ED) from her nursing home. She developed abdominal pain two days ago and had her last bowel movement 4 days ago. Today she regurgitated her lunch about an hour after eating and is febrile. The ED physician listens to her abdomen with a stethoscope for bowel sounds and hears sounds of hyperactivity in the upper half of the abdomen, but hears almost nothing in the lower half of the abdomen. She has marginal kidney function for a CT with contrast so an abdominal MRI with vascular rendering is ordered because the ED physician suspects which one of the following conditions?

a. Aortic aneurysm
b. Cirrhosis of the liver
c. Diverticulosis
d. Ischemic colitis
e. Psoas abscess

387. Regions of the gastrointestinal tract that are at junctions between different developmental regions often have dual blood supply. The inferior end of the gastrointestinal tract joins the anus, a somatic structure. Occlusion of the inferior mesenteric artery will not result in mucosal necrosis of the rectum for which one of the following reasons?

a. Arterial supply to the rectum is from anastomotic connections from the superior mesenteric artery.
b. Arterial supply to the rectum is from the left colic artery with anastomoses to branches of the internal iliac artery.
c. The inferior mesenteric artery does not supply the rectum.
d. A principal branch of the external iliac artery is a major source of arterial blood to the rectum.
e. The middle rectal artery, a branch of the internal iliac artery, supplies the rectum.

388. Sympathectomy may occasionally relieve intractable pain of visceral origin, since visceral afferent pain fibers run along the sympathetic pathways in the abdomen. The autonomic control of peristalsis in the descending colon should not be affected by bilateral lumbar sympathectomy for which one of the following reasons?

a. The descending colon is controlled chiefly by parasympathetic innervation from the pelvic splanchnic nerves.
b. The descending colon receives its parasympathetic innervation from the vagus nerve.
c. The descending colon receives its sympathetic innervation from thoracic splanchnic nerves.
d. Lumbar splanchnics from L1, L2, and L3 only innervate the pelvic viscera via the hypogastric nerve.
e. Only presynaptic sympathetic fibers have been severed.

389. A 36-year-old man was the victim of a superficial knife wound to the lower left abdomen during a barroom brawl. At 56 he develops a direct inguinal hernia on the left side. Damage to which one of the following nerves is most likely responsible for the predisposing weakness of the abdominal wall?

a. Genitofemoral nerve
b. Ilioinguinal nerve
c. The subcostal nerve
d. Pelvic splanchnic nerves
e. The nerve of the tenth intercostal space (T10)

390. A multiparous mother brings her 18-month-old second son, to his pediatrician because she has noticed blood (sometimes red, one time "currant jelly") in his stools. Although the toddler is trying new foods, she doesn't think the blood is associated with anything in his diet. Physical examination, including a digital rectal examination, is normal. An upper GI barium swallow with small bowel follow through is ordered. The radiological report describes a 2-inch-long diverticulum, pointing toward the umbilicus, in the ileum, about 2 ft from the ileocecal valve. The blood is most likely from which one of the following sources?

a. An appendix that must be removed
b. A Meckel (ileal) diverticulum
c. Active diverticulitis
d. Internal hemorrhoids
e. A duodenal ulcer

391. A 34-year-old woman gave birth to her second daughter who was born at 40 weeks of gestation. The father, who was present for the birth, just about fainted when the baby girl came out of the vagina with a large protruding projection about 4 cm high and 6 cm in circumference bulging from her anterior abdominal wall where the umbilical cord was attached. A clear membrane covered what seemed to be a portion of the small intestine. The baby girl was otherwise normal. What is the name of this congenital dysmorphology?

a. Omphalocele
b. Bochdalek hernia
c. Gastroschisis
d. Meckel diverticulum
e. Nephroptosis

392. A middle-aged woman describes flushing, severe headaches, and a feeling that her heart is "going to explode" when she gets excited. At the beginning of a physical examination her blood pressure (130/85 mm Hg) is not significantly above normal. However, on palpation of her upper left quadrant, the examining physician notices the onset of sympathetic signs. Her blood pressure (200/135 mm Hg) is abnormally high. A subsequent CT scan confirms the suspected tumor of the left adrenal gland. The patient is scheduled for surgery. Her symptoms that correlate with the onset of excitement are most likely due to neural stimulation of the adrenal glands. The adrenal medulla receives its innervation from which one of the following?

a. Preganglionic sympathetic nerves
b. Postsynaptic sympathetic nerves
c. Preganglionic parasympathetic nerves
d. Postganglionic parasympathetic nerves
e. Somatic nerves

393. A 27-year-old man presents to his family practice physician with a mass within his left testicle. Upon physical examination it is confirmed that his left testicle is about twice the size of his right testicle. A CT scan of his abdomen and pelvis is ordered. Which structure on the CT below receives blood from the left testicle?

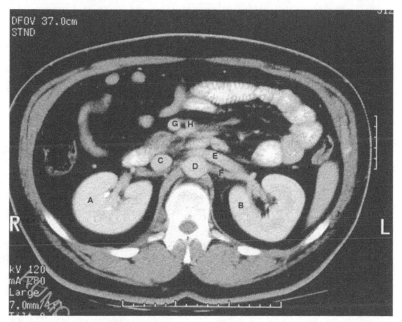

(Image 4204-028 used with permission from the Radiological Anatomy web site, University of Kansas, School of Medicine, http://classes.kumc.edu/som/radanatomy/.)

a. A
b. B
c. C
d. D
e. E
f. F
g. G
h. H

394. A 78-year-old man is brought to the emergency department by his wife. The man is doubled over with sudden onset of lower abdominal pain after eating dinner at an "all-you-can-eat" buffet. The man's abdomen is distended, with vague lower left abdominal pain and he states that he cannot pass any gas. Bowel sounds are extensive in the upper abdomen, but are lacking in the left lower abdomen. The on-call GI fellow is asked to bring a sigmoidoscope. What condition does this patient have and how might a sigmoidoscope help?

a. Colitis; the sigmoidoscope will be able to visualize the lining of the rectum and colon and confirm the diagnosis.
b. Peptic ulcer; the sigmoidscope would show a normal colon.
c. Diverticulosis; the sigmoidoscope will be able to visualize the multiple diverticula, thus confirming the diagnosis.
d. Meckel diverticulum; the sigmoidoscope will be able to visualize the typically 2 inch long diverticulum.
e. Sigmoid volvulus; the sigmoidoscope may actually be used to help straighten the sigmoid colon if it has twisted on itself.

395. While moving furniture, an 18-year-old teenager experiences excruciating pain in his right groin. A few hours later he also develops pain in the umbilical region with accompanying nausea. At this point he seeks medical attention. Examination reveals a bulge midway between the midline and the anterior superior iliac spine, but superior to the inguinal ligament. On coughing or straining, the bulge increases and the inguinal pain intensifies. The bulge courses medially and inferiorly into the upper portion of the scrotum and cannot be reduced with the finger pressure of the examiner. It is decided that a medical emergency exists, and the patient is scheduled for immediate surgery. Nausea and diffuse pain referred to the umbilical region in this patient most probably are due to which one of the following?

a. Compression of the genitofemoral nerve
b. Compression of the ilioinguinal nerve
c. Dilation of the inguinal canal
d. Ischemic necrosis of a loop of small bowel
e. Ischemic necrosis of the cremaster muscle

396. A 77-year-old woman complains to her doctor about left-sided chest pain, difficulty swallowing, and the sensation that food is stuck in her esophagus. "Antacids don't seem to help much." The symptoms seem to get worse if she lies down shortly after a meal and she often has some small reflux of acidic stomach contents. A barium swallow study is performed and one of the late images taken is illustrated below.

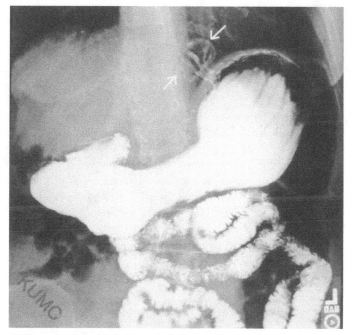

(Image 4910 used with permission from the Radiological Anatomy web site, University of Kansas, School of Medicine, http://classes.kumc.edu/som/radanatomy/.)

Based on the history and radiological image which of the following is the most likely diagnosis?

a. Sliding hiatal hernia
b. Para esophageal hiatal hernia
c. Congenital Bochdalek hernia
d. Pylorospasm
e. Congenital hypertrophic pyloric stenosis

397. A concerned mother called her family practice office about her 3-week-old baby boy. This is her first child. The baby boy keeps regurgitating immediately after breast-feeding. The emesis has always been milky in color and never green. The vomit seems to come violently from the boy's stomach. The baby has become quite cranky and the mother wants to bring the boy in because she is worried that he is becoming dehydrated. The family's physician has the mother come in immediately and orders an ultrasound because which one of the following conditions is likely present?

a. Duodenal atresia
b. Diverticulosis
c. Intestinal ischemia
d. Psoas abscess
e. Pyloric stenosis

398. A full-term 7 lb 15 oz baby girl has a slight barrel chest yet relatively shallow and small abdomen. The baby's breathing is labored, but the girl is handed over to the new first time mother who is anxious to hold her child. About 3 or 4 minutes later, the baby girl is not as pink as she should be and appears to be breathing rapidly. There are no lung sounds on the left side, and the rapid heart sounds are all shifted to the right. As supplemental oxygen and a sonogram are ordered for the baby what is the working diagnosis?

a. Diaphragmatic hernia
b. Splenic rupture
c. Tetralogy of Fallot
d. Tracheoesophageal fistula
e. Transposition of the great arteries

399. A 62-year-old woman has renal failure as a result of Alport syndrome. While she is currently on dialysis, she is hoping to receive a kidney transplant. She asks the nephrologists and the transplant surgeon to describe the procedure. Which one of the following is the best description of the procedure?

a. The right kidney is always removed since it is more inferior and the newly transplanted kidney will replace it.

b. The left kidney will be removed because it is easier to move the descending colon out of the way and the newly transplanted kidney will replace it.

c. She will keep both of her kidneys, and the newly transplanted kidney will be placed on the left posterior wall just inferior to her left kidney since the left kidney is higher and will leave more space for the transplant.

d. The newly transplanted kidney will be placed in the iliac fossa in the greater pelvis, attached to branched iliac vessels and the ureter connected directly to the bladder.

e. Both right and left kidneys will be removed and the new kidney transplanted into either place.

400. The patient is a 30-year-old bachelor who frequents "singles" bars. He is cautious and always uses a condom in his sexual encounters. Recently, he has felt "off," experiencing a sore throat, malaise, and a slight fever. When he is seen by his internist, he has a few swollen lymph nodes and has a large palpable structure in the left upper abdomen indicated by the asterisk in the accompanying radiograph. He has a positive monospot test and an elevated sedimentary rate. The structure palpated by his physician is best described as which one of the following?

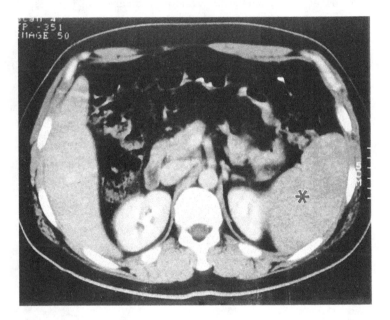

   a. Hepatomegaly
   b. Splenomegaly
   c. The stomach
   d. A tumor of the liver
   e. Liver cirrhosis

401. A patient complained of severe abdominal pain on several occasions, but no cause could be identified. She was recently diagnosed with polyarteritis nodosa so an abdominal arteriogram is ordered to determine whether there are abdominal vascular changes that would explain her abdominal pain. On her arteriogram there is a tortuous large diameter vessel indicated by the arrow. What is this vessel?

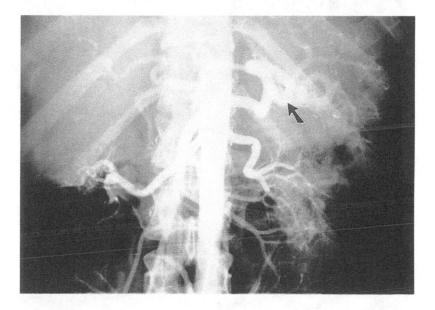

a. Left gastric artery
b. Superior mesenteric artery
c. Splenic artery
d. Right gastric artery
e. Right gastro-omental artery

402. A 21-year-old man presents with severe epigastric pain that radiates to his back. His father died of a pancreatic cancer at age 60. An abdominal CT with IV contrast was performed. Which one of the following is structure 20 in the axial CT of the abdomen?

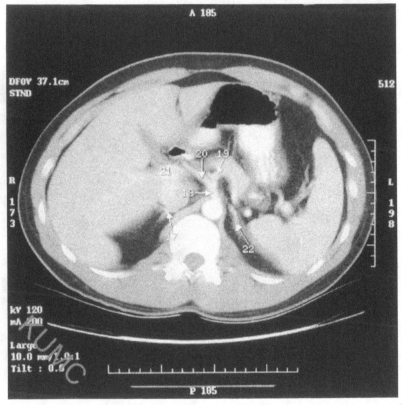

(*Image 4201-009 used with permission from the Radiological Anatomy web site, University of Kansas, School of Medicine, http://classes.kumc.edu/som/radanatomy/.*)

a. Celiac trunk (artery)
b. Common hepatic artery
c. Left crus of diaphragm
d. Splenic artery
e. Superior mesenteric artery

403. Pathology within some abdominal organs can occasionally cause referred pain in the shoulder and neck regions, C3 to C5, because the diaphragm receives its motor and afferent innervation from this level as a result of its cranial embryonic development. Which one of the following abdominal organs causes unilateral shoulder/neck pain and which side of the body is affected?

a. Liver; left side
b. Gallbladder; right side
c. Pancreas; right side
d. Spleen; right side
e. Appendix; left side

404. A 58-year-old man presents to the emergency department with fatigue and weakness. Although he has a slight cough, his lungs sound clear, and his heart sounds are normal. His sclerae are icteric. He has a solid mass extending 6 cm inferior to the right inferior costal margin and there are extensive veins radiating from his umbilicus, especially inferiorly. He admits to consuming alcohol daily for more than 20 years. What is the name of the radiating varicose veins on the anterior abdominal wall and in what other locations might one expect to find varicose veins?

a. Ascites; esophageal varices and hemorrhoids
b. Caput medusa; esophageal varices and hemorrhoids
c. Cirrhosis; esophageal varices and lymphedema
d. Diverticulosis; esophageal varices and lymphedema
e. Diverticulosis; lymphedema and hemorrhoids

405. A 50-year-old man schedules a physical so he can attend a boy scout camp with one of his sons. You suggest a colonoscopy after he returns from camp. He agrees, but wants you to describe the procedure and potential risks and complications. You explain that the goal of a colonoscopy is to look at the entire length of the large intestine from the anus to the small intestine (ileocecal junction), observing polyps or diverticuli with a flexible fiber optic colonoscope inserted through the anus. There is a small risk of perforating the bowel especially when the colon takes a sudden turn or twists on itself at regions where it is intraperitoneal rather than attached to the posterior abdominal wall (retroperitoneal). During colonoscopy which of the following regions of the colon generally poses the greatest risk for perforation?

a. Rectum, sigmoid colon, and descending colon
b. Sigmoid colon, descending colon, and splenic flexure
c. Sigmoid colon, splenic flexure, and descending colon
d. Sigmoid colon, splenic flexure, and hepatic flexure
e. Descending colon, transverse colon, and ascending colon

406. A 63-year-old woman presents with lethargy and unremitting epigastric pain. She is 5 ft 6 in tall and weighs 170 lb and has smoked for 44 years. She has lost 5 lb in the last week despite eating normally. She reports that her skin and eyes have started to yellow. She has midline epigastric pain, which also radiates to her back. The pain sometimes gets worse with eating but has become unbearable and interferes with her sleeping. What nerves likely carry her pain and what diagnosis should she fear the most?

a. Greater splanchnic nerves; ascites from cirrhosis
b. Greater splanchnic nerves; duodenal ulcer
c. Greater splanchnic nerves; pancreatic adenocarcinoma
d. Lesser splanchnic nerves; gallstones
e. Lesser splanchnic nerves; gastric carcinoma

407. A 42-year-old slightly overweight woman presents to her primary care physician complaining of recent blood in her stool. She has no fever and feels well otherwise. She generally has one or two bowel movements daily with no change in frequency or consistency. She describes an absence of painful hemorrhoids and no pain on defecation. Prior to examining the patient what should be her physician's list of potential causes of blood in the stool?

a. Diverticulitis and colorectal cancer
b. Diverticulitis and internal hemorrhoids
c. Diverticulosis and external hemorrhoids
d. External hemorrhoids and fissures, and diverticulitis
e. Diverticulosis, internal hemorrhoids, and colorectal cancer

408. During the physical examination of a 52-year-old man for a life insurance policy, internal hemorrhoids are noted. The man had noticed occasional bright red blood on some of his larger, well-formed stools. Which of the following arteries could be the source of his rectal bleeding?

a. Superior mesenteric artery
b. External iliac artery
c. Internal pudendal artery
d. Inferior gluteal artery
e. Superior, middle, and inferior rectal arteries

409. Three major anatomic structures pass through the openings in the diaphragm: inferior vena cava (labeled A); esophagus (labeled C); aorta (labeled E). Which one of the following lettered openings normally transmits the azygos vein?

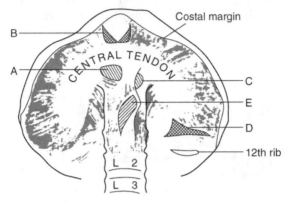

Diaphragm–inferior surface.

a. A
b. B
c. C
d. D
e. E

410. A 73-year-old man presents to his geriatrician for ongoing control of his hypertension (155/90). His physician notes that he has lost about 5 lb since his last visit. The patient reports that he does not "have as much room for food or as much of an appetite." He states that he is getting tired of the food at his nursing home. His physician palpates his abdomen and notes that there is a mid-line pulse, which is initially mistaken for a heartbeat, but it is slightly delayed. His physician is concerned about the pulsating abdominal mass and orders an abdominal CT with IV contrast because his physician suspects that he has which one of the following?

a. A hiatal hernia
b. Splenomegaly
c. Cirrhosis of the liver
d. An aortic aneurysm
e. A horseshoe kidney

411. Most direct inguinal hernias occur in older men as the conjoint tendon weakens with increased abdominal pressure, often a complication of excessive abdominal weight gain. In contrast, most indirect inguinal hernias occur in which one of the following?

a. Teenage females
b. Multiparous women
c. Newborn boys
d. Teenage males
e. Skinny middle-aged men

412. Colorectal carcinoma at the splenic flexure of the colon is diagnosed in a 55-year-old man following endoscopy and frozen and paraffin section pathology. About a foot-long section of large intestine is removed, which includes part of the transverse and descending colon. The surgeon reattaches the cut ends to each other, reconnects a major artery, and collects numerous lymph nodes. Which one of the following major arteries will be reconnected and which lymph nodes will be collected?

a. Aorta; splenic and suprarenal lymph nodes
b. Splenic artery; splenic and suprarenal lymph nodes
c. Marginal artery; splenic and superior mesenteric lymph nodes
d. Marginal artery; superior and inferior mesenteric lymph nodes
e. Sigmoid artery; left colic and sigmoidal nodes

413. When examining a 48-year-old woman for the first time at a free clinic her physician notes that she is quite slender with prominent veins both on her anterior abdominal wall and her nose. Abdominal palpation reveals a fairly large firm organ that extends well below the right costal margin during both inspiration and expiration. There is no abdominal tenderness. Which one of the following is the most likely explanation for your physical findings?

a. Splenomegaly
b. Hepatomegaly
c. Appendicitis
d. Cholecystitis
e. Abdominal aortic aneurysm

Abdomen

Answers

369. The answer is d. (*Moore, pp 258-260. Sadler, p 228.*) During the first month of development, the midgut communicates with the yolk sac. The midgut undergoes rotation during the second month as it rotated around the vitelline duct (yolk stalk, omphalomesenteric duct). At about the ninth week, the midgut moves back into the abdominal cavity as the anterior abdominal wall closes. The vitelline duct always attaches to the ileum. Failure of closure of the anterior abdominal wall or apoptosis of the omphalomesenteric duct may result in a persistent vitelline fistula, vitelline cysts, or simply an ileal diverticulum (of Meckel). A vitelline ligament and any attached ileal diverticulum would normally be surgically removed to reduce the chances of future problems. Other regions (**answers a, b, c, and e**) of the gastrointestinal tract are unlikely to be attached to the anterior abdominal wall.

370. The answer is a. (*Moore, pp 278-280, 286-287, 301-304.*) Visceral afferent pain fibers from the gallbladder travel through the celiac—along the greater splanchnic nerves to levels T5 to T9 of the spinal cord. Therefore, pain originating from the gallbladder will be referred to the dermatomes served by T5 to T9, which include a band from the infrascapular region to the epigastrium. If the gallbladder enlarges sufficiently, then pain could be carried by the phrenic nerve (**answer c**), but this would refer pain to the neck. Intercostal nerves (**answer b**) would course above the diaphragm and thus are not involved. The vagus (**answer d**) generally does not transmit pain information. Pelvic splanchnics (**answers e**) receive pain information from pelvic organs and are therefore not involved.

371. The answer is b. (*Moore, pp 277-280.*) The gallbladder lies on the inferior surface of the liver between the right and quadrate lobes (not **answer a**). The caudate lobe lies posteriorly between the right and left lobes. The falciform ligament, a portion of the lesser omentum, attaches to the liver at the incisura between the quadrate and left lobes as well as along the fissure for the round ligament. Toward the superior surface of the liver, the falciform ligament (**answer c**) splits to form the left and right coronary ligaments, which define the bare area of the liver. The coronary ligaments (answer e) come together again to form the gastrohepatic ligament of the lesser omentum (answer d).

372. The answer is c. (*Moore, pp 278-280, 286-287.*) Obstruction of any portion of the biliary tree will produce symptoms of gallbladder obstruction. If the common hepatic duct (answer b) or bile duct (answer a) is occluded by stone or tumor, biliary stasis with accompanying jaundice occurs. In addition, blockage of the duodenal papilla (of Vater), distal to the juncture of the bile duct with the pancreatic duct (answer e), can lead to complicating pancreatitis. If only the cystic duct is obstructed, jaundice will not occur because bile may flow freely from the liver to the duodenum. Bile duct obstruction also may arise as a result of pressure exerted on the duct by an external mass, such as a tumor in the head of the pancreas. Answer d is not anatomically correct.

373. The answer is d. (*Moore, pp 212-214.*) The newborn boy has a hydrocele. The testicles develop on the posterior abdominal wall and are guided out of the abdominal cavity by the gubernaculum. The final descent through the inguinal canal does not generally occur until the ninth month in utero. The testis remains a retroperitoneal organ behind the fluid-filled space (tunica vaginalis), which is connected to the abdominal cavity by the processus vaginalis. In this case the testicles successfully migrated into the scrotum on both sides (so he did not have cryptorchid testes [answer b]), but rather the processus vaginalis failed to seal itself off from the abdominal cavity. Congenital hydrocele normally resolves itself after 2 to 3 months without any intervention. An abdominal hernia (answer a) is a defect on the anterior abdominal wall and is not present. Varicoceles (answer c) are a stasis of venous blood around the testicle and often present as a bluish scrotal mass. Femoral hernias (answer e) are defects in both the femoral sheath and fascia lata and present on the anterior thigh below the inguinal ligament.

374. The answer is c. (*Moore, pp 193, 198-199.*) The cutaneous nerve which is at risk with this type of incision is the iliohypogastric nerve (L1). The thoracoabdominal (intercostal) nerve T10 (answer a) generally supplies the dermatome that includes the umbilicus, while the skin over the inguinal ligament is generally served by the L1 spinal level. T11 (answer b) is also too cranial to be at risk of injury. Both the subcostal nerve T12 (not listed as a choice) and the iliohypogastric nerves are likely cut during the Pfannenstiel incision. The ilioinguinal nerve **(answer d)** tends to course about an inch superior to the inguinal ligament, and would most likely not be cut. The lateral (femoral) cutaneous nerve of the thigh (from L2-L3; **answer e**) runs across the iliacus muscle and under the inguinal ligament lateral to the femoral sheath to serve the anterolateral aspect of the thigh, and should not be at risk.

375. The answer is b. (*Moore, pp 199, 259-260.*) Rebound tenderness over McBurney point is the characteristic symptom for the diagnosis of appendicitis. McBurney point is located one-third of the way along a line drawn between the patient's right (thus left and **answer c** is wrong) anterior superior iliac spine and the umbilicus. This is the approximate location of the ileocecal junction where the appendix would lie deep to the anterior abdominal wall. The history of first umbilical pain and nausea and vomiting is consistent with appendicitis, not kidney stones **(answers d and e)**. The inguinal ligament courses between the anterior superior iliac spine and the pubic tubercle, which is the lateral portion of the pubic crest. While kidney stones are very painful they are not always associated with vomiting, nor does the pain refer to either the umbilical region or McBurney point. Gallbladder pain often presents with rebound tenderness at the right costal margin at the mid-clavicular line **(answer a)**.

376. The answer is d. (*Moore, pp 282-283.*) The likely cause of the elevated conjugated bilirubin is a blocked pancreatic and bile duct at the duodenal papilla. This is known as obstructive jaundice and is a form of post-hepatic jaundice. Other forms are pre-hepatic and hepatic (see question and feedback for question 217). Pancreatic cancer (usually ductal adenocarcinoma) frequently arises from the head of the pancreas where it blocks the normal flow of bile out of the liver via the hepatic duct. Bile flows from the gall bladder through the cystic ducts which join to form the (common) bile duct that passes through the substance of the head of the pancreas. There it joins the main pancreatic duct just before forming the hepatopancreatic ampulla at the second portion of the duodenum. Blockage of the cystic duct **(answer b)** may just lead to a gallbladder enlargement/inflammation. Viral hepatitis **(answer a)** would normally not be associated with pancreatic cancer, but would cause jaundice (hepatic) with normal or increased unconjugated bilirubin. Portal hypertension (**answer c**) induced by cirrhosis may also lead to elevated unconjugated serum bilirubin levels. Gilbert syndrome (**answer e**) is due to mild, chronic unconjugated hyperbilirubinemia and is not involved.

377. The answer is j. (*Moore pp 239-241.*) Number 34 is the second or descending portion of the duodenum, which is the location of the entrance of the pancreatic duct and common bile duct into the small intestine. Number 1 is the right lobe of the liver, number 2 is the abdominal aorta, number 5 is the inferior vena cava, number 16 is the right kidney, number 17 is the left kidney, number 19 is the left lobe of the liver, number 31 is the gallbladder, number 32 is the superior mesenteric artery, number 33 is the superior mesenteric vein anterior to the body of the pancreas, and number 34 is the second portion of the duodenum.

378. The answer is c. (*Sadler, pp 231.*) Hirschsprung disease is generally a loss of functional peristalsis of the distal large intestine due to lack of autonomic innervation. Hirschsprung disease or congenital aganglionic megacolon affect about 1 in 5000 newborns with a male to female ratio of 4:1. A 30 cm or less section of the sigmoid colon or rectum is often affected. A biopsy of the suspected region of the colon can be used to confirm the lack of autonomic innervation due to failure of neural crest cell migration. Surgical resection of the non-innervated section of the colon and anastomosis is possible in many cases. Sometimes the disease is less severe and leads to chronic constipation and lower GI problems that often go undiagnosed for years. Crohn disease and ulcerative colitis (**answers a and b**) are not congenital diseases. The physical examination of the boy stated that the anus was functional, so imperforate anus is not possible (**answer d**). Pyloric stenosis (**answer e**) results from hypertrophy of the stomach musculature with narrowing of the pyloric lumen, thus obstructing normal feeding. Omphalocele is a herniation of the abdominal viscera which may include the small and large bowel, liver, and spleen (**answer f**). Also see answer for Question 205.

379. The answer is b. (*Moore, pp 301-305.*) The surgeon will inject 50% ethanol to kill nerve cells around the celiac trunk. Palliative pain relief for pancreatic cancer is called chemical splanchnicectomy. The purpose is to kill afferent pain fibers which detect free ATP (from dying cells) and stretch receptors for the foregut area, affected by the cancer. This is best accomplished by injecting ethanol around the celiac trunk at the posterior abdominal wall in the region of the celiac plexus. Injection of each subcostal nerve T6 to T8 (**answer a**) would cause a loss of sensation on the upper anterior abdominal wall, but would not cover the complete area to which pain is referred. The lateral epigastric folds (**answer c**) are inferior and only house inferior epigastric blood vessels, not nerves. The coronary ligament (**answer d**) holds the liver to the undersurface of the diaphragm. The lateral arcuate ligaments (**answer e**) are connective tissue structures on the posterior abdominal wall that allow the psoas muscles to pass inferiorly. The Whipple procedure (not performed in this case) removes the head of the pancreas and much of the duodenum and attaches the gallbladder to the descending portion of the duodenum to relieve the back up of bile.

380. The answer is b. (*Moore, pp 415-416.*) The hematoma was contained by the superficial perineal space. This is a typical "straddle" injury to the perineum. The blood is collecting in the superficial perineal space, which houses the erectile tissue and is created by the superficial membranous fascia, which is called Scarpa on the anterior abdominal wall (where it is attached half way up to the rectus abdominis muscle sheath) and is called Colles fascia in the perineum. The membranous fascia attaches (deep) to the perineal membrane posteriorly and to the fascia lata of thigh and inguinal ligament. In males the membranous fascia has three names: Scarpa (anterior abdominal wall); Dartos on penis and scrotum; and Colles on perineum. Following straddle injuries, blood does not enter the inguinal canal (**answer e**), femoral sheath (**answer d**), and ischioanal fossa (**answer a**). The deep perineal space (**answer c**) is deep to the perineal membrane.

381. The answer is e. (*Moore, p 318.*) The psoas muscle originates from the sides of the vertebral bodies and transverse processes of T12 to L5 and inserts onto the lesser trochanter of the femur and as such serves as a major flexor of the thigh. Abscesses of the psoas muscle are more common in countries where tuberculosis is common, but also occur in the United States and are caused by a variety of bacteria. Pain associated with flexing the thigh would be typical for a psoas abscess and at times there may also be low back pain referred to the upper anterior thigh by a lumbar nerve passing by the muscle. Aortic aneurysms (**answer a**) would pulsate and would more likely produce back pain. Pain from appendicitis (**answer b**) would be in the lower right quadrant, not on the left. Cirrhosis of the liver (answer c) does not produce lower abdominal pain. Diverticulosis (answer d) is simply the presence of multiple diverticula, typically within the sigmoid colon. If the diverticula become inflamed, then diverticulitis would be present possibly with similar symptoms. Generally, diverticulosis presents without any referred pain to the anterior upper thigh and the patient would be less likely to feel pain upon flexing of just one leg.

382. The answer is a. (*Moore, p 257. Sadler, pp 229, 230.*) The diagnosis is duodenal atresia. Barium fills the stomach and passes through the pyloric valve into the first portion of the duodenum, but not distally. Duodenal atresia occurs in about 1 in 6000 births, with equal numbers of males and females. Polyhydramnios occurs in approximately half of duodenal atresia cases and is due to blockade of the intestinal lumen and back-up of swallowed amniotic fluid. If esophageal atresia (answer b) were present, the barium would not be present in the stomach. Pyloric stenosis (answer c) would not allow barium into the duodenum at all. Volvulus of the ileum or jejunum (answer d and e) would have allowed barium into the entire duodenum and is not usually associated with polyhydramnios. (Also see answer for Question 21.)

383. The answer is b. (*Moore, p 281.*) The spleen is a large blood-filled organ with a relatively thin capsule that can rupture upon sudden deceleration, causing bleeding into the peritoneal cavity. Appearing pale, the positional hypotension and tachycardia would be consistent with bleeding into the peritoneal cavity, leading to generalized abdominal pain, and guarding. A ruptured gallbladder (answer c) does not fit with the blood loss symptoms. Neither diverticulitis (answer d) nor hemorrhoids (answer e) would cause the set of symptoms listed. A lacerated kidney (answer a) is less likely to bring on the sudden onset of symptoms.

384. The answer is b. (*Sadler, pp 106, 206, 207.*) Polyhydramnios is associated with the VACTERL constellation of congenital anomalies: vertebral, anal atresia, cardiac, tracheoesophageal fistula, renal, and limb. When swallowed amniotic fluid cannot pass through the small intestine, then excess amniotic fluid accumulates (polyhydramnios). Lung hypoplasia is associated with too little amniotic fluid (oligohydramnios [answer a]). Limb defects (answers c and e) such as clubfoot are more frequently associated with too little amniotic oligohydramnios. Neither inguinal nor femoral hernia (answer d) is associated with polyhydramnios. (Also see answer for Question 21).

385. The answer is e. (*Moore, pp 199-200, 285, 288.*) Because of an enlarged liver and the history of excessive alcohol consumption, you suspect cirrhosis of the liver, which resulted in portal hypertension. Because the blood is bright red, suggesting that it has not been exposed to duodenal or gastric secretions, the most likely source would be esophageal varices, as blood is trying to return from the portal system to the systemic circulatory system. Hemorrhoids (**answer a**) are commonly associated with cirrhosis of the liver, but at the other end of the GI tract. Colon cancer (**answer b**) does not present with upper GI bleeding, rather lower GI bleeding. Neither duodenal (**answer c**) nor gastric ulcers (**answer d**) present with bright red blood.

386. The answer is d. (*Moore, p 258. Fauci, pp 1910-1912.*) Ischemic colitis is uncommon, but more common in elderly patients and those who are diabetic and tend to have clotting problems. Ischemic colitis usually presents with crampy abdominal pain and bloody stools. If the condition does not improve with bowel rest (liquid diet) then surgical resection may be necessary to prevent gangrene. Aortic aneurysms (**answer a**) would pulsate and would more likely produce back pain. Cirrhosis of the liver (**answer b**) does not produce lower abdominal pain. Diverticulosis (**answer c**) is the simple presence of multiple diverticula, typically within the sigmoid colon. If the diverticula become inflamed, then diverticulitis may present with similar symptoms. Pain associated with a psoas abscess (**answer e**) occurs with straightening and flexing of the thigh.

387. The answer is e. (*Moore, pp 280, 409-413.*) The rectum receives blood from the superior rectal (hemorrhoidal) artery and from the paired middle and inferior rectal arteries. The superior rectal artery is a direct continuation of the inferior mesenteric artery, but the middle and inferior rectal arteries are branches of the internal iliac artery and continue to supply the distal rectum despite occlusion of the inferior mesenteric artery. It should be noted that Sudeck's point, between the last sigmoidal artery and the rectosigmoid artery, is an area of potentially weak arterial anastomoses, but that is further cranial. The superior mesenteric artery (**answer a**) distributes arteries to the small intestine right and middle colic arteries, that supply blood as far distal as the splenic flexure of the transverse colon. The left colic artery (**answer b**) anastomoses with the sigmoidal arteries. The inferior mesenteric artery supplies the superior rectal artery, so **answer c** is not correct. The principal branch of the external iliac artery is the femoral artery (**answer d**).

388. The answer is a. (*Moore*, *pp 301-305.*) The descending colon is controlled chiefly by parasympathetic innervation from the pelvic splanchnic nerves. Control of peristalsis is principally a function of the parasympathetic division of the autonomic nervous system. Although removal of the lumbar sympathetic chain (lumbar sympathectomy) does sever the sympathetic fibers innervating the descending colon as well as the pelvic viscera, (not thoracic splanchnics [**answer c**]) the action of sympathetic fibers to the descending colon is mostly confined to vasoconstriction. Because the parasympathetic innervation to the descending colon is derived from the sacral outflow (S2-S4) through the pelvic splanchnic nerves (nervi erigentes; not by the vagus [**answer b**]) peristalsis will occur normally after lumbar sympathectomy. Lumbar splanchnics do not include L3 (**answer d**). The **answer e** is not anatomically correct.

389. The answer is b. (*Moore, pp 212-213.*) The ilioinguinal nerve innervates the portion of the internal oblique muscle inserting in the lateral border of the conjoint tendon. Paralysis of those fibers would create weakness in the conjoint tendon, allowing herniation to occur medial to the inferior epigastric vessels. The genitofemoral nerve (**answer a**) supplies sensory innervation to the skin of the femoral triangle and scrotum/labia majora. The subcostal nerve (T12; **answer c**) supplies lower portions of the external abdominal oblique muscle. The pelvic splanchnic nerves (**answer d**) supply autonomic (parasympathetic) innervation to the pelvic viscera. The tenth thoracic spinal nerve (T10; **answer e**) supplies abdominal muscles superior to the inguinal region.

390. The answer is b. (*Moore, pp 258-259. Sadler, p 228.*) Meckel (ileal) diverticuli are the most common congenital abnormality of the digestive system. They are a remnant of the herniation and rotation of the midgut and at times the diverticulum remains attached to the umbilicus by a connective tissue stalk, as is mostly likely the case here. The rule of "two" helps remind one of the characteristics of Meckel diverticulum. The diverticulum generally extends 2 in from the ileum; about 2 ft from the ileocecal valve and usually manifests itself by bleeding prior to the first 2 years of life. There may be two types of ectopic tissues present in the diverticulum: either acid secreting epithelium (stomach; detected with radioactive technetium injected into the venous blood stream which then accumulates within the diverticulum) or pancreatic epithelium. The appendix (**answer a**) is a diverticulum off the cecum, not the ileum. Diverticuli **(answer c)** can cause blood in the stool but would be extremely rare in a toddler. Internal hemorrhoids **(answer d)** would generally be detected in a rectal examination, especially in a toddler and is not associated with "currant jelly" stools. The blood would more likely be black if a duodenal ulcer **(answer e)** were present, which would also be very rare in a toddler.

391. The answer is a. *(Sadler, pp 224-227, Moore, pp 298, 317.)* An omphalocele occurs when the intestines, which normally move outside the abdominal cavity at about sixth to tenth week and normally return to inside the anterior abdominal wall at about the eleventh week, fail to completely return to the abdominal cavity. About 2.5 babies out of 10,000 are born with an omphalocele. It is important to check for other congenital chromosome defects as about 50% of omphalocele babies have other developmental dysmorphism. This omphalocele sounds relatively small, so often repair of the anterior abdominal wall is very successful with few long-term consequences. Bochdalek hernia **(answer b)** is a defect in the left posterior portion of the diaphragm, which can allow abdominal contents into the space normally occupied by the left lung. A gastroschisis **(answer c)** is similar to an omphalocele, but the intestines are not covered with peritoneal lining and are directly exposed to amniotic fluid. Generally gastroschisis occurs in the anterior abdominal wall to the right of the umbilical cord. Meckel diverticulum **(answer d)** is an internal remnant of the intestines leaving and returning to the abdominal cavity during development and is generally a 2 inch long appendage which is often 2 ft from the ileocecal junction. It may contain two ectopic tissue types: gastric and pancreatic tissues. Nephroptosis **(answer e)** is a dropping of the kidney inferiorly (more than the normal 3 cm) within the renal fascia (of Gerota) upon standing.

392. The answer is a. *(Moore, pp 294-296.)* The adrenal medulla is innervated from thoracic levels of the spinal cord mediated by preganglionic sympathetic nerve fibers traveling in the lesser and least splanchnic nerves, with some contribution from the greater splanchnic and lumbar splanchnic nerves (thus not **answer b**). Because both the adrenal medulla and postganglionic sympathetic neurons are adrenergic and derived from neural crest, the homology of the chromaffin cells and postganglionic sympathetic neurons is apparent. There is no parasympathetic innervation **(answers c and d)** to the adrenal medulla or cortex. There is no somatic (**answer e**) innervation of the adrenal medulla, by definition a visceral organ.

393. The answer is e. (*Moore, p 356.*) The letter "E" marks the left renal vein. The left testicular vein drains blood into the left renal vein, while the right testicular vein drains blood into the inferior vena cava. A is the right kidney, B is the left kidney, C is the inferior vena cava, D is the abdominal aorta, E is the left renal vein, F is the left renal artery, G is the superior mesenteric vein, and H is the superior mesenteric artery.

394. The answer is e. (*Moore, pp 260, 261. Fauci, p 1914.*) The sigmoido-scope may be used for treatment as well as diagnosis. The sigmoidscope can be used specifically to straighten the sigmoid colon if it has twisted on itself. Volvulus is a twisting of the bowel on itself, cutting off its blood sup-ply and blocking luminal passage. Volvulus can occur along the small intestine or, next most frequently, at the sigmoid colon. This man has early symptoms of sigmoid volvulus. Surgery may be needed to untwist the sig-moid colon before necrosis sets in. Colitis (**answer a**) is inflammation of the colon and rectum and normally would be diagnosed in someone in their thirties, not seventies. In diverticulosis (**answer c**), multiple divertic-ula can be seen with a sigmoidoscope since they are often located within the sigmoid colon, but do not produce pain unless inflamed. Meckel diver-ticulum (**answer d**) will typically occur within 2 ft of the ileocecal junction and may contain two other tissue types: pancreas and gastric tissues would be too proximal in the GI tract to be seen with a sigmoidoscope. Peptic ulcer is not consistent with the clinical findings (**answer b**).

395. The answer is d. (*Moore, pp 212-213.*) The diffuse central abdomi-nal pain in the patient presented is probably referred pain from the loop of small bowel incarcerated within the herniated peritoneal sac that then undergoes ischemic necrosis. Compression of the bowel results in compro-mise of the blood supply and subsequent ischemic necrosis (thus not **answer e**). The visceral afferent fibers from the distal small bowel travel along the blood vessels to reach the superior mesenteric plexus and lesser splanchnic nerves, which they follow to the T10 to T11 levels of the spinal cord. The pain, therefore, is referred to (appears as if originating from) the T10 to T11 dermatomes, which supply the umbilical region. Because the gut develops as a midline structure, visceral pain tends to be centrally located regardless of the adult location of any particular region of the gut. As a result of dilation (answer c) of the inguinal canal by the hernial sac, however, the patient also experiences localized somatic pain mediated by the iliohypogastric, ilioinguinal (answer b), and genitofemoral nerves (answer a), but this was not what the question asked.

396. The answer is a. (*Moore, pp 254-255.*) This patient has a sliding hiatal hernia. Sliding hiatal hernias are more common than paraesophageal hiatal hernias (answer b). Sliding hiatal hernias are generally acquired in middle age and lead to chest pain, difficulty swallowing food, and acid reflux. A congenital Bochdalek hernia (answer c) is unlikely since they usually allow much of the small intestine to enter the left pleural cavity and are a medical emergency in newborns. Neither pylorospasm (answer d) nor congenital hypertrophic pyloric stenosis (answer e) is likely since barium is reaching the small intestine.

397. The answer is e. (*Moore, pp 254-255. Sadler, p 218.*) Congenital pyloric stenosis is most common in first born boys, occurring to 1 of every 150 newborn boys and 1 of 750 newborn girls. While the condition is often called congenital (or infantile) hypertrophic pyloric stenosis, it normally doesn't develop until 3 to 12 weeks after birth. While IV hydration of the newborn may be needed, in most instances surgical treatment is performed laparoscopically to cut open the pyloric smooth muscle to allow stomach contents to pass into the duodenum. Duodenal atresia (answer a) would not permit even a second feeding, but does produce projectile vomit. Diverticulosis (answer b) does not occur in infants. Intestinal ischemia (answer c) can produce vomiting, but occurs mainly in a much older population. A psoas abscess (answer d) is painful and does not produce projectile vomiting.

398. The answer is a. (*Sadler, pp 162-163. Moore, p 317.*) Congenital diaphragmatic hernias (CDHs) are a common (1/2,000), often fatal, congenital dysmorphology and are caused by the failure of the pleuroperitoneal membranes to close the pleuroperitoneal canals. In the most common manifestation (over 90%) of CDH, the abdominal viscera enter the pleural cavity through a defect which is called the foramen of Bochdalek and the hernia of the same name, Bochdalek hernia. This CDH is characterized by a hole in the posterolateral corner of the diaphragm which allows passage of the abdominal viscera into the pleural cavity on the left side of the diaphragm. Newborns are typically cyanotic, with rapid breathing, lung hypoplasia and pulmonary hypertension because of compression of the lungs by the misplaced abdominal viscera. The heart is often shifted to the right. Splenic rupture (**answer b**) in newborns is very rare and would not explain breathing difficulty. Tetralogy of Fallot (**answer c**) often goes undetected for weeks after birth. Tracheoesophageal fistula (**answer d**) would typically present with aspiration after feeding. Transposition of the great arteries (**answer e**) would present with cyanosis, but generally the heart is not displaced toward the right and lung sounds should be heard in both pleural cavities.

399. The answer is d. (*Moore, p 298.*) The newly transplanted kidney will be placed in the iliac fossa in the greater pelvis, attached to branched iliac vessels (thus **answer c** is not correct). The ureter is usually connected directly to the bladder. Generally, unless the kidneys are infected the host kidneys are left in place (thus not **answers a, b, and e**). Often the internal iliac artery is connected to the renal arteries. Normally, anastomotic connections across the midline from the opposite internal iliac artery provide pelvic organs with enough blood to maintain proper function. The transplanted renal vein is often connected to the external iliac vein, not the internal iliac vein, since it is typically larger and thus easier to establish anastomoses.

400. The answer is b. (*Moore, p 281.*) The patient in the scenario has infectious mononucleosis, a virus-induced illness, leading to swollen lymph nodes and spleen. The splenomegaly is diagnosed by the very rounded contours of the organ. Infectious mononucleosis can exhibit liver involvement; however, the organ indicated is not the liver (**answers a, d, and e**), but the spleen in the upper left hypochondrium. The bright organ between it and the vertebra is the left kidney. The liver is on the opposite side of the abdominal cavity. The stomach (**answer c**) is not seen in the radiograph.

401. The answer is c. (*Moore, pp 264-265.*) The splenic artery originates from the celiac trunk and courses tortuously along the posterior aspect of the pancreas. The left gastric artery (**answer a**) is a separate branch of the celiac trunk and courses along the lesser curvature of the stomach where it anastomoses with the right gastric artery **(answer d)**, a branch of hepatic artery. The right gastro-omental (gastroepiploic) artery **(answer e)** is a branch of the gastroduodenal artery and courses along the greater curvature of the stomach. The superior mesenteric artery **(answer b)** is located more inferiorly and is seen running to the right side of the patient.

402. The answer is b. *(Moore, p 265.)* Structure 20 is the common hepatic artery. The celiac (18; **[answer a]**) artery (trunk) gives off the splenic (19; **[answer d]**) artery (to the patient's left) and the common hepatic (20; **[answer b]**) artery (to the patient's right). Other labeled structures are as follows: 17, right adrenal gland; 21, portal vein; and 22, left adrenal gland. The crus of the diaphragm **(answer c)** is seen covering each side of the abdominal aorta. The superior mesenteric artery **(answer e)** is not seen in this image and would be located further inferiorly with the abdomen.

403. The answer is b. *(Moore, pp 286-287, 317.)* Enlargement of the gallbladder is a common complication of gallstone development. If the gallbladder enlarges sufficiently and becomes inflamed, then it can contact the inferior surface of the diaphragm, leading to right-sided shoulder/neck pain. The liver, if inflamed, would also produce right-sided shoulder/neck pain (thus not **answer a**). The pancreas **(answer c)** is mainly a midline organ that is retroperitoneal, thus even when infected and inflamed it is unlikely to contact the center of the diaphragm (that portion which carries afferent information back to cervical levels of the spinal cord). An enlarged spleen could cause left-sided shoulder/neck pain (thus not **answer d**). Normally, the appendix **(answer e)** is too inferior in location to contact the diaphragm and would cause pain on the right, not the left side.

404. The answer is b. *(Moore, pp 280, 281, 285, 288.)* Varicose veins radiating from the umbilicus are called caput medusae. Caput medusae typically present as a result of portal hypertension, secondary to cirrhosis of the liver, caused by excessive alcohol consumption. There are three classic locations for portal caval anastomoseis that develop varicose veins: on the anterior abdominal wall (caput medusa); at the anus leading to hemorrhoids; and at the esophagus leading to esophageal varices. The 58-year-old man presents with an enlarged liver (solid mass extending inferior to right costal margin) as a consequence of years of excessive alcohol consumption and has presumably developed cirrhosis of the liver. Ascites (answer a) is an abnormal accumulation of fluid in the peritoneal cavity and would occur with late stage cirrhosis of the liver. This patient more than likely would have ascites but the question asked is about the varicose veins. Cirrhosis (answer c) of the liver leads to increased resistance to blood flow through the liver, which produces portal hypertension. Diverticulosis (answers d and e) is the presence of multiple outpocketings of the mucosa of the large intestine and is not relevant to cirrhosis of the liver.

405. The answer is d. *(Moore, pp 247-253.)* The colon normally has two regions where it is retroperitoneal: the ascending and descending colon. There are also two normal points of flexure: the hepatic (right) and splenic (left) flexures. Therefore, the sigmoid colon, splenic flexure, and hepatic flexure are the regions where the gastroenterologist has the greatest difficulty passing the fiberoptic scope, and thus present the greatest risk of bowel perforation. This is perhaps most easily visualized by looking at Fig. 2.57 on p 253 of Moore, Dalley and Agur's *Clinically Oriented Anatomy.* Other answers (answers a, b, c, and e) are not correct.

406. The answer is c. *(Moore, pp 283, 318. Fauci, pp 586-589.)* Foregut-derived organs; stomach, liver, pancreas, and proximal half of the duodenum are all innervated by greater splanchnic nerves (T5-T9) and generally refer pain to the epigastric region. The patient in the vignette appears to have pancretic adenocarcinoma with only a 5% survival rate 5 years after diagnosis. The lesser splanchnic nerves (answers d and e) innervate midgut derived organs, distal duodenum, jejunum, ileum, and ascending and two-thirds of transverse colon. Cirrhosis of the liver (answer a) may be treated by liver transplantation. Duodenal ulcer (answers b) can generally be treated medically or surgically, if needed. Gallstones (answer d) are generally treated surgically or endoscopically. Gastric carcinomas (answer e) have a 5 year survival rate of 60% to 90% survival for stage I; 30% to 50% survival for stage II; and 10% to 25% survival for stage III cancers.

407. The answer is e. *(Moore, pp 260-261, 417. Fauci, pp 257-260. Kumar pp 814-826.)* Potential causes of blood in the stool (hematochezia) without external hemorrhoids (answer c), include diverticulosis, internal hemorrhoids, and colorectal cancer. The patient is afebrile and feels well so answers a, b, and d cannot be correct. Diverticular disease mainly affects middle age and older adults. It is an outpocketing of the lining of the colon, occurring most frequently in the sigmoid colon. Diverticular disease may be caused by lack of fiber in the diet. If the diverticula get large, they may rupture blood vessels and bleed. Internal hemorrhoids are dilated (varicose) veins that develop above the pectinate line within the internal rectal venous plexus. They can develop as a consequence of hepatic cirrhosis, which could cause portal hypertension as blood resistance within the liver increases. Venous blood within the portal system backflows down the superior rectal veins and into the inferior rectal veins that are part of the systemic venous system that does not have to pass through the liver. Most colorectal cancers initially develop as polyps, which continue to grow and differentiate and in later stages develop increased vascularity and bleed. External hemorrhoids and fissures may result in blood in the stool, but are generally painful (thus not **answers c and d**).

408. The answer is e. (*Moore, pp 410-414, 417.*) The rectum receives blood from three different arteries, which come from three different major branches: superior rectal artery off the inferior mesenteric artery, middle rectal artery off the internal iliac artery, and inferior rectal artery off the internal pudendal artery. **Answers a, b, and c** are not anatomically correct and the inferior gluteal artery (**answer d**) does not supply blood to the rectum. There are also three sets of veins: superior rectal veins, which drain into the hepatic portal system; middle rectal veins, which drain into the internal iliac veins (part of the systemic venous system); and inferior rectal veins, which drain into internal pudendal veins (also part of the systemic venous system). Because the internal rectal venous plexus is a potential site of portal-systemic anastomoses, internal hemorrhoids may be an indication of liver pathology.

409. The answer is e. (*Moore, pp 308-309.*) The azygos vein passes through the diaphragm along with the aorta, and thoracic duct. The diaphragm possesses three principal hiatuses shown in the diagram accompanying the question: the hiatus for the inferior vena cava (**answer a**), the esophageal hiatus (**answer c**), and the aortic hiatus (**answer e**). Potential diaphragmatic developmental defects include the foramen of Morgagni (**answer b**), just lateral to the xiphoid attachment of the diaphragm, and the pleuroperitoneal canal of Bochdalek (**answer d**), which is the most common site for congenital hernias. The inferior vena cava and frequently small branches of the right phrenic nerve pass through a hiatus (**A**) slightly to the right of the midline at the T8 level. The left phrenic nerve usually passes through the central tendon of the diaphragm on the left side to innervate the left hemidiaphragm from below. The esophageal hiatus (C) just to the left of the midline at the T10 level transmits the esophagus, the left and right vagus nerves, and the esophageal branches of the left gastric artery and vein. An acquired hiatal hernia usually is the consequence of a short esophagus or of a weakened esophageal hiatus.

The two diaphragmatic crura are joined superiorly by the median arcuate ligament to form an opening (E) at the T12 level. The aortic hiatus transmits the aorta, thoracic duct, and a continuation of the azygos vein into the abdomen. The splanchnic nerves penetrate the crura on each side of the aortic hiatus to reach the abdomen.

410. The answer is d. (*Moore p 338.*) This patient may have an abdominal aortic aneurysm. Risk factors for the development of an abdominal aortic aneurysm include hypertension, excessive weight, and smoking. Males are about five times more likely to have an aortic aneurysm than females. About 5% of men over 60 years of age have abdominal aortic aneurysms. Ninety percent of the time abdominal aortic aneurysms develop inferior to the renal arteries. About two-third of the time they extend inferiorly to include one of the common iliac arteries. (What blood vessel comes from the aorta inferior to the renal arteries and superior to the bifurcation into common iliac arteries? Answer: gonadal and inferior mesenteric arteries.) Despite the retroperitoneal location of the abdominal aorta, the high pressure in the vessel typically means that rupture of abdominal aortic aneurysms is fatal. Blood fills the peritoneal cavity and the individual bleeds to death. If discovered prior to rupture they are typically repaired if greater than about 5.5 cm in diameter. Currently they tend to be repaired intravascularly by placing a 6-in Dacron tube with metal-mesh cylinder into the aorta via the femoral artery. Anecdotally, abdominal aortic aneurysms have been known to rupture with straining, such as during defecation. None of the other conditions, a hiatal hernia (**answer a**), splenomegaly (**answer b**), cirrhosis of the liver (**answer c**), nor a horseshoe kidney (**answer e**) would normally pulsate.

411. The answer is c. (*Moore, pp 212-213.*) Most indirect inguinal hernias are congenital (present at birth; thus not **answers d and e**). Indirect inguinal hernias recapitulate the passage of the testis through the abdominal wall, and as such, originate lateral to the inferior epigastric vessels and reopen the processus vaginalis if it separated from the peritoneal cavity. Large indirect inguinal hernias need to be repaired to prevent intestinal organs from being strangulated within the inguinal canal and the processus vaginalis needs to be closed to prevent abdominal peritoneal fluid from accumulating in the scrotum, causing swelling upon increased intraabdominal pressure. Only about 1 in 20 inguinal hernias occur in females (thus not **answers a and b**); 95% therefore occur in males.

412. The answer is d. (*Moore, pp 249-253, 315-316.*) The major artery that is going to be reconnected is the marginal artery and the superior and inferior mesenteric lymph nodes will be collected. About a foot long section of the splenic flexure along with the marginal artery (of Drummond) and vein, paracolic lymph nodes and adjacent mesentery would all be surgically removed. The splenic flexure receives blood from the marginal artery. Blood from the splenic flexure portion of the marginal artery comes from both the middle colic artery, which is a branch off the superior mesenteric artery and from the left colic, which is a branch of the inferior mesenteric artery. Thus, it is essential to collect lymph nodes from the base of both the superior mesenteric and inferior mesenteric arteries. Neither the splenic artery (**answers b and c**) nor aorta (**answer a**) would be sectioned. The sigmoid artery (**answer e**) serves the sigmoid colon and would remain intact.

413. The answer is b. (*Moore, pp 283, 285-286.*) The findings are consistent with hepatomegaly. There are two pieces of physical evidence that point toward an enlarged liver as being the likely cause of the physical findings. While the liver lies in the upper right quadrant of the abdomen it is generally well covered by the costal margin. Enlargement of the liver can be caused by chronic alcohol consumption. In addition, the prominent veins on the anterior abdominal wall of the patient in the vignette (called caput medusae) may be a sign of portal hypertension as blood backs up within the hepatic portal system and uses alternative routes, rather than through the liver, to return to the systemic circulatory system. In addition to prominent abdominal veins, portal hypertension may also cause esophageal varices and hemorrhoids. Splenomegaly (**answer a**) would be palpated on the left side. While both the gall bladder and appendix are on the right side of the abdomen, both cholecystitis (**answer d**) and appendicitis (**answer c**) should result in abdominal pain, which is absent in this patient. An abdominal aortic aneurysm (**answer e**) would normally appear in the midline and pulsate.

Pelvis

Questions

414. A 15-year-old adolescent fails to start menstruating, but has monthly cramping and pain. She has normal physical characteristics for her age including breast development, and axillary and pubic hair. Estradiol, FSH, and LH are all within normal limits. She appears to have a normal vulva, but a vagina that is only 2 inches deep with no detectable cervix. A pelvic ultrasound identifies normal ovaries, uterine tubes, a slightly enlarged uterus, and a septum separating the proximal and distal ends of the vagina from each other, thus trapping menses in the uterus and upper half of the vagina. What embryonic structure(s) failed to develop, fuse, or regress during the development of the teenager's reproductive system?

a. The left and right mesonephric ducts failed to meet in the midline and fuse with each other.
b. The left and right paramesonephric ducts failed to meet in the midline and fuse with each other.
c. The sinovaginal bulbs failed to fully fuse with the fused paramesonephric ducts.
d. The mesonephric ducts failed to undergo complete apoptosis.
e. The metanephric buds failed to form.

415. A young couple goes to an urologist because of inability to conceive a child after 1 year of unprotected sex. The wife had already undergone a gynecological workup, including testing for 3 months showing a normal ovulation profile as confirmed by an ovulatory kit. The primary care physician describes the husband's physical examination as normal and had already ordered a semen analysis and had forwarded the results to the urologist. The semen volume was 0.5 mL, pH 6.8, and azoospermic without any fructose. The husband has a brother, with one child who is confirmed to have cystic fibrosis, but the brother has never been specifically tested. The husband was sent for cystic fibrosis (CF) testing and for a pelvic MRI to test for which one of the following?

a. Bilateral abdominal testicles
b. Hypospadias
c. Congenital absence of ejaculatory ducts and vas deferens
d. Congenital hydrocele
e. Congenital absence of the prostate gland

416. The gubernaculum is a continuous mesenchymal condensation extending inferiorly from the caudal pole of each gonad through the inguinal canal to the labioscrotal swelling. In males, the testicles normally migrate into the scrotum. In females gubernaculum becomes which of the following?

a. Canal of Nuck
b. Median umbilical ligament
c. Medial umbilical ligaments and lateral umbilical (epigastric) folds
d. Round ligament of the uterus and the ligament of the ovary or proper ligament of the ovary
e. Suspensory ligament of the ovary

417. Parts of human skeletal remains are brought to the county coroner of a rural community. The pelvis is complete, yet the individual bones of the pelvis, the ilium, ischium, and pubis have just started to fuse. The subpubic angle is estimated at 60° and the pelvic brim has a distinctive heart-shaped appearance. On the basis of this information, the remains are most likely from which one of the following?

a. 3-year-old boy
b. 4-year-old girl
c. 14-year-old adolescent boy
d. 30-year-old woman
e. 80-year-old man

418. A 37-year-old woman is undergoing her first round of 5 injections of 75 IU of FSH for induced ovulation for in vitro fertilization (IVF). During the ultrasound examination several days later to determine the number of Graafian follicles, a mass between the ovary and the broad ligament is observed. The day of the oocyte collection by laparoscopy, the obstetrician biopsies the unidentified structure in addition to collecting 18 eggs. The IVF is successful and 3 blastocysts are returned to her uterus and 15 are frozen for future reproductive cycles, if needed. The biopsied structure is identified as an epoöphoron. What does the obstetrician tell the patient?

a. Epoöphoron is a benign remnant of the pronephric duct that normally undergoes apoptosis during embryonic development and there is little reason for concern.
b. Epoöphoron is a benign remnant of the mesonephric duct that normally undergoes apoptosis during embryonic development and there is little reason for concern.
c. Epoöphoron is a benign remnant of the metanephric duct that normally undergoes apoptosis during embryonic development and there is little reason for concern.
d. Epoöphoron is a benign remnant of the paramesonephric duct that normally undergoes apoptosis during embryonic development and there is little reason for concern.
e. Epoöphoron is a malignant remnant of the paramesonephric duct that normally undergoes apoptosis during embryonic development and that the pregnancy should be terminated in order to start chemotherapy.

419. During an obstetrics rotation a third year medical student delivers her fourth baby of the week. She clamps and then allows the father to cut the umbilical cord as she clears mucus from the crying face of the 7 lb baby girl. The student notes that she has a slightly underformed anus. In private the student tells the obstetrician about the problem. A few hours later the baby girl passes meconium, but the nurse reports that it has come from the newborn's vagina rather than the anus. The baby girl urinates while the nurse cleans up the meconium, so the urinary system appears normal. What is the working diagnosis?

a. Cloacal agenesis
b. Hypospadias
c. Rectovaginal fistula
d. Rectourethral fistula
e. Urovaginal fistula

420. A 36-year-old man complains to his primary care physician of occasional dull, throbbing pain associated with the right testis and scrotum. Examination indicates a varicocele of the pampiniform plexus. The physician remarks that in all probability the patient had this condition since adolescence and should not be bothered by it. The patient is emphatic that the condition has arisen within the last few months and sought a second opinion from a urologist. The urologist orders abdominal and pelvic CT. Factors that the urologist considers include which one of the following in regard to varicocele of the pampiniform plexus on the right side?

a. It is very uncommon.
b. It occurs as frequently as on the left side.
c. It may be the result of testicular torsion.
d. It may be associated with a long, redundant mesorchium.
e. It may result from a hydrocele.

421. A 19-year-old female college student presents to the emergency department at 10:30 PM on a Friday night with severe left-sided flank and pelvic pain. While she has never had similar pain, she states that she thinks she has a kidney stone. The pain started in her mid back about a week ago and then subsided and now the pain has increased and moved inferiorly along her flank and also extends down into her labia majora. She is taking birth control pills, but is not currently sexually active. She is having her period, but denies the pain is menstrual. Abdominal and pelvic CT are ordered. What two specific locations will one look for in the CTs for obstructing calculi?

a. At the junction of the renal papilla with the minor calyx and junction of the renal papilla with the major calyx
b. As the ureter leaves the kidney and as the ureter forms the infundibulum
c. As the ureter crosses the edge of the false pelvis and as the ureter crosses the edge of the true pelvis
d. As the ureter crosses the external iliac artery at the pelvic brim and as the ureter passes through the wall of the bladder
e. As the ureter passes through the wall of the bladder and as the ureter passes through the center of the trigone of the bladder

422. A full-term baby boy receives an Apgar score of 9 out of 10. The obstetrician notes that his scrotum is rather large compared to his penis and when he cries and strains, the scrotum gets even bigger. The physician palpates for testes and epididymides which are present and does not feel any abnormal structures. The obstetrician tells the parents the newborn has which one of the following?

a. Cryptorchidism
b. Direct inguinal hernia
c. Varicocele
d. Hydrocele
e. Klinefelter syndrome

423. While on an obstetrics rotation, a third year student delivers a term 8 lbs 2 oz baby boy by vaginal delivery. While performing the initial assessments, all appears normal including the two testicles within his scrota and the presence of a normal penis. The baby both breast-feeds normally, wets his diaper, and passes his meconium, so the baby and mother are released from the hospital about 30 hours after delivery. The parents are instructed to dampen the umbilical stalk with alcohol until it falls off. About a week later the mother brings the child back to the hospital and delivery service because the boy's umbilical cord is still slightly moist and there appears to be fluid coming from it. What is the tentative diagnosis and what does the physician tell the mother?

a. Hypospadia; the boy is urinating when having an erection and thus keeps wetting the umbilical cord stump; nothing needs to be done.

b. Epispadia; the boy's urine is passing upwards within the diaper, thus keeps wetting the umbilical cord stump; nothing needs to be done.

c. Exstrophy of the bladder; the boy's bladder wall failed to form properly from the urogenital sinus/allantois which connects to the umbilicus, thus urine is seeping through the skin and wetting the umbilical cord stump; this can be surgically repaired.

d. Normal; the boy's urine fills his diaper and thus keeps wetting the umbilical cord stump; nothing needs to be done.

e. Urachal fistula; the boy's bladder developed from the urogenital sinus/allantois which connects with the umbilicus and the urachus has failed to completely close, so he is leaking urine at the umbilicus; this can be surgically repaired.

424. An obstetrician delivers the fourth child of a hairdresser who has previously delivered one boy and two girls. The mother goes into labor during her 39th week and delivers a 7 lbs and 6 oz baby boy who is 21 inches long. While clamping the umbilical cord and drying off the baby, it is noted that his penis does not have a urethral opening within the glans, but rather has an elongated opening along the mid-shaft of the penis on the ventral surface. Both testicles are within the scrotum. What is the most appropriate characterization of the congenital dysmorphology and what will the physician tell the parents?

a. Epispadias; right and left urethral folds failed to meet in the midline. There is no need for surgical repair; he can sit on the toilet to urinate.

b. Epispadias; right and left urethral folds failed to meet in the midline and that surgical repair should be performed and his foreskin can be used for the repair.

c. Hypospadias; right and left urethral folds failed to meet in the midline and surgical repair should be performed and his foreskin may be used for the repair.

d. Hypospadias; the genital tubercle split during development. There is no need for surgical repair; but he should be circumcised.

e. Urachal fistula; the genital tubercle split during development. There is no need for surgical repair; he can sit on the toilet to urinate.

425. In this CT of the pelvis, the structure indicated by the arrow is which one of the following?

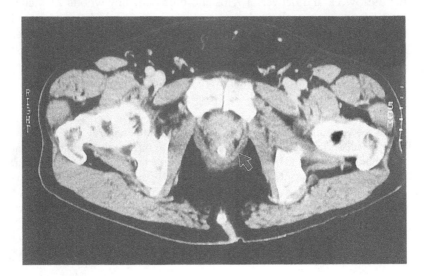

a. Sphincter urethrae/urogenital diaphragm
b. Levator ani/pelvic diaphragm
c. Obturator internus
d. Obturator externus
e. Seminal vesicle

426. A 62-year-old man presents with weak urine flow, increased difficulty initiating urination, and increased frequency of urination since his bladder often is not fully emptied. In benign disease, those symptoms are most often associated with enlargement of which one of the following?

a. Entire prostate gland
b. Lateral/posterior lobes of the prostate gland
c. Mucosal and submucosal regions of the prostate gland
d. Anterior region of the prostate gland
e. Prostatic utricle

427. A rectal cancer that occurs within the anal canal penetrates the mucosa and basement membrane. Which nodes would the colorectal surgeon harvest at the same time she/he resected the rectum?

a. Superior mesenteric and external iliac nodes
b. Right colic and external iliac nodes
c. Superficial inguinal, internal iliac, and preaortic inferior mesenteric nodes
d. Middle colic, right colic, and ileocolic nodes
e. External iliac, epicolic, and left colic nodes

428. An obstetrician follows the third pregnancy of a 28-year-old mother who has a BMI of 28. She goes into labor during her 36th week and the labor is difficult because she has an android-shaped pelvis. While drying off and evaluating the 6 lb 13 oz 22 in baby boy, the obstetrician notes that the right testicle is missing from the scrotal sac while the left testicle is scrotal. There is a bulge in the right, but not the left inguinal canal. The physician notes on the chart that the baby boy has a right cryptorchidism. The undescended testis is most likely to descend in which one of the following time frames?

a. The first 3 postnatal months
b. The first 18 months after birth
c. The first 3 years after birth
d. Immediately before puberty
e. Once puberty begins and testosterone levels are augmented

429. A 24-year-old woman seeking assistance for apparent infertility has been unable to conceive despite repeated attempts in 5 years of marriage. She reveals that her husband fathered a child in a prior marriage. Although her menstrual periods are fairly regular, they are accompanied by extreme lower back pain. The lower back pain during menstruation experienced by this woman probably is referred from the pelvic region. The pathways that convey this pain sensation to the central nervous system involve which of the following?

a. Hypogastric nerve → L1 and L2
b. Lumbosacral trunk → L4 and L5
c. Pelvic splanchnic nerves → S2 to S4
d. Pudendal nerve → S2, S3, and S4
e. Genitofemoral nerve → L1 and L2

430. While on a medical mission to rural Haiti a physician sees a 24-year-old mother of one who is complaining of right lower quadrant pain. Initially the physician examines her for rebound tenderness over McBurney point; however, the pain is lower and more pelvic. She tells the physician that she thinks she is about 2 months pregnant. A urine dipstick confirms that she is pregnant, so a pelvic examination is completed since ultrasound is unavailable. What is the most likely, potential deadly condition the young mother might have and what procedure will the physician use during the pelvic examination to support her/his hypothesis?

a. Eclampsia; confirmed by vaginally observing that the external os of the cervix is closed tightly
b. Peritoneal ectopic pregnancy; confirmed by placing one hand in the vagina and one hand in the rectum palpating the rectouterine pouch of Douglas
c. Preeclampsia; confirmed by vaginally observing the appearance and nature of the external os of the cervix
d. Tubal ectopic pregnancy; confirmed by placing one hand in her vagina and one hand gently pressing on her anterior abdominal wall
e. Twin pregnancy; confirmed by estimating the size of the uterus with one hand in her vagina and one hand gently pressing on her anterior abdominal wall in the midline

431. A 50-year-old associate professor is scheduled for a routine physical examination for increased life insurance coverage. He has never had a digital rectal examination or PSA level determined so the physician recommends both to him. The physician has him hop off the examination table, turn away and face the table, then bend at the waist while she gently inserts a lubricated gloved finger into his anus. Typically what part of three reproductive organs can a physician palpate through the anterior wall of the rectum during a digital rectal examination?

a. Ejaculatory ducts, main peripheral portion of the prostate gland, prostatic utricle
b. Ejaculatory ducts, main peripheral portion of the prostate gland, seminal colliculus
c. Main peripheral portion of the prostate gland, seminal vesicles, ampulla of the vas deferens
d. Main peripheral portion of the prostate gland, seminal vesicles, epididymal ducts
e. Seminal vesicles, periurethral portion of the prostate gland, prostatic utricle

432. One of the new staff members at a skilled nursing facility asks the physician to examine a 92-year-old woman. She has suddenly developed a very large cylindrical mass between her legs. The woman tells the physician that she has 7 children and 22 grandchildren and has been constipated lately. Upon examining the woman she appears to have a perineal procidentia, with no rectal involvement. What is the correct list of structures that were compromised to produce this condition?

a. Stretching of the cardinal and round ligaments of the uterus and suspensory ligaments of the ovary
b. Stretching of the urachus, medial and lateral umbilical ligaments/folds
c. Stretching of the median, medial and lateral umbilical ligaments/folds
d. Stretching of the cardinal ligaments of the uterus, the round ligament of the ovaries, and the suspensory ligament of the ovaries.
e. Stretching of the vaginal wall, cardinal and round ligaments of the uterus

433. A 22-year-old woman presents at the free clinic with pelvic pain "that just won't quit." She states that she has been trying to get pregnant with her new husband, who just got a job, but the health care benefits don't start until after 6 months on the job. Her last menses were about 7 weeks ago. She denies any spotting of blood. A pregnancy test is positive. During the initial palpation she has tenderness in the left inferior quadrant. During a bimanual pelvic examination you note some softening and flexibility of her uterus and cervix, but she is quite tender to palpation and manipulation. Ultrasound equipment is not available. What procedure will you perform and how will it help to determine if she may have an ectopic pregnancy?

a. Amniocentesis; by collecting amniotic fluid for analysis to determine if peritoneal fluid is present along with amniotic fluid
b. Amniocentesis; by collecting amniotic fluid for analysis to determine if the fetus is a male or a female, as males are more likely to be ectopic than females
c. Chorionic villous sampling; by collecting parts of the chorionic villi of the placenta by a catheter placed through the vagina and cervix and into the uterus to determine if the fetus carries genes for ectopic pregnancy
d. Culdocentesis; by collecting peritoneal fluid with a needle passing through the anterior fornix of the vagina to determine if unclotted blood is present
e. Culdocentesis; by collecting peritoneal fluid with a needle passing through the posterior fornix of the vagina to determine if unclotted blood is present

434. A full-term baby girl presents with a bulge over the right inguinal region extending into her right labial majora. When the neonatologist gently presses in one area of the inguinal region or labial majora, the opposite area bulges, suggesting that a cystic structure is being palpated. What congenital dysmorphology does the baby girl likely have?

a. Cryptorchidism
b. Cyst in the canal of Nuck
c. Direct inguinal hernias
d. Exstrophy of the bladder
e. Indirect inguinal hernia

435. The patient is a 45-year-old man with a history of anal fistulas. He complains of fever with pain and swelling in the rectal area. You are concerned that the anal fistula may have become infected and ruptured into the space indicated by the asterisk in this CT scan. Which one of the following is correct regarding the indicated space?

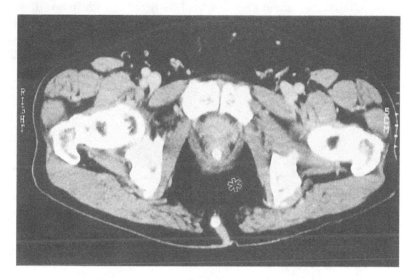

a. It is called the paracolic gutter.
b. The space is largely filled with muscle.
c. The space is located superior to the pelvic diaphragm.
d. Pus from the anal fistula in that space can extend anteriorly deep to the perineal membrane, but inferior to the urogenital diaphragm.
e. Pus from the anal fistula in that space can extend superiorly, anterior to the sacrum.

436. A 13-year-old adolescent is brought into his pediatrician's clinic by his concerned mother. The boy was slow to meet physical milestones such as sitting up, crawling, and walking. He is shy. He has now grown tall and skinny, with small testicles and penis, and slight breast development. The boy has a great deal of trouble both reading and expressing himself in school. The mother would like the school district to provide him with special educational resources. The school district claims he is no different than lots of other inattentive boys. A blood test is ordered to determine his karyotype. What abnormal karyotype do you suspect the boy will have and what do you call this genetic condition?

a. 45X; Turner syndrome
b. 45Y; Turner syndrome
c. 47XXY; Klinefelter syndrome
d. 47XYY; super male syndrome
e. 48XYYY; super male syndrome

437. A couple comes to the reproductive endocrinology infertility clinic because they have been unable to conceive a child after 1 year of trying. Physical examination of the man reveals a darkish mass and fullness of the left scrotum/spermatic cord that feels like a bag of worms. The physician suggests that he follow up with a urologist because of suspicion of which one of the following?

a. Undiagnosed cryptorchidism of the right testicle
b. Acquired varicocele
c. Acquired left femoral hernia
d. Acquired right direct femoral hernia
e. Congenital absence of the pampiniform plexus on the right side

438. A 24-year-old woman is having her third prenatal check. This is her first pregnancy and she states that she hopes to deliver the child vaginally, but thinks she might want some pain relief. The obstetrician discusses the options of a caudal epidural or a pudendal nerve block. Which of the following is the most accurate description of the pain relief afforded by a pudendal nerve block?

a. Sensation from the vulva is reduced.
b. Sensation from the vulva and perineum is reduced.
c. Sensation from the perineum, cervix, and uterus is reduced.
d. Sensation below the umbilicus is reduced.
e. Sensation above the umbilicus is reduced.

439. Both the autonomic and vascular systems need to function properly for successful male sexual function. Which one of the following statements concerning erection, emission, and ejaculation in the male is correct?

a. Contraction of the internal urethral sphincter is under control of the parasympathetic nervous system.
b. The parasympathetic nerves stimulate closure of helicine arteries.
c. Sympathetic neurons stimulate the helicine arteries to dilate and increase blood flow to the corpora cavernosum.
d. Parasympathetic innervation stimulates emission of seminal fluid.
e. Contraction of the bulbospongiosus muscles impedes the drainage of blood from the corpus spongiosum.

440. A 45-year-old man is riding a snowmobile and hits a snow-covered rocky outcropping. When standing for the first time after the accident, he slips and falls on the outcropping and now is experiencing pain in his gluteal region. His injury involves the dark linear structure indicated by the arrow on the accompanying CT scan. What is that structure?

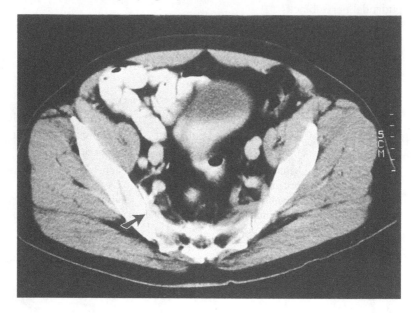

a. A fracture of the sacral body
b. The sacrococcygeal joint
c. A spinal nerve
d. The superior gluteal artery
e. The inferior gluteal artery

441. A 24-year-old woman has been married for 2 years and is trying to have a child. Her husband had a semen analysis, which suggests he may be marginally fertile. Since she was treated for gonorrhea while in college, she is concerned about the condition of her Fallopian tubes. In order to determine if her uterine tubes were patent, she underwent a hysterosalpingography. In the hysterosalpingogram below, the dye at C is within which one of the following?

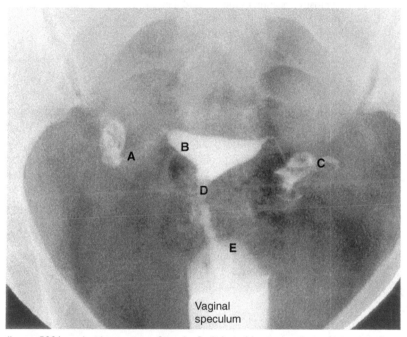

(Image 5001 used with permission from the Radiological Anatomy web site, University of Kansas, School of Medicine, http://classes.kumc.edu/som/radanatomy/.)

a. Ovary
b. Peritoneal cavity
c. Isthmus of the oviduct
d. Uterus
e. Vagina

442. A 19-year-old woman has been admitted through the emergency department to the obstetrics service because she is in stage I of labor. She is about 38 weeks into the pregnancy, but she has not had any previous contact with healthcare other than obtaining some prenatal vitamins. She is in a great deal of pain and requests pain relief, but still wants to fully and actively participate in labor despite never delivering or attending birthing classes before. The obstetrician decides on a pudendal nerve block. What landmarks would be used to perform the procedure in this woman?

a. Ischial tuberosity; location of the pudendal canal
b. Ischial spine; location of the pudendal nerve
c. Sacrotuberous ligament; location of the pudendal nerve
d. Pubic symphysis; location of the pudendal canal
e. Tip of the coccyx; location of the pudendal nerve

443. A 32-year-old woman is in stage I of labor. This will be her fourth child and the other three have all been delivered vaginally, but with pudendal nerve blocks. During the beginning of stage II labor the obstetrician wants to give her a pudendal nerve block. The obstetrician asks the rotating medical student to provide a complete list of the major structures that are attached to the ischial spines. Which of the following is the correct response?

a. Sacrotuberous ligament, inferior gemellus muscle and quadratus femoris muscle
b. Piriformis muscles
c. Abdominal wall muscles
d. Coccygeus muscle, the sacrospinous ligament, and the tendinous arch of the levator ani muscles
e. Lateral attachment of the inguinal ligament

444. A Cesarean section (C-section) delivery of the third child of a 32-year-old mother is scheduled. The mother had C-sections for the birth of all of her children because of an android pelvis. Because this mother had a long history of menstrual cramps and she already has both a boy and a girl at home, she had indicated that she wanted a hysterectomy (including removal of her cervix) immediately after the C-section. During the C-section the physician carefully confirms the location of both the right and left ureters prior to ligating the uterine arteries. Twelve hours after the delivery of a 7 lb 8 oz term baby girl, the mother complains of severe left-sided back pain that radiates toward her labia majora. A CT with contrast that is excreted by the kidneys is ordered. The right kidney and ureter look normal. What congenital anomaly does the mother have that the obstetrician forgot to consider while performing the hysterectomy?

a. The mother had a didelphus uterus and only one was removed.
b. The mother had a duplication of the ureters on the left side, one of which was sutured closed while ligating the left uterine artery.
c. The mother had an urachal fistula which leaked urine after it was cut during the initial incisions for the C-section and subsequent hysterectomy.
d. The mother had a horseshoe-kidney.
e. The mother had a left tubal pregnancy.

445. A 32-year-old lawyer is about to have her first child. At the beginning of her third trimester she takes birthing classes in which they taught her how to do Kegel exercises. Which muscles is she exercising while she practices the Kegel maneuver?

a. Ischiocavernous muscles
b. Piriformis and obturator internus muscles
c. Puborectalis, pubococcygeus, and iliococcygeus muscles
d. Piriformis, puborectalis, pubococcygeus, and iliococcygeus muscles
e. Obturator internus, puborectalis, pubococcygeus, and iliococcygeus muscles

446. Episiotomies are performed to control tearing that can occur during a vaginal delivery. When performing a mediolateral episiotomy, an obstetrician will likely cut through several structures of the perineum. What perineal structures must be sutured back together following a typical mediolateral episiotomy?

a. Vaginal wall, pubococcygeus, and piriformis muscles
b. Vaginal wall, pubococcygeus, and iliococcygeus muscles
c. Vaginal wall, bulbospongiosus, and superficial transverse perineal muscles
d. Vaginal wall, prepuce, and rectus abdominis muscle
e. Vaginal wall, sacrospinous, and sacrotuberous ligaments

447. A man comes to his physician's office because of bilateral pain in his inguinal region which he attributes to bilateral hernias. Upon physical examination he does not have either a direct nor indirect inguinal hernia, but does have bilateral palpable superficial inguinal lymph nodes, which are tender. A differential diagnosis of locations from which lymph drains into the superficial inguinal lymph nodes is formulated. Which anatomical region or structure does not drain into the superficial inguinal lymph nodes is and thus should be excluded from the differential diagnosis list?

a. Penis
b. Scrotum
c. Testicles
d. Anus
e. Epididymides

448. A 57-year-old man comes to the clinic for a physical examination for his life insurance. While he denies having either erectile difficulties or problems with urination, a digital rectal examination is performed. The prostate is enlarged, but was neither nodular nor excessively firm, so blood was drawn for prostate specific antigen (PSA) levels and he is sent to have a plain pelvic film obtained. The PSA is 3 ng/dL (within normal range). The radiology report states that there are some small calcifications within the enlarged prostate and pelvic calcifications consistent with phleboliths. What should the physician tell her patient?

a. Return in a year because he has prostate cancer that is slowly growing and currently confined to his prostate.
b. Return immediately because he has prostate cancer that has spread locally within the pelvis.
c. Return immediately for biopsy of the calcified concretions and phleboliths.
d. Return in 5 years for follow up of the phleboliths.
e. Return in a year because calcified prostatic concretions and pelvic vein phleboliths are of little concern and he needs to return for normal follow up.

449. A 50-year-old multiparous woman comes to her gynecologist's office to rule out cancer. She reports a growing mass or fullness on the anterior wall of her vagina. Upon physical examination a soft, bulging, and a very compressible mass is detected on the anterior surface of the vagina. When her physician pushes on the bulging mass she feels the need to urinate. A CT is ordered because of suspicion of which one of the following?

a. Rectocele
b. Cystocele
c. Cervical cancer
d. Didelphic uterus
e. Indirect inguinal hernia

450. A 24-year-old man is in a single car accident when he falls asleep at the wheel on a two-lane highway, striking a tree on the side of the road. A passerby finds him unconscious and seat belted. On the ambulance ride into the emergency department he regains consciousness and complains of pelvic and penile pain as he thinks his pelvis slammed into the lower edge of the steering wheel when he hit the tree. A CT of his pelvis is shown in the accompanying radiological image. Which lettered structure is the corpus spongiosum?

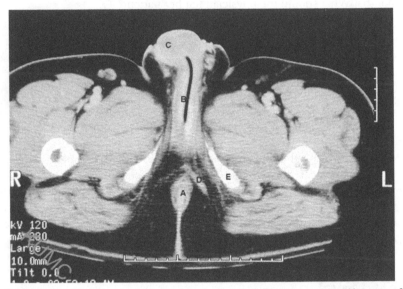

(Image 4204-065 used with permission from the Radiological Anatomy web site, University of Kansas, School of Medicine, http://classes.kumc.edu/som/radanatomy/.)

a. A
b. B
c. C
d. D
e. E

Pelvis

Answers

414. The answer is c. *(Sadler, pp 249-254.)* The sinovaginal bulbs failed to fully fuse with the fused paramesonephric ducts. The vagina is formed from two embryonic structures: the sinovaginal bulbs and the caudal ends of the paramesonephric (Müllerian) ducts, which fuse in the midline. Normally the paramesonephric ducts form the uterine tubes, fusing to form a single uterus, cervix, and upper portion of the vagina. During normal female development, the cells of the mesonephric ducts undergo apoptosis **(answer a)**, as these structures in males are rescued by androgens and form the vas deferens and epididymis. If the left and right paramesonephric ducts fail to meet and fuse in the midline **(answer b)**, then a didelphus uterus with two cervices and two vaginas will form. Failure of mesonephric duct cells to undergo apoptosis **(answer d)** results in epoöphoron and paroöphoron structures embedded in the broad ligament. The nephron portion of the kidneys develops from the metanephric buds which are essential for normal kidney development. If the buds fail to form **(answer e)**, the result would be renal agenesis.

415. The answer is c. *(Fauci, p 1634. Casals, pp 1476-1483.)* If the brother has a child with CF, then the brother must be a carrier of the cystic fibrosis gene, and there is a 25% chance that the husband has CF. Five percent of patients with CF are diagnosed as adults. Congenital absence of the ejaculatory ducts/ductus deferens occurs in up to 95% of males with CF. If the ejaculatory ducts are absent, then there should be no sperm from the vas deferens (normally 0.5 mL of the semen volume) and no products of the seminal vesicles (normally 2.0 mL of the semen volume). The seminal vesicles are responsible for fructose normally present in the ejaculate. Prostatic secretions are normally slightly acidic. The normal physical examination of the husband rules out hypospadias **(answer b)**, bilateral cryptorchidism **(answer a)**, and hydrocele **(answer d)**. The congenital absence of the prostate gland is extremely rare **(answer e)**.

416. The answer is d. (*Moore, pp 205-206. Sadler, p 250.*) In the female, the gubernaculum becomes the round ligament of the uterus and the proper ligament of the ovary. The gubernaculum, which runs from the gonadal anlage to the sexually undifferentiated labioscrotal fold, guides the descent of the testes into the scrotum in the male and the descent of the ovary into the true pelvis in the female. In the female, the developing uterus grows into the gubernacular tract and divides it into the proper ligament of the ovary and the round ligament of the uterus. Thus, the proper ligament of the ovary runs within the broad ligament from the medial pole of each ovary to the uterus. It then continues within the broad ligament as the round ligament of the uterus into the deep inguinal ring. It thereby gains access to the canal of Nuck, the female homologue of the inguinal canal (**answer a**) to insert into the major labial folds. The suspensory ligament of the ovary (**answer e**) contains the ovarian arteries and veins. The median umbilical ligament (**answer b**) is derived from the urachus. The medial umbilical ligaments are the obliterated umbilical arteries (**answer c**). The lateral umbilical (epigastric) folds (**answer c**) are the peritoneal folds overlying the inferior epigastric vessels. Those ligaments and folds are not derivatives of the gubernnaculum.

417. The answer is c. (*Moore, pp 329, 331.*) The pelvis is most likely that of a 14-year-old adolescent boy. Because the subpubic angle is about 60° and the pelvic brim is heart shaped, so the pelvis is from a male and not from a female (**answers b and d**). The bones of the pelvis arise from three different centers of ossification and generally fuse between puberty and the twenty-third year. Therefore, you know you are looking at a 14-year-old adolescent boy, not a 3-year-old boy (**answer a**; would have three separate pelvic bones) nor an 80-year-old man (**answer e**; pelvic bones would be fused).

418. The answer is b. (*Sadler, pp 249-250.*) Epoöphoron is a benign remnant of the mesonephric duct that normally undergoes apoptosis during embryonic development and there is little reason for concern. The epoöphoron that remains in the adult will normally form a cyst or benign adenoma, not a malignant adenocarcinoma (**answer e**). There would only be concern if it enlarged and blocked the uterine tube or ovarian function. The pronephric ducts (**answer a**) normally undergo spontaneous apoptosis during embryonic development. The metanephric ducts (**answer c**) become the ureters that drain urine into the bladder. The paramesonephric (Müllerian) ducts (**answer d**) form the uterine tubes, uterus, and upper portion of the vagina.

419. The answer is c. *(Sadler, pp 230-233.)* Rectovaginal fistula is the failure of the rectovaginal urorectal septum (formed from both Rathke and Tourneux folds) to completely separate the cloaca into an urovaginal sinus anteriorly and anorectal canal posteriorly. If the cloaca (**answer a**; a common embryonic "receptacle" for both fluids and solids) fails to form, then either the bladder and urethra or the rectum also fail to form. This is not the case for this newborn infant. Hypospadia (**answer b**) is a condition of baby boys in which the urethra opens on the ventral surface of the penis rather than at the distal end of the glans. A rectourethral fistula (**answer d**) would be a connection between the rectum and the urethra, which would be a more severe defect and is not consistent with normal urinary function. A urovaginal fistula (**answer e**) would be a failure of the urethra to separate from the vagina. The nurse observes normal urinary function, so this condition is not consistent with the physical findings.

420. The answer is a. *(Moore, p 215.)* Varicocele on the right side is very uncommon. It usually occurs on the left side (~95%) and is rarely found on the right (**answer b**). Left varicocele results from local venous congestion caused by compression of the testicular vein as it passes beneath the usually full sigmoid colon. Testicular torsion (**answer c**), wherein a long mesorchium (**answer d**) is a contributing factor, strangulates the testicular artery, and produces testicular ischemia, not varicocele. Testicular torsion is a medical emergency which normally presents in adolescents as sudden testicular pain. Hydrocele (**answer e**) is not relevant to varicocele.

421. The answer is d. *(Moore, pp 292-294, 300.)* As the ureter crosses the external iliac artery at the pelvic brim and as the ureter passes through the wall of the bladder. Renal and ureteric calculi (lay term: kidney stones) generally are formed in the kidneys and then lodge at one of three locations: (1) at the junction of the renal pelvis with the ureter; (2) as the ureters cross the external iliac vessels at the pelvic brim; and (3) as the ureters pass through the wall of the bladder (see Fig. 2.82, p 294 Moore et al.). Calculi occasionally form in the minor (**answer a**) or major calyces or in the renal pelves and infundibula (**answer b**), but those so called "staghorn" calculi, would produce mid-back pain. Renal calculi rarely become stuck as the ureter crosses the edge of the false pelvis (**answer c**). The ureter does not pass through the center of the trigone (**answer e**), but rather opens at the superior lateral edge of the trigone. The referred pain from ureteric calculi is usually described as from "loin to groin" in that it often starts in the mid back then over the kidney and extends in a band toward the labia majora or scrotum (from T11-L2). Normally the pain is intermittent and comes and goes in waves and may change in location, generally moving inferiorly. Since the ureters undergo peristaltic movement, the calculi often move with time. Depending on the chemical composition and shape of the calculi they may either block urine flow or if spiky, stick into the wall of the ureter. Kidney stone pain is often described as being worse than labor pain. Treatments include pain relief and drinking lots of fluids, and either lithotripsy (use of ultrasound waves to break up the stone) or physical removal (surgical) of the stone in severe cases.

422. The answer is d. (*Moore, pp 212-214.*) The newborn boy has congenital hydrocele. As the testicles migrate from the posterior abdominal wall to the anterior abdominal wall through the inguinal canal, they bring along a process of the peritoneal lining, the processus vaginalis, which is filled with fluid and is connected to the peritoneal cavity. Normally, this processus vaginalis disconnects from the abdominal cavity and forms the tunica vaginalis. Sometimes due to the late migration of the testes, the processus vaginalis does not lose its connection with the peritoneal cavity, so that during straining and coughing or crying the scrotum swells. Normally this condition spontaneously corrects itself a few months after birth. Cryptorchidism (**answer a**) is the failure of the testes to migrate down into the scrotum, but the physical examination indicates the testes are in the scrotum. A direct inguinal hernia (**answer b**) is very rare in newborns. Congenital varicocele (**answer c**) would generally appear bluish and would feel like a bag of worms. Klinefelter newborn (**answer e**) would have normal-sized testicles and is not related to a hydrocele.

423. The answer is e. (*Sadler, pp 245-246.*) The boy's bladder developed from the urogenital sinus/allantois which connects to the umbilicus and the urachus has failed to completely close, so is leaking urine at the umbilicus. The bladder develops from the allantois. Normally the intraembryonic portion undergoes atrophy and closes and loses its fluid connection to the umbilicus. A urachal fistula allows urine to exit the body through the umbilicus, and thus keeps the umbilical stump moist. Both epispadias (**answer b**) and hypospadias (**answer a**) are problems with the penis and there is no indication of any problem with the penis in this boy. Umbilical cord stumps normally fall off after just a few days. Exstrophy of the bladder (**answer c**) is a much more severe condition resulting from failure of the anterior abdominal wall and anterior bladder wall to form normally. It is not normal (answer d) to leak fluid from the umbilicus.

424. The answer is c. (*Sadler, pp 255-257.*) The baby boy has second degree hypospadia; right and left urethral folds failed to meet in the midline. Surgical repair should be performed and may utilize his foreskin for the repair, so he should not be circumcised (answer d). Since the urethral opening is on the ventral surface (remember an erect penis is in the "anatomical" position) the child has a hypospadia. Note that epispadia (answers a and b) results in a urethral opening on the dorsal surface of the penis and is much more rare (1/100,000 boys). Hypospadias are present in about 1 in 125 to 250 boys and may be on the rise due to environmental estrogens. Hypospadias are twice as frequent in offspring of mothers exposed to high concentrations of hairspray (the mother was a hairdresser). Hypospadia is caused by a failure of the right and left urethral folds to fully fuse in the midline during the first trimester. A first degree hypospadia is an abnormal opening of the urethra within the glans and is generally only of cosmetic concern. A second degree hypospadia is an abnormal opening of the urethra along the shaft of the penis. A third degree hypospadia is an abnormal opening of the urethra within the scrotum. Urachal fistula (answer e) would allow urine from the bladder to leak out the umbilicus.

425. The answer is b. (*Moore, pp 338-343, 435.*) The muscle indicated is attached to the pubic bone and extends around the rectum. It is the puborectalis portion of the levator ani (pelvic diaphragm). The puborectalis is responsible for fecal continence. The urogenital diaphragm (answer a) is positioned inferior to the pelvic diaphragm and includes the deep transverse perineal muscle. The obturator internus (answer c) covers the lateral wall of the lesser pelvis. The obturator externus (answer d) is found in the deep thigh. The seminal vesicles (answer e) would be in a section more cranial to this section.

426. The answer is c. (*Moore, pp 377-381. Kumar, pp 994-996.*) The patient in the vignette is diagnosed with benign prostatic hypertrophy/hyperplasia (BPH). BPH is the result of enlargement of the mucosal and submucosal (median) region, which may compress the prostatic urethra leading to urinary retention (thus not answer a). This hypertrophic tissue may also protrude into the urinary bladder to prevent complete emptying. The lateral/posterior lobes (answer b) are commonly associated with malignant transformation. The anterior region (answer d) tends to be asymptomatic due to its mainly fibrous nature. BPH is not associated with enlargement or benign change in the prostatic utricle (answer e).

427. The answer is c. (*Moore, pp 400, 413-414.*) Lymph from the anal region is drained into three different regions because its blood supply is derived from those same three regions. Superior to the pectinate line the lymph drains into the internal iliac nodes and preaortic inferior mesenteric nodes (along the path of the superior rectal artery, a branch off the inferior mesenteric artery). Inferior to the pectinate line the lymph drains into the superficial inguinal nodes. Thus the external iliac, superior mesenteric, right colic, middle colic, ileocolic, epicolic, and left colic (**answers a, b, d, and e**) nodes are not an immediate concern in the harvesting of lymph nodes in this patient.

428. The answer is a. (*Sadler, p 262. Moore, p 211.*) About 3% of the time, newborn boys have undescended testes. Up to 30% of premature boys have an undescended testicle, but normally those will spontaneously descend into the scrotum by the 3rd month (thus **answers b, c, d, and e** are not correct). About 1% of the time descent does not occur at all (**answer e**). The testicle initially develops along the posterior abdominal wall between fetal weeks 7 and 12. The gubernaculum normally aids the descent of the testicles into the pelvis so that by the seventh month the testicles are at the cranial end of the inguinal canal. Testicles normally migrate through the inguinal canal and into the scrotum in the last 2 months of pregnancy. Abdominal testicles need to be surgically moved into the scrotum in a orchiopexy procedure prior to one year of age as there is an increased (4-40 fold) incidence of testicular cancer developing in the cryptorchid testicle.

429. The answer is a. (*Moore, pp 389-390.*) The visceral afferent fibers that mediate sensation from the fundus and body of the uterus, as well as from the oviducts, tend to travel along the sympathetic nerve pathways (via the hypogastric nerve and lumbar splanchnics) to reach the upper lumbar levels (L1 and L2) of the spinal cord. Thus, uterine pain will be referred to the upper lumbar dermatomes and produce backache. The visceral afferent fibers that mediate sensation from the cervical neck of the uterus travel along the parasympathetic pathways (via the pelvic splanchnic nerves [*nervi erigentes*]; **answer c**) to the midsacral levels (S2, S3, and S4) of the spinal cord. In this instance, pain originating from the cervix will be referred to the midsacral dermatomes and produce pain that appears to arise from the perineum, gluteal region, and legs. Neither the lumbosacral trunk to L4 and L5 (answer b) nor the pudendal and genitofemoral nerves (answers d and e) should be involved.

430. The answer is d. (*Sadler pp 51-53. Moore, pp 392-393.*) Tubal ectopic pregnancy; confirmed with bimanual palpation by placing one hand in her vagina and one hand gently pressing on her anterior abdominal wall. Using this method, the physician would likely be able to determine the approximate location of a tubal ectopic pregnancy. About 1% of pregnancies are ectopic with greater than 95% of ectopic pregnancies being tubal pregnancies (see question 9 and feedback). Fertilization normally occurs within the ampullar region of the Fallopian (named after Gabriel Fallopius) tubes. If there has been damage to the tube, most often due to pelvic inflammatory disease (PID, see questions 252 to 254 and feedback), then the fertilized egg may not be carried to the uterus, the normal site of implantation of the blastocyst. Less than 5% of ectopic pregnancies are intraperitoneal (answer b). Peritoneal ectopic pregnancy can occur in the peritoneal cavity, specifically within the rectouterine pouch of Douglas, which can be palpated by a rectovaginal examination; however this is much less likely than an ectopic tubal pregnancy. Preeclampsia (answer c) and eclampsia (answer a) are complications of pregnancy that only occur within the third trimester and are not diagnosed by a vaginal examination. A twin pregnancy (answer e) is not a life threatening condition and generally could not be detected by bimanually estimating uterine size at 2 months.

431. The answer is c. (*Moore, pp 378, 381.*) In most males, during a digital rectal examination, one can palpate the main peripheral portion of the prostate gland, then just a little more cranially, both the seminal vesicles and ampulla of the vas (ductus) deferens if one has a long enough finger. The main goal of the digital rectal examination is to palpate the backside of the prostate gland which is the main peripheral portion of the gland; the site of most prostate cancer growth. An additional screening tool is the PSA level within blood. Generally the PSA level should be below 2.5 ng/mL. Elevated levels of PSA, however, can also indicate inflammation of the prostate in addition to cancerous growth. Both the prostatic utricle (answers a and e) and seminal colliculus (answer b) are internal structures found deep within the prostate gland, a blind outpocketing from the prostatic urethra, and thus cannot be palpated. The epididymal ducts **(answer d)** are in the scrotum, thus cannot be palpated during a digital rectal examination.

432. The answer is e. *(Moore, pp 392-393.)* The uterus is stabilized by the cardinal and round ligaments in conjunction with the sacrouterine ligaments. Perineal procidentia is also known as uterine prolapse and is caused by stretching of the vaginal wall and cardinal and round ligaments of the uterus. Generally, the term perineal procidentia is synonymous with descent of the uterus fully into the vagina causing its complete eversion. Uterine prolapse is common in multiparous women. There are several stages of uterine prolapse. Stage I (first degree) uterine prolapse is the descent of the cervix and uterus into the vagina to any point above the hymen. Stage II (second degree) uterine prolapse is descent of the cervix to the hymen. Stage III (third degree) uterine prolapse is descent beyond the hymen. The folds/ligaments on the interior surface of the anterior abdominal wall (urachus/median, medial, and lateral umbilical; **answers b and c)** would not be involved or stretched during uterine prolapse. While the round ligament of the ovary and suspensory ligaments of the ovaries **(answers a and d)** would be stretched during stage IV prolapse, generally these ligaments stabilize the ovaries within the broad ligament. They generally do not stabilize the uterus.

433. The answer is e. *(Moore, p 397.)* Ectopic pregnancy may be diagnosed by culdocentesis; by collecting peritoneal fluid with a needle passing through the posterior fornix of the vagina to determine if unclotted blood is present. Culdocentesis can be performed with relatively simple equipment likely to be found in a free clinic: a speculum to expand the vagina and allow full visualization of the cervix and fornices; forceps to pull the cervix upwards and a long large gauge (19G) needle attached to a syringe to insert through the posterior fornix and into the rectouterine pouch of Douglas to collect fluid. If the fluid is filled with erythrocytes then bleeding from an ectopic pregnancy is suspected. Since 95% of ectopic pregnancies are tubal, blood often leaks out to the end of the Fallopian tube and into the cul-de-sac of Douglas, the most dependent portion of the pelvic cavity. Chorionic villous sampling **(answer c)** is generally performed in the screening of genetic diseases at about 10 to 12 weeks and is always performed under ultrasound guidance to determine proper location for sampling. Amniocentesis **(answers a and b)** is generally performed even later in pregnancy (between the 15th and 20th week) and again requires ultrasound guidance for proper location of the needle. While the risk of ectopic pregnancy may have a minor genetic component, specific genes have yet to be identified in most cases. Male embryos are not more likely to be ectopic than female embryos **(answer b)**.

434. The answer is b. *(Sadler, pp 260-263. Moore, pp 212-214.)* The baby girl has a cyst in the canal of Nuck, a remnant of the processus vaginalis. The canal of Nuck is the name given to the processus vaginalis if it remains beyond the fetal period. Both male and female infants develop a processus vaginalis, at about the sixth month of fetal development, that extends through the anterior abdominal wall into the future scrotum in males and future labia majora in females. In males, the processus vaginalis lies just anterior to the gubernaculum, which normally aids testicular descent through the inguinal canal and into the scrotum. In females, the processus vaginalis also lies just anterior to the gubernaculum, but the ovaries do not descend into the labia majora. Normally the processus vaginalis involutes in females and closes its communication with the peritoneal cavity in males. Thus, a cyst in the canal of Nuck is the female equivalent of a male congenital hydrocele. Cryptorchidism **(answer a)** is a hidden (non-scrotal) testicle and only occurs in males. Direct inguinal hernias **(answer c)** result from a defect in the anterior abdominal wall medial to the inferior epigastric vessels, typically occurring in elderly males. Exstrophy of the bladder **(answer d)** is a failure of the proper development of the bladder and anterior abdominal wall. Bladder exstrophy literally means that the bladder is essentially inside out and exposed on the outside of the abdomen. While a cyst in the canal of Nuck might predispose one to develop an indirect inguinal hernia.

435. The answer is d. *(Moore, p 416.)* Pus from an anal fistula in the ischioanal fossa can extend anteriorly deep to the perineal membrane, but inferior to the urogenital diaphragm. The ischioanal fossa (asterisk on CT accompanying the question) is a fat-filled space (thus not muscle [**answer b**]) that extends from below the levator ani muscle (puborectalis, pubococcygeus, and iliococcygeus muscles). It also extends anteriorly in the area between the pelvic diaphragm (superiorly) and the perineal membrane (inferiorly). It cannot extend superiorly above the pelvic diaphragm (thus not **answer c**) and, therefore, cannot extend superiorly anterior to the sacrum **(answer d)**. The paracolic gutter **(answer a)** is not on the image.

436. The answer is c. (*Sadler, pp 20, 258. Fauci, pp 2340-2341.*) Individuals with Klinefelter syndrome have an extra X chromosome compared to other males and this condition is common. It occurs about 1 in 500 to 1000 male births. At birth, Klinefelter boys appear no different than boys with XY chromosomes. Klinefelter is sometimes detected in elementary school due to learning (language in particular) disabilities. Klinefelter boys are more often detected at puberty when they fail to undergo complete masculinization and may develop gynecomastia. Less often Klinefelter males are discovered during work up for infertility as adults. 45, X, Turner syndrome females are infertile with a single X chromosome. Physically, Turner syndrome females have shortened stature, with webbed neckline and small, wide set breasts. Super male syndrome may be 47, XYY or 48, XYYY. Those individuals are tall with language learning disabilities, but at puberty they have typical male development and are more likely to suffer from acne due to excess androgens.

437. The answer is b. (*Moore, p 215.*) A dark mass within the scrotum would most likely be one of two diagnoses: varicocele or indirect inguinal hernia. Varicoceles are a stasis of blood within the pampiniform plexus (often described as a "bag of worms") and occur most frequently on the left side because the testicular vein on the left drains into the higher pressure left renal vein, whereas the right testicular vein drains into the inferior vena cava. The presence of a varicocele is associated with reduced fertility. A femoral hernia (**answers c and d**) would not end up in the scrotum, rather within the thigh. Cryptorchidism (**answer a**), that is an undescended testicle, on the right side does not fit the physical examination findings. The right side is normal (thus not **answer e**).

438. The answer is b. (*Moore, pp 397-399.*) A pudendal nerve block reduces sensation from somatic structures, mainly the vulva and perineum (not just vulva, **answer a**). Generally the woman would still feel uterine contractions, actively participate in the labor process, and participate in the pushing phase. Pudendal nerve blocks can be delivered while the woman is supine. A caudal epidural block must be administered ahead of time and requires that the mother be able to turn onto her side to perform the procedure. Caudal epidural blocks reduce sensation from the perineum, vagina, and cervix (**answer c**). A lumbar spinal block would reduce sensation below the umbilicus (**answer d**), not above (**answer e**). After a spinal block most women are completely unaware of uterine contractions and thus watch a monitor, which tracks uterine contractions so as to know when to push.

439. The answer is e. (*Moore, pp 423-424.*) The bulbospongiosus muscle is innervated by the pudendal nerve (S2-S4) and its contraction helps to keep blood within the shaft of the penis. Contraction of the internal urethral sphincter is under control of the sympathetic nervous system (thus not **answer a**). Concomitant with dilation of the helicine arteries under parasympathetic innervation (thus not **answers b and c**), which allows increased blood to flow into the cavernous spaces. Contraction of the bulbospongiosus and ischiocavernosus muscles at the base of the cavernous bodies reduces blood from leaving, resulting in engorgement and penile (or clitoral) erection. Emission of seminal fluid, prostatic secretions, and sperm from the vas deferens is due to contraction of smooth muscle under sympathetic control (thus not **answer d**). Sympathetic discharge is also responsible for closing the internal urethral sphincter muscle at the neck of the bladder, thus preventing retro-ejaculation into the bladder. Ejaculation is largely a reflex response of the bulbospongiosus muscle (innervated by S2-S4) to semen in the lumen of the urethra. Note, the external urethral sphincter (innervated by S2-S4) must relax to allow semen to move past.

440. The answer is b. (*Moore, pp 330-332.*) The indicated line represents the sacroiliac joint, seen bilaterally between the alae of the sacrum and the ilia. The body of the sacrum (**answer a**) is in the midline and normal. The sacroiliac ligaments might have been sprained by the trauma of the fall. The pathway for spinal nerves (**answer c**) is through foramina of the sacrum, not through long bony canals. Similarly, the pathway for the gluteal arteries (**answers d and e**) is through the greater sciatic foramen between the ilium and the sacrum.

441. The answer is b. (*Moore, p 391, Kumar, p 1038.*) The purpose of performing a hysterosalpingogram is to determine if the Fallopian tubes are patent (open) and thus potentially capable of transporting sperm and eggs for conception which normally occurs within the ampulla of the tube. The dye is generally introduced via a catheter placed through the cervix and injected into the uterus. In this case the dye is spilling into the peritoneal cavity at ends of each Fallopian tube, which suggests she should be capable of conceiving naturally. The dye would pass the isthmus of the oviduct next to the body of the uterus. Within the image (**E**) is the vagina, (**D**) is the isthmus of the cervix, (**B**) is the body of the uterus, and (**A**) is the ampulla of the oviduct just proximal to the infundibulum out of which dye is flowing as curling wisps.

442. The answer is b. (*Moore, pp 398, 433.*) Transvaginally palpate the ischial spine and inject local anaesthetic at this site just after passing through the sacrospinous ligament. That is where the pudendal nerve wraps around the external surface of the sacrospinous ligament. The neurovascular bundle of the pudendal nerve, and the internal pudendal artery and vein pass just external (not internal) to the sacrospinous ligament which must be penetrated in order to gain access to the nerve. The ischial tuberosity can be palpated transperineally (**answer a**) and it is true that the pudendal canal which contains the pudendal nerve runs on the medial surface of the obturator internus muscle near here, but this is not where pudendal nerve blocks are performed. The sacrotuberous ligament (**answer c**) is located superficial to the course of the pudendal nerve, but it is not used as a landmark for pudendal nerve blocks. The pudendal canal runs along the obturator internus muscle not near the pubic symphysis (**answer d**). The tip of the coccyx can be palpated rectally but is not the location of the pudendal nerve (**answer e**).

443. The answer is d. (*Moore, pp 339-343.*) Coccygeus muscle, the sacrospinous ligament and the tendinous arch of the levator ani muscle all take their origin from the ischial spine. The sacrotuberous ligament, inferior gemellus muscle, and the quadratus femoris muscle all arise just superior to the ischial tuberosity (**answer a**). The piriformis muscle (**answer b**) arises from the anterior surface of the sacrum. The abdominal wall muscles arise from the iliac crest (**answer c**). The lateral attachment of the inguinal ligament (**answer e**) arises from the anterior superior iliac spine.

444. The answer is b. (*Sadler, pp 240-241.*) The mother has a duplication of the ureters on the left side, one of which was accidentally sutured closed while ligating the left uterine artery. The second left ureter, which had been carefully identified and protected during surgery, was intact. Duplication of the ureter occurs in about 1% of the population and up to 10% of children who are diagnosed with urinary tract infections. Duplication of the ureter is caused by a splitting or duplication of the ureteric bud off the mesonephric duct. Complete duplication of the ureter often leads to improper trigone formation, which may result in structures more susceptible to infections. A didelphus uterus (**answer a**) would easily be discovered during the hysterectomy and would not produce pain. The symptoms and findings are not consistent with urachal fistula (**answer c**). A horseshoe-kidney (**answer d**) generally remains in the lower abdomen as it is "caught" on the inferior mesenteric artery as the kidney "rises" within the abdominal cavity. Generally a tubal pregnancy (**answer e**) cannot be carried to term and would have been discovered during the C-section.

445. The answer is c. (*Moore, p 349.*) Puborectalis, pubococcygeus, and iliococcygeus muscles make up the levator ani muscles that are exercised during Kegel exercises. Kegel exercises are designed to strengthen the levator ani muscles so they can better support the added weight of the growing fetus and placenta and stronger muscles are less likely torn during the birthing process. The ischiocavernous muscles (**answer a**) contracts and forces blood into the body of the clitoris during sexual arousal. Both the piriformis (**answer b and d**) and obturator internus (**answer b and e**) muscles have their origins in the pelvis; both act on the femur to laterally rotate the leg and have nothing to do with Kegel exercises.

446. The answer is c. (*Moore, pp 414-415.*) The structures are the vaginal wall, bulbospongiosus, and superficial transverse perineal muscles. Both the pubococcygeus and iliococcygeus muscle (**answers a and b**) are part of the pelvic diaphragm and are much deeper muscles and thus would not be cut. The prepuce and rectus abdominis muscle (**answer d**) are superior and lateral to the vagina and an episiotomy is performed in a posterior mediolateral direction. Both the sacrospinous and sacrotuberous ligaments (**answer e**) are much deeper structures, which stabilize the pelvis and never cut during an episiotomy.

447. The answer is c. (*Moore, p 400.*) Lymph drains from the testicles to preaortic nodes, because the blood supply for the testicles comes directly off the abdominal aorta, where the testicles first develop, prior to their inferior migration into the scrotum. All the other pelvic structures: penis (**answer a**), scrotum (**answer b**), anus (**answer d**), and epididymides (**answer e**) have lymphatic drainage to the superficial inguinal nodes. The anus and rectum have drainage to three sites: superficial inguinal nodes, internal iliac nodes, and inferior mesenteric preaortic nodes.

448. The answer is e. (*Moore, p 381. Fauci, p 595.*) The patient should be told that he probably has calcified prostatic concretions and pelvic vein phleboliths which are of little concern and that he needs to schedule an appointment for annual follow up. Prostatic concretions that undergo calcification are quite common. If the prostate is generally enlarged, then it is more likely due to BPH, rather than prostate cancer **(answers a and b)**. If the prostate gland were hard and nodular, then prostate cancer would be suspected and biopsy would be recommended, especially if PSA levels were above 4 ng/dL. Phleboliths are calcifications in the wall of pelvic veins, not in the prostate **(answer d)** and they are quite common in Western society as one ages. However, 5 years is too long to wait for follow up with a PSA in the high normal range and considering that the patient is approaching 60 years of age. Phleboliths are of little health concern **(answer c)**.

449. The answer is b. (*Moore, pp 373-374.*) Bulges in the anterior wall of the vagina are most likely due to the bladder falling posteriorly into the anterior vaginal wall. A bulge on the posterior wall of the vagina would most likely be a rectocele **(answer a)**. Cervical cancer **(answer c)** generally would not present as described. A didelphic uterus **(answer d)** is a duplication of the uterus as result of failure of the right and left paramesonephric ducts to fuse in the midline. An indirect inguinal hernia **(answer e)** would generally present as a mass within the labia major.

450. The answer is b. (*Moore, pp 419-421, 436.*) The corpus spongiosum surrounds the urethra (the black curving line) at the base of the penis next to the letter **B** above. The right corpus cavernosum is letter **C**. **A** is the anus, **D** is the left ischiocavernosus muscle, and **E** is the left ischial tuberosity.

Extremities and Spine

Questions

451. A 13-year-old adolescent is brought to the family practice clinic by his mother, because he can barely walk. He has been trying out for a soccer team for the last 2 weeks, but in the last few days has developed right knee pain and swelling. Upon examination the pain is below the knee joint along the tibia where the patellar tendon attaches. What is the most likely source of the problem?

a. Anterior cruciate ligament (ACL) strain
b. Bursitis
c. Osteochondritis of the tibial tubercle
d. Prepatellar bursitis
e. Quadriceps tendonitis

452. During icy conditions on a lightly traveled rural road, a teenager in a pickup truck passes another vehicle. Just as the truck passes it starts to fishtail and rolls over several times and lands on the driver's side door. The driver is pinned under the overturned truck with a very badly gashed anterior forearm and profuse bleeding. Where should the emergency mobile technician compress the man's arm to stop the blood flow to the severely lacerated forearm?

a. At the brachial artery as it crosses the first rib in the neck
b. At the brachial artery as it crosses under the bicipital aponeurosis in the cubital fossa
c. At the brachial artery as it courses medial to the humerus in the arm
d. At the radial artery just lateral to the flexor carpi radialis tendon as it crosses the wrist
e. At the ulnar artery just medial to the flexor digitorum profundus tendon as it crosses the wrist

453. A 47-year-old radiology professor suddenly notices that he can no longer hit his normal three-point shot in basketball on his driveway. He also notes a diminished ability to do his usual pushup regimen. He presents to his family physician's office where it is learned that he has been suffering some mild neck pain of 6 weeks' duration. In addition, he describes right arm pain down the back of his right arm and extending to the dorsal surface of his hand, including his middle finger. A diminished triceps tendon reflex is noted on the right side only. His physician orders which of the following because of concern that his patient has herniated which intervertebral disk?

a. Lateral x-ray; C6 to C7
b. Cervical MRI; C6 to C7
c. Cervical MRI; C8 to T1
d. CT; C5 to C6
e. CT; C8 to T1

454. A 49-year-old motorcycle rider was brought into the emergency department unconscious having been found at the side of the highway. He was breathing on his own and his heartbeat was regular. Upon physical examination he has both biceps and triceps reflexes, but his anal tone is weak and he has neither patellar tendon nor Achilles tendon reflexes. He is noted to have a displacement of the spinous process of his mid-to-lower back. An x-ray is taken and is shown below. If and when the 49-year-old man regains consciousness what should his physician tell him about his spinal injury?

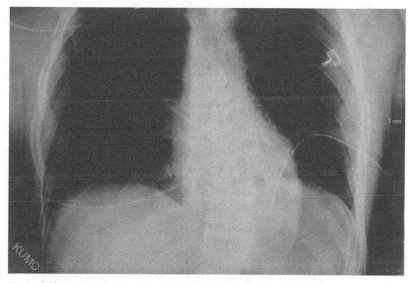

(Image 2133 used with permission from the Radiological Anatomy web site, University of Kansas, School of Medicine, http://classes.kumc.edu/som/radanatomy/.)

a. Your injury is at T5 and sensation and most movements below your neck have been lost.
b. Your injury is at T7 and sensation from your umbilicus inferiorly has been lost.
c. Yourinjury is at T7 and most movements from below your umbilicus inferiorly have been lost.
d. Your injury is at T10 and sensation and most movements below your umbilicus have been lost.
e. Your injury is at L2 but you should be able to walk with a cane since the injury is inferior to where the spinal cord extends.

455. A patient presents in her fifth pregnancy with a history of numbness and tingling in her right thumb and index finger during each of her previous four pregnancies. Currently, the same symptoms are constant, although worse in the early morning. Symptoms could be somewhat relieved by vigorous shaking of the wrist. Neurologic examination revealed atrophy and weakness of the abductor pollicis brevis, the opponens pollicis, and the first two lumbrical muscles. Sensation was decreased over the lateral palm and the volar aspect of the first three digits. Numbness and tingling were markedly increased over the first three digits and the lateral palm when the wrist was held in flexion for 30 seconds. The symptoms suggest damage to which one of the following?

a. The radial artery
b. The median nerve
c. The ulnar nerve
d. Proper digital nerves
e. The radial nerve

456. A 52-year-old man is brought to the emergency department (ED) after being found in the park, where apparently he had lain overnight after a fall. He complains of severe pain in the left arm. Physical examination suggests a fractured humerus that is confirmed radiologically. The patient can extend the forearm at the elbow, but supination appears to be slightly weak; the hand grasp is very weak compared with the uninjured arm. Neurologic examination reveals an inability to extend the wrist (wrist-drop). Because these findings point to apparent nerve damage, the patient is scheduled for a surgical reduction of the fracture. The observation that extension at the elbow appears normal, but supination of the forearm appears weak, warrants localization of the nerve lesion to which one of the following?

a. Posterior cord of the brachial plexus in the axilla
b. Posterior divisions of the brachial plexus
c. Radial nerve at the distal third of the humerus
d. Radial nerve in the midforearm
e. Radial nerve in the vicinity of the head of the radius

457. Wrist-drop (flexion) results in a very weak hand grasp. This is why self-defense classes teach students to flex the wrist of an attacker holding an object to loosen their grip on that object. The strength of the hand grasp is greatest with the wrist in the extended position for which one of the following reasons?

a. Flexor digitorum superficialis and profundus muscles are stretched when the wrist and metacarpophalangeal joints are extended.
b. Lever arms of the interossei are longer when the metacarpophalangeal joints are extended.
c. Lever arms of the lumbrical muscles are longer when the metacarpophalangeal joints are extended.
d. Line of action of the extensor digitorum muscle is most direct in full extension.
e. Radial half of the flexor digitorum profundus muscle is paralyzed because it is innervated by the radial nerve.

458. A 13-year-old adolescent is brought to the pediatrician's office by his mother. He has a body mass index (BMI) of 29 and he is limping significantly as he walks due to left knee and hip pain. He does not recall any specific incident; he just woke up early this week in pain. Physical examination reveals that his left leg is shorter than the right and an increase in the gluteal skin fold is noted. He carries his left leg turned slightly outward. Flexion, extension, and rotation of the left leg is limited, with guarding. What is the pediatrician's working diagnosis as she orders a plain film evaluation of the hip joint?

a. Developmental dysplasia of the hip
b. Avascular necrosis of the femoral head
c. Pelvic fracture
d. Slipped capital femoral epiphysis
e. Trendelenburg gait

459. A 28-year-old mother delivered her first child vaginally, a 7 lb 14 oz full-term baby girl. After the mother and father had held the girl for a few minutes and after the placenta had been successfully delivered, the obstetrician asks to take the baby girl back to weigh her, determine her length and perform appropriate tests. The physician places the baby girl on her back and holds each leg while flexing both the hip and the knee at 90° as he first abducts her legs then pushes each leg toward the pelvis as he moves the girl's leg around in small circular movements. For which one of the following conditions is the physician testing?

a. Avascular necrosis of the hip
b. Clubfoot
c. Developmental dysplasia of the hip
d. Osteochondritis of the tibial tubercle
e. Slipped capital femoral epiphysis

460. If a compound fracture of the humerus in the region marked Z on the accompanying radiograph occurs, then there is likely to be a severe injury to a major nerve that passes on the dorsal aspect of the bone. Which one of the following is most likely to occur as a result of such an injury?

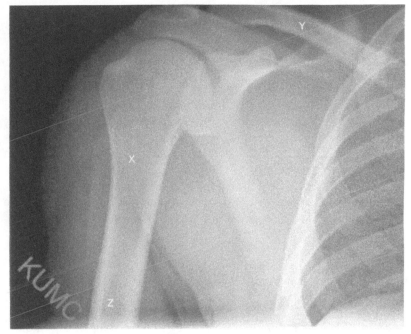

(Image 6101, used with permission from the Radiological Anatomy web site, University of Kansas, School of Medicine, http://classes.kumc.edu/som/radanatomy/.)

a. Wrist-drop palsy
b. Total clawing of the hand
c. Waiter's tip palsy
d. Clawing of digits 4 and 5
e. Dupuytren contracture

461. Fractures of the humerus in different regions have the potential to damage different nerves. What muscle innervation may be compromised by a fracture of the humerus at the "surgical neck"?

a. Subscapularis
b. Pectoralis major
c. Teres major
d. Deltoid
e. Suprascapularis

462. A 12-year-old boy was riding his bicycle across an intersection when an elderly woman tried to pull out into the busy street just as the boy was riding in front of her, hitting the boy. Fortunately the boy landed on the hood of the car, but the bumper struck the boys legs just below the knees and created a very large cut. The boy presents to the ED bleeding and walking with a distinct left foot-drop. The boy has also lost most of his ability to flex his left ankle or evert his left foot and he has lost sensation on the lateral side of his leg distal to the cut. Plain films show that there are no broken bones and examination of the knee reveals that it is intact. A plastic surgeon is consulted to reanastomose which one of the following?

a. Sciatic nerve
b. Tibial nerve
c. Common fibular (peroneal) nerve
d. Deep fibular (peroneal) nerve
e. Obturator nerve

463. A 45-year-old plumber presents in the clinic complaining of long-standing pain in the elbow. Subsequent examination reveals normal flexion/extension at both the elbow and the wrist, but weakened abduction of the thumb and extension at the metacarpophalangeal joints of the fingers. Those symptoms are found to be caused by entrapment of the posterior interosseus nerve. Which one of the following muscles could itself cause that entrapment?

a. Extensor carpi ulnaris
b. Extensor indices
c. Anconeus
d. Extensor digitorum
e. Supinator

464. A 67-year-old woman slipped on a scatter rug and fell with her right arm extended in an attempt to ease the impact of the fall. She experienced immediate severe pain in the region of the right clavicle and in the right distal arm. Painful movement of the right arm was minimized by holding the arm close to the body and by supporting the elbow with the left hand. There is marked tenderness and some swelling in the region of the clavicle about one-third of the distance from the sternum. The examining physician can feel the projecting edges of the clavicular fragments. The radiograph confirms the fracture and shows elevation of the proximal fragment with depression and subluxation of the distal fragment. Traction by which one of the following muscles causes the most subluxation with the distal fragment underriding the proximal fragment?

a. Deltoid muscle
b. Pectoralis major muscle
c. Pectoralis minor muscle
d. Sternocleidomastoid muscle
e. Trapezius muscle

465. Internal bleeding can be a rare complication of a broken clavicle if the broken bone fragment becomes significantly displaced and tears a vessel and punctures the pleura. Normally the subclavius muscle protects the underlying vessels. Which one of the following vascular structures is particularly vulnerable in a displaced clavicular fractures?

a. Subscapular artery
b. Cephalic vein
c. Lateral thoracic artery
d. Subclavian vein
e. Thoracocervical trunk

466. A 72-year-old woman trips over the edge of the carpet and falls forward onto the floor. A common reflex reaction to tripping and falling forward is to extend ones hands to ease the impact of striking the floor. She presents to the ER holding her left arm with her right hand. There is an obvious posterior displacement of the left distal wrist and hand that looks like a dinner fork. Which bone(s) is/are likely involved in a classic Colles fracture?

a. Always the ulna and sometimes the radius
b. Always the radius and sometimes the ulna
c. Always the ulna and sometimes the scaphoid
d. Always the radius and sometimes the trapezium
e. Only the ulna

467. A 36-year-old man fell while playing soccer one week earlier. He fell on his left hand and "didn't think he broke anything," but he has a palmar mass, weakened ability to grasp with that hand, and has tingling in his thumb and index finger. He has no pain when his physician presses on the anatomical snuffbox. Which one of the following carpal bones is most likely dislocated anteriorly and causing a form of carpal tunnel syndrome?

a. Capitate
b. Hamate
c. Lunate
d. Navicular
e. Scaphoid

468. A third year medical student on cardiology service receives a transfer patient from the ED. The 52-year-old woman is having chest pain and her cardiac enzymes and ECG suggest that she may have had a myocardial infarction. The attending cardiologist is about to perform a cardiac catheterization to inject dye into her coronary arteries. He prepares her right inguinal region for insertion of the catheter into her femoral artery. The attending cardiologist asks the medical student, "what are the landmarks for finding the femoral artery just under the inguinal ligament and what is on each side of it if we miss?" Which of the following is the best answer?

a. Halfway between the anterior superior iliac spine and the pubic tubercle, with the femoral nerve medial and the femoral vein lateral to the femoral artery
b. Halfway between the anterior superior iliac spine and the pubic tubercle, with the femoral nerve lateral and the femoral vein medial to the femoral artery
c. Two-thirds of the way between the anterior superior iliac spine and the pubic tubercle, with the femoral nerve lateral and the femoral vein medial to the femoral artery
d. Halfway between the anterior inferior iliac spine and the pubic tubercle, with the femoral nerve medial and the femoral vein lateral to the femoral artery
e. Halfway between the anterior inferior iliac spine and the pubic tubercle, with the femoral nerve lateral and the femoral vein medial to the femoral artery

469. Which bone on the plain film below is most likely fractured when falling on an outstretched hand?

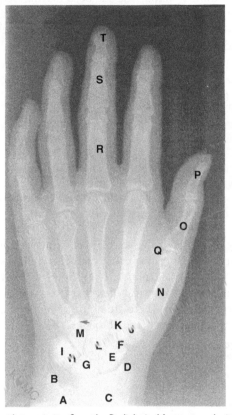

(Image 6107 used with permission from the Radiological Anatomy web site, University of Kansas, School of Medicine, http://classes.kumc.edu/som/radanatomy/.)

a. A
b. G
c. EF
d. HI
e. M

470. A 3-year-old girl is brought into the family practice office. The girl is holding her left arm pronated and bent across her abdomen with her right hand. The girl still has some elbow movement, just very painful, especially on the lateral portion. Yesterday she had been playing "red-rover" when an older child slammed into her, pulling her arm in a linear fashion in relation to its long axis at the elbow joint. What is the most likely diagnosis and treatment based on the history of the injury?

a. Bruising of the coronoid fossa at the distal end of the humerus; recommend rest, icing the elbow twice daily while elevating it, and NSAIDs
b. Subluxation of the head of the radius from the annular ligament; relocation by flexing the elbow at 90° and supernating the hand
c. Subluxation of the head of the radius from the annular ligament; relocation by hyperextending the elbow 5° beyond 180° and gently applying proximal pressure
d. Subluxation of the radius from the trochlea at the distal end of the humerus; relocation by flexing the elbow at 90° and pronating the hand
e. Dislocation of the ulna at the olecranon fossa of the distal end of the humerus; pain relief prior to forceful relocation

471. After a night of fraternity parties, a 21-year-old college junior came to the ED the following morning complaining that she could not raise her wrist. There is no history of trauma. On examination, the patient cannot extend her fingers or wrist but can flex them. She can also both flex and extend her elbow normally. There are no other motor deficits. The symptoms suggest damage to which one of the following?

a. Median nerve
b. Ulnar nerve
c. Radial nerve
d. Axillary nerve
e. Musculocutaneous nerve

472. An 8-year-old boy returns to the pediatric clinic because he has a "pain in his butt" and walks with a limp. He just visited the clinic a few days ago for a normal summer checkup and an update on his vaccinations. When the physician asks how this happened, the boy says that the pain started when the nurse gave him his booster shot in his left buttock. When he walks, he drops his right hip as he places all the weight on his left leg and swings his right leg forward. When lying prone on the examination table both legs flex normally with equal strength, and he can extend his thigh at the hip well, but there is flaccidity of his muscles just under the iliac crest only on the left side. The pediatrician tells the boy and his mother that the booster shot he received a couple of days ago likely damaged which one of the following?

a. Lateral cutaneous nerve of the thigh causing his pain
b. Superior gluteal nerve partially paralyzing his gluteus medius muscle
c. Superior gluteal nerve partially paralyzing his gluteus maximus muscle
d. Inferior gluteal nerve partially paralyzing his gluteus medius muscle
e. Sciatic nerve partially paralyzing his hamstring muscles

473. A woman falls on an icy sidewalk and complains of her "thumb hurting." The ED physician orders an x-ray (see below) and shows the patient that there are no fractures. However, she asks the ED physician to identify the small light circles (arrow) on the x-ray. He explains that they are sesamoid bones in the tendon of which one of the following?

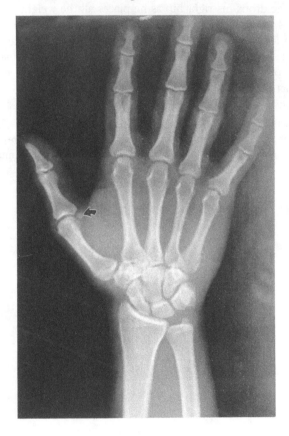

a. Flexor pollicis longus
b. Flexor pollicis brevis
c. Adductor pollicis
d. Abductor pollicis longus
e. Abductor pollicis brevis

474. A workman accidentally lacerates his wrist as shown in the ac panying diagram. On exploration of the wound, a vessel and nerve found to be severed, but no muscle tendons are damaged. From the ina cated location of the laceration and loss of sensation, the involved nerve is which one of the following?

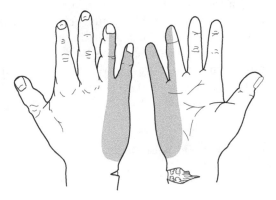

a. Median nerve
b. Recurrent branch of the median nerve
c. Superficial branch of the radial nerve
d. Ulnar nerve
e. Radial nerve

475. A 71-year-old grandmother falls halfway down the basement stairs while carrying a laundry basket. She does not lose consciousness, but sits at the bottom of the stairs "gathering her wits" and the scattered laundry. She Halfway does not think she fractured any bones as she can move all her limbs. Her husband, who hears the noise helps her stand up. It is then that she feels a slight pain in her left hip on weight bearing. She limps for the rest of the day. The next morning her husband brings her into their family physician's office where it is noted that she walks with her pelvis tilted as if her left leg is slightly shorter than the right. She still has left hip pain. A plain film is ordered of the left femur from hip to the knee expecting to find which one of the following?

a. Femoral neck fracture with compression
b. Femoral neck fracture with complete displacement
c. A spiral fracture of the femoral shaft
d. A transverse supracondylar fracture
e. An intercondylar fracture

9. A 10-year-old boy is brought into his pediatrician's office by his mother. The boy is supporting his left arm at the elbow by using his right hand because he thinks he has "broken his arm." The 10-year-old was playing tag and tripped over the curb and landed on the grass, catching himself with his hands. Upon physical examination, the pediatrician notes a slight drooping of the left shoulder when unsupported, and tenderness over the mid-clavicular region but no palpable fracture or displacement. The jugular notch appears symmetrical. The shoulder has normal movement, but the boy is unwilling to lift his hand above his head because it hurts. Otherwise, hand and arm movements are relatively normal with normal sensation. Anteroposterior and lateral x-rays of the thorax and upper arm are ordered because of suspicion of which one of the following?

a. Colles fracture
b. Scaphoid fracture
c. Fracture of the surgical head of the humerus
d. Dislocated sternoclavicular joint
e. Greenstick fracture of the clavicle

477. A 16-year-old girl is brought into the orthopedic clinic because she fell off her bicycle while riding down a steep hill. The orthopedic surgeon examines her left arm and palpates a displaced mid-shaft break of her humerus. It is noted that she cannot extend her wrist, but there are no distal broken bones. She has limited ability to extend and abduct her arm at the shoulder. Her left forearm and hand feel slightly colder than her right arm and she seems to have lost some sensation on the posterior lateral portion of her left hand, though she says she can feel with all her fingertips. The physician is concerned that she has damaged which of the following?

a. Axillary nerve
b. Axillary nerve and posterior humeral circumflex artery
c. Radial nerve
d. Radial nerve and deep artery of the arm
e. Median nerve and brachial artery

478. Hip fractures, especially in the elderly, often do not heal adequ
As a result broken femurs often lead to complete hip replacement with ε
ficial parts. What type of femoral fracture in adults is most likely to resu
in avascular necrosis of the femoral head?

a. Acetabular
b. Cervical
c. Intertrochanteric (between the trochanters)
d. Subtrochanteric
e. Midfemoral shaft

479. Paresthesia, hyperesthesia, or even painful sensation in the anterolateral region of the thigh may occur in obese persons. It results from an
abdominal panniculus adiposus that bulges over the inguinal ligament and
compresses which one of the following underlying nerves?

a. Femoral branch of the genitofemoral nerve
b. Femoral nerve
c. Iliohypogastric nerve
d. Ilioinguinal nerve
e. Lateral femoral cutaneous nerve

.. A 40-year-old man started jogging in the evening for exercise and complains to his family physician that after less than a mile or so his left leg begins to hurt. A physical examination finds that he has widespread pain throughout his left lower limb. An arteriogram from the patient in the vignette is shown below. Based on the location of the constriction of the artery (indicated by the arrow), which compartment or movement would most likely be normal or unaffected by the reduced arterial blood flow?

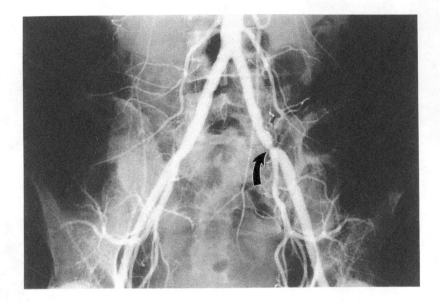

a. Gluteal region
b. Flexion of the thigh
c. Extension of the leg
d. Posterior thigh
e. Plantar flexion of the foot

481. How would a physician test for the destruction of structure 9 in the sagittal MRI of the knee shown below?

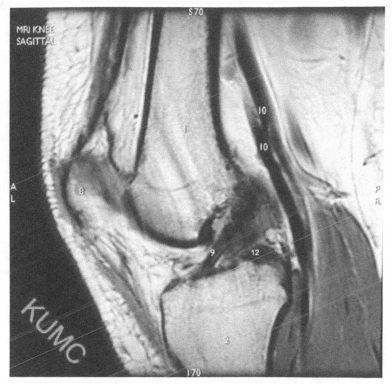

(Image 7304, used with permission from the Radiological Anatomy web site, University of Kansas, School of Medicine, http://classes.kumc.edu/som/radanatomy/.)

a. Excess ability to displace a flexed leg posteriorly
b. Excess ability to displace a flexed leg anteriorly
c. Excess ability to displace the ankle medially
d. Excess ability to displace the ankle laterally
e. Excess ability to displace the leg medially

482. A 12-year-old boy is brought to the ED by his mother after being pushed out of the neighbor's tree house, about 10 ft off the ground. He can walk but his right heel hurts every time he puts weight on it. When his foot is examined, it is found to be tender to pressure on both the medial and lateral aspects of the heel inferior to the tibia. Plain films of his right lower extremity are ordered because of suspicion that he has fractured which one of the following?

a. Calcaneus
b. Fibula
c. Tibia
d. Navicular
e. Cuneiform

483. A 40-year-old man presents to the emergency department barely able to walk. He finds it painful to sit down. He was waterskiing and was trying to learn to water ski backwards when his left ski caught the water "wrong" and he fell. He has intense pain in the left gluteal region. Examining him in the prone position, a bulging of the left hamstring muscles is noted with significant pain upon palpation of the left ischial tuberosity. An avulsion of the hamstring muscles from their origin on the ischial tuberosity is suspected. Which three muscle origins most likely avulsed a piece of bone from the ischial tuberosity when his ski caught the water?

a. Adductor longus, adductor magnus, and biceps femoris
b. Adductor longus, adductor magnus, and gracilis
c. Semitendinosus, semimembranosus, and adductor magnus
d. Semitendinosus, semimembranosus, and biceps femoris.
e. Semitendinosus, semimembranosus, and gracilis

484. A 22-year-old man who belongs to a weekend football league presents the ED. He was running with the ball when a defender tackled him in th. midthigh. The patient reports that when he got up, his thigh hurt, so he sat out the rest of the game. When walking to the car, his posterior thigh was extremely painful and swollen. After his shower, he noticed it was becoming discolored with increased swelling. There is concern about the presence of a hematoma and disruption of the arterial blood flow to the hamstring muscles. An arteriogram is performed and the vessels in question (arrows) show good filling by contrast. What is the name of those blood vessels?

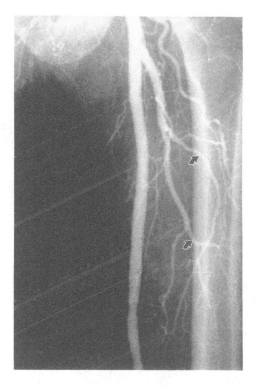

a. Descending branches of the inferior gluteal artery
b. Perforating branches of the deep femoral artery
c. Perforating branches from the obturator artery
d. Perforating branches of the femoral artery
e. Obturator artery

485. A patient experiences a prolonged stay in one position during a recent surgery and postoperative recovery that results in compression of the common fibular (peroneal) nerve against the fibular head. Which one of the following motor deficits would most likely occur?

a. Loss of extension at the knee
b. Loss of plantar flexion
c. Loss of flexion at the knee
d. Loss of eversion
e. Loss of medial rotation of the tibia

486. A 34-year-old woman is brought into the ED following a car accident in which she hit a patch of ice and slammed into the back of a trash truck. She is unable to walk because she has intense pain in her left knee and hip. She thinks her knee hit the left side of the dashboard as she twisted under the seat belt when she was thrown forward. She reports severe pain as the physician moves her hip. A plain film of the leg up to the pelvis is ordered and it shows no broken bones, but posterior displacement of the head of the femur out of the acetabulum. She is sedated in order to forcefully relocate the femoral head back into the acetabulum. Despite successful relocation there is concern that she has damaged which one of the following nerves, which may take several months to regain function?

a. Obturator
b. Pudendal
c. Sciatic
d. Femoral
e. Superior gluteal

487. A 19-year-old is brought by ambulance to the emergency department following a farm accident. He had been trying to unjam a wheat thrasher when his right arm was crushed in the equipment. The radius is cleanly fractured and could be pinned, but the ulna is crushed in the middle with a 3-in section of missing bone. Which long bone is the best replacement for the destroyed section of ulna?

a. Distal portion of tibia
b. Iliac crest on left side
c. Left body of the mandible
d. Medial edge of right scapula
e. Middle portion of fibula

488. A 19-year-old woman was dancing in clogs in an ethnic street fe_
val when she inverted her left foot. She presents to the clinic the next da_
with a swollen foot, but mainly complains about tenderness on the lateral
aspect of the foot along the plantar surface. Her foot is carefully palpated
and it is determined that she has tenderness over the tuberosity of the fifth
metatarsal bone. What muscle has avulsed from its insertion onto the
tuberosity of the fifth metatarsal?

a. Abductor digiti minimi
b. Fibularis (peroneus) brevis
c. Fibularis (peroneus) longus
d. Tibialis anterior
e. Tibialis posterior

489. The bone marked B in the lateral plain film of the right foot is which
one of the following?

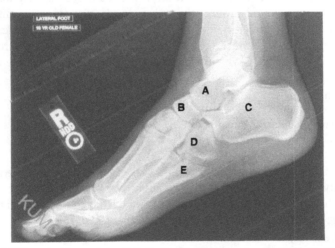

(Image 7107, used with permission from the Radiological Anatomy web site, University of
Kansas, School of Medicine, http://classes.kumc.edu/som/radanatomy/.)

a. Talus
b. Navicular
c. Calcaneus
d. Cuboid
e. Fifth metatarsal

90. While some people continue to increase in height through their teenage years, most change very little in height for decades. However, many elderly men and women often lose height as a result of which one of the following?

a. Lordosis
b. Scoliosis
c. Kyphosis
d. Osteoarthritis
e. Rheumatoid arthritis

491. A 27-year-old man receives a neurologic evaluation following a gunshot wound received 5 days previously. A 9-mm bullet had passed through both the medial and lateral heads of the gastrocnemius muscle. The exit wound on the lateral head of the muscle was somewhat deeper than the entrance wound in the medial head. The bullet did not strike bone or significant arteries although significant tissue damage, suppuration, and swelling were found around the exit wound. Neurologic examination reveals losses of dorsiflexion and eversion of the left foot. The patient cannot feel pinprick or touch on the dorsum of the left foot or anterolateral surface of the left leg. Which nerve was most likely involved in the injury?

a. Sciatic nerve
b. Femoral nerve
c. Sural nerve
d. Common fibular (peroneal) nerve
e. Tibial nerve

492. In a presurgical patient, the great saphenous vein is cannulated in the vicinity of the ankle. During the procedure, the patient experiences severe pain that radiates along the medial border of the foot. Which one of the following nerves was accidentally included in a ligature during this procedure?

a. Medial femoral cutaneous nerve
b. Saphenous nerve
c. Superficial fibular nerve
d. Sural cutaneous nerve
e. Tibial nerve

493. As one grows older peripheral vascular disease may develop. Because it is a long distance from the heart the pulse of the dorsalis pedis artery is often evaluated. The pulse in the dorsalis pedis artery may be palpated in which one of the following locations in the foot?

a. Between the tendons of the extensor digitorum longus and fibularis (peroneus) tertius muscles
b. Between the tendons of the extensor hallucis and extensor digitorum muscles
c. Between the tendons of the tibialis anterior and extensor hallucis longus muscles
d. Immediately anterior to the lateral malleolus
e. Immediately posterior to the medial malleolus

494. At the annual recital for a ballet school, a wide variety of dancers perform, from about 4 years of age to adulthood. One ballerina in particular is noticed because her spine seems to curve slightly to the left of her mid back. When this student bends away from the audience, her right scapula is somewhat lower that her left. What is the term for this dysmorphology and in what age group does it most often first present itself?

a. Kyphosis; 16 to 20 years old
b. Lordosis; 4 to 8 years old
c. Lordosis; 6 to 10 years old
d. Scoliosis; 4 to 8 years old
e. Scoliosis; 10 to 14 years old

Questions 495 and 496 refer to the radiograph below.

495. A 43-year-old father of three boys presents to his family practice physician Monday morning with severe back pain. He had been roughhousing with his three sons in the living room when his back twisted and popped. What pathological condition is illustrated in this plain film of the lumbosacral spine?

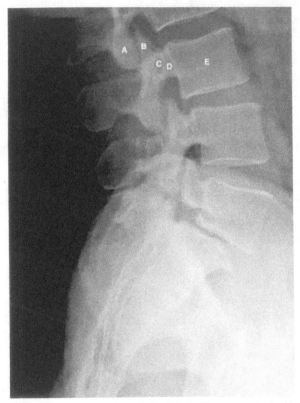

(Image 2115 used with permission from the Radiological Anatomy web site, University of Kansas, School of Medicine, http://classes.kumc.edu/som/radanatomy/.)

a. Kyphosis
b. Scoliosis
c. Lordosis
d. Spondylolisthesis
e. Sacral fracture

496. In the film shown in Question 495, p. 612, which part of the vertebra would connect to the three other parts: the body, the lamina, and the transverse process?

a. Inferior articular facet
b. Superior articular facet
c. Lamina
d. Pedicle
e. Body

97. A 22-year-old man who belongs to a weekend football league was running with the ball when a defender tackled him mid-lower limb from the side. After the tackle, his knee is injured and he presents to the ED. From the MRI of the knee shown, the lateral meniscus is uniformly black; however, the medial meniscus has a tear (lucent area within the meniscus). Which one of the following is the reason why the medial meniscus is more susceptible to damage than the lateral meniscus?

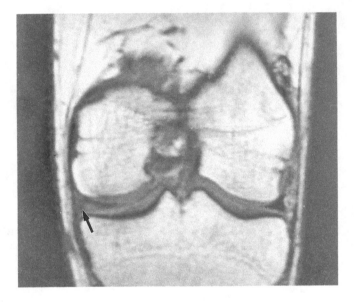

a. The medial meniscus is attached to the popliteus muscle tendon, making it more susceptible.
b. The medial meniscus is attached to the medial (tibial) collateral ligament, which holds it relatively immobile, making it more susceptible.
c. The medial meniscus is attached to the anterior cruciate ligament, which holds it relatively immobile, making it more susceptible.
d. The only reason the medial meniscus is more susceptible to damage is that the knee usually gets hit laterally, causing more torsion on the medial meniscus.
e. The medial meniscus is attached to the medial condyle of the femur.

498. A 64-year-old woman presents with a new complaint of back pai. She was previously diagnosed with rheumatoid arthritis, and is managed with antirheumatic and non-steroidal anti-inflammatory drugs (NSAIDs). The back pain is worse after activity, such as square dancing. Examination reveals no muscular pain with a little muscle guarding within the erector spinae muscles. The spinous process and supraspinous ligament are all pain free. Her physician can elicit back pain up and down the spinal column, lateral to the spinous processes, but medial to the transverse processes when the patient twists. Bending and flexing of the spinal column is less painful than standing and twisting and there is no radicular pain. What are the most likely nerves that perceive the pain?

a. Anterior rami of the spinal nerve
b. Articular branches of the dorsal rami
c. Meningeal branches of the ventral rami of spinal nerves
d. Recurrent meningeal nerves that innervate the intervertebral disks
e. Referred pain from cervical nerves that innervate the nuchal ligament

499. A physician examines a patient who complains of pain and paresthesia in the left leg. The distribution of the pain, running down the lateral aspect of the leg and the dorsal surface of the foot, is suggestive of a herniated intervertebral disk. The physician links the distribution of symptoms with nerve L5 and concludes that herniation has occurred at which location?

a. L3 to L4 intervertebral disk
b. L4 to L5 intervertebral disk
c. L5 to S1 intervertebral disk
d. S1 to S2 intervertebral disk
e. Insufficient data to determine

500. A 25-year-old woman is brought to the ED by her roommate because she has a fever of 102°F, stiff neck, and the "worst headache of her life." The fundus of her eyes shows no evidence of papilledema. In addition to collecting blood to be sent to the lab for evidence of sepsis, the attending recommends a spinal tap to obtain CSF for evidence of infection. What landmarks and ligaments need to be remembered when performing a spinal tap?

a. The umbilicus, which is a landmark for dermatome T10, and the sacrococcygeal ligament, which must be penetrated.

b. The posterior superior iliac crest, which is parallel with the spinous process of L4, supraspinous and intraspinous ligaments, and ligamentum flavum, which must be penetrated prior to piercing the dura and arachnoid membranes.

c. The anterior superior iliac crest, which is parallel with the spinous process of L2, supraspinous and intraspinous ligaments, and the ligamentum flavum, which must be penetrated prior to piercing the dura and arachnoid membranes.

d. The sacral cornu, which demarcates the sacral hiatus, and the sacrococcygeal ligament, which must be penetrated to gain access to the extradural space.

e. The posterior superior iliac crest, which is parallel with spinous process of S2, supraspinous and interspinous ligaments, and ligamentum flavum, which must be penetrated prior to piercing the dura and arachnoid membranes.

Extremities and Spine

Answers

451. The answer is c. (*Moore, pp 528, 646, 662-665.*) The diagnosis is osteochondritis of the tibial tubercle (Osgood-Schlatter disease) which is a disruption of the patellar tendon insertion into the tibial tuberosity. It is an overuse injury caused by repetitive avulsion of the secondary ossification center of the tibial tubercle. Chronic avulsion can cause separation of the proximal patellar tendon insertion from the tibial tubercle, which results in an elevation of the insertion. Osgood-Schlatter disease typically presents in athletic adolescents going through their growth spurt and whose epiphysial plates are still open. ACL strain (**answer a**) could be reproduced with the anterior drawer test. Bursitis (**answer b**) would present with swelling of the synovial membrane of the knee, which extends cranially as the suprapatellar bursa under the quadriceps tendon and patella. Prepatellar bursitis (**answer d**) is a small subcutaneous bursa that is just anterior to the patella and most commonly becomes irritated by kneeling. The quadriceps tendon (**answer e**) runs between the quadriceps muscle and the patella, thus would produce pain above the knee joint.

452. The answer is c. (*Moore, p 742.*) Blood to the forearm can best be limited by compressing the brachial artery as it runs medial to the humerus in the arm. It is the subclavian artery not the brachial artery (**answer a**) that crosses the first rib along the brachial plexus. There is extensive anastomosis around the elbow; stopping blood at the cubital fossa (**answer b**) is not likely to be very successful. Stopping blood within either the radial (**answer d**) or ulnar (**answer e**) arteries at the wrist is unlikely to significantly reduce bleeding in the forearm since there are arterial arches that connect radial and ulnar arteries in the hand.

453. The answer is b. (*Moore, pp 474-475.*) Herniations of intervertebral disks occur most frequently at L4 to L5, L5 to S1, and C6 to C7. The diminished triceps function in the right arm, as indicated by the inability to shoot three-point shots and do pushups, points to a weakened triceps. The triceps tendon reflex is principally mediated by C7. Spinal nerve C7 exits between the sixth and seventh cervical vertebrae (thus not **answer c**) and is most likely compromised by herniation at the C6 to C7 disk. The dermatomal pattern of pain down the posterior surface of the arm and hand and onto the middle finger is also consistent with C7. MRI (thus not **answers a, d, and e**) is the most useful radiological imaging study for viewing soft tissue structures such as herniated disks. CT is much less useful at visualizing soft structures.

454. The answer is d. (*Moore, p 507.*) The spinal column is displaced between T10 and T11 with both the 11th and 12th thoracic vertebrae displaced to the patient's left, severing the spinal cord at this level. The motorcycle rider would have no sensation below the umbilicus, which marks the 10th thoracic (T10) dermatome, and little leg movement other than some flexion at the hip. A severed spinal cord at T5 **(answer a)** would result in no movement nor sensation just below the nipples. A spinal cord break at T7 **(answer b and c)** would result in no motor nor sensory function below the xiphoid process. While a spinal column break below L2 **(answer e)** often does not damage the spinal cord since the cord terminates at L1 or higher in most individuals, the x-ray of the motorcycle rider shows a break at T10.

455. The answer is b. (*Moore, pp 790-791.*) The patient has a classic case of carpal tunnel syndrome, in which the median nerve is compressed as it passes through the carpal tunnel formed by the flexor retinaculum in the wrist. Evidence for involvement of the median nerve is weakness and atrophy of the thenar muscles (abductor pollicis brevis, opponens pollicis) and lumbricals 1 to 3. Sensory deficits also follow the distribution of the median nerve. The median nerve enters the hand, along with the tendons of the superficial and deep digital flexors, through a tunnel framed by the carpal bones and the overlying flexor retinaculum. Symptoms are worse in the early morning and in pregnancy because of fluid retention, resulting in swelling that entraps the median nerve. Flexing the wrist for an extended period exaggerates the paresthesia ("Phalen" sign) by increasing pressure on the median nerve.

Neither the ulnar nerve **(answer c)**, radial nerve **(answer e)**, nor radial artery **(answer a)** passes through the carpal tunnel. The ulnar nerve supplies the third and fourth lumbricals and only the short adductor of the thumb. The radial nerve innervates mostly long and short extensors of the digits and the dorsal aspect of the hand. Proper digital nerves **(answer d)** lie distal to the carpal tunnel, but are only sensory.

456. The answer is c. (*Moore, pp 684-685, 743.*) The clinical signs a findings in the patient vignette indicate radial nerve damage. The evidenc that extension (triceps brachii muscle) at the elbow appears normal while supination appears weak is used to localize the lesion. The innervation to the medial and long heads of the triceps brachii, principal extensor of the arm, arises from the radial nerve (in the axilla) as the medial muscular branches. The innervation to the lateral head, and to a smaller portion of the medial head, arises from the radial nerve as it passes along the musculospiral groove at mid-humerus. The supinator muscle is innervated by muscular twigs from the deep branch of the radial nerve in the forearm, just before the radial nerve reaches the supinator muscle. Thus, paralysis of the supinator muscle, but not of the triceps brachii (thus not **answers d and e**), localizes the fracture to the distal third of the humeral shaft between the elbow and musculospiral groove. Damage to the posterior cord (**answer a**) or division (**answer b**) of the brachial plexus would also affect the axillary nerve that innervates the deltoid, which is not affected.

457. The answer is a. (*Moore, pp 771-772.*) Muscles are most powerful (disregarding leverage factors) when slightly stretched by extension of the joint(s) over which they pass, because this places the sarcomeres at the optimum tension-producing length in the length-tension relationship. Thus, hand grasp is strongest when the wrist joint and metacarpophalangeal joints are extended, which stretches the digitorum superficialis and profundus flexors to their optimum position (thus not **answer d**). Paralysis of the radial nerve with subsequent wrist-drop will weaken hand grasp because the extrinsic flexor muscles are compelled to operate in a nonoptimum region. The lever arms of the lumbricals (**answer c**) and interossei (**answer b**) are greatest when the metacarpophalangeal joints are flexed, a consideration that does not apply to the patient presented in the question. The median nerve innervates the radial side of the flexor digitorum profundus (thus **answer e** is irrelevant to the vignette).

458. The answer is d. (*Moore, pp 526-527.*) Slipped capital femoral epiphysis is the dislocation of the articular head of the femur at the epiphysial plate. It occurs in about 1 in 10,000 children, with boys affected about 2.5 times more often than girls and in left hip more frequently than the right hip. Slipped capital femoral epiphysis often presents with knee pain, even though the problem is with the hip joint. It is most commonly seen in verweight boys from 10 to 16 years of age and teenage girls from 12 to 14 years of age. It requires surgical realignment and securing of the head of the femur with a screw placed through the neck of the femur. Developmental dysplasia of the hip (DDH) **(answer a)** is a dislocation of the hip joint that is present at birth. Avascular necrosis of the femoral head **(answer b)** or Legg-Calve-Perthes disease is the idiopathic necrosis of the femoral epiphysis leading to degenerative hip disease. It most often occurs in children 5 to 12 years of age, with male frequency 4 to 5 times that of females. Pelvic fractures **(answer c)** can occur at any age, but almost always are associated with a history of trauma. Trendelenburg gait **(answer e)** is a dropping of the pelvis on the unaffected side typically due to loss of the superior gluteal nerve to the gluteus medius and gluteus minimus muscles.

459. The answer is c. *(Moore, p 660.)* The developmental dysplasia of the hip (congenital hip dislocation) is a common congenital condition (about 1 per 1,000 births) occurring most frequently in firstborn, breech babies and about 8 times more frequent in girls than boys. The procedure being described is called the Ortolani test. A clicking noise and instability of the hip joint would confirm developmental dysplasia of the hip. The Barlow test is a deliberate dislocation of the hip followed by relocation and is also used to examine for developmental dysplasia of the hip joint. Avascular necrosis of the hip **(answer a)** does not occur in newborns, but is seen in children, teenagers, and even young adults. While clubfoot **(answer b)** is thought to be due to a malposition of the limbs in utero such as present in firstborn, that is not the condition for which the physician is testing. Osteochondritis of the tibial tubercle **(answer d)** or Osgood-Schlatter disease is a failure of the insertion of the patella tendon into the tibial tuberosity that occurs in young adolescents. Slipped capital femoral epiphysis **(answer e)** is most commonly seen in overweight boys from 10 to 16 years of age and girls from 12 to 14 years of age.

460. The answer is a. *(Moore, pp 685, 743.)* The area marked Z points to the approximate location of the spiral (radial) groove. That shallow depression, on the posterior (dorsal) aspect of the humeral shaft, accommodates the radial nerve and the deep (profunda) brachial vessels. A midline fracture of the humerus may rupture blood vessels, causing a hematoma that would compress and impair the ability of the radial nerve to conduct information to the extensor muscles of the wrist and digits. A more severe fracture may transect the radial nerve, causing paralysis of the same mu: cles, resulting in wrist-drop. Those muscles include the following: brachioradialis, extensor carpi radialis longus, extensor carpi radialis brevis, extensor digitorum communis, extensor digiti minimi, extensor carpi ulnaris, supinator, abductor pollicis longus, extensor pollicis longus, extensor pollicis brevis, and the extensor indicis. The causes of other palsies listed in this question are injuries due to the nerves within brackets: total claw hand palsy (median and ulnar nerves; **[answer b]**); clawing of digits 4 and 5 (ulnar nerve; **[answer d]**); waiter's tip palsy (C5, C6 roots of the brachial plexus; upper trunk of the brachial plexus; **[answer c]**); and Erb-Duchenne palsy. Dupuytren contracture **(answer e)** is caused by a thickening of the palmar aponeurosis and occurs more frequently in diabetics.

461. The answer is d. *(Moore, pp 684-685.)* The surgical neck of the humerus is the narrow area located just distal to the head and anatomical neck of the humerus (the area marked X in the radiograph for Question 460). The posterior (dorsal aspect) of the surgical neck is traversed by the axillary nerve (C5, C6; posterior/dorsal cord of the brachial plexus) and the accompanying posterior circumflex humeral vessels. A fracture of the surgical neck may rupture the posterior circumflex humeral vessels, causing either the compression of the axillary nerve or transection of the same nerve. Injury to this nerve causes weakness (paresis) or paralysis of the deltoid and teres minor muscles. The nerve supply to the other muscles mentioned is shown in brackets: subscapularis (upper and lower subscapular nerves; **[answer a]**); pectoralis major (medial and lateral pectoral nerves; **[answer b]**); teres major (lower subscapular nerve; **[answer c]**); and supraspinatus (suprascapular nerve; **[answer e]**).

462. The answer is c. *(Moore, p 605.)* The common fibular (peroneal) nerve wraps around the fibular shaft just distal to its proximal head. This places it close to the skin, where it is easily damaged. The common fibular nerve then divides into the deep fibular nerve, which innervates the anterior compartment leg muscles and the superficial fibular nerve, which innervates the lateral compartment leg muscles. Both of these nerves also have cutaneous distribution as well. The inability to dorsiflex the ankle and evert the foot is consistent with the boy's clinical presentation. The sciatic **(answer a)** and obturator **(answer e)** nerves are in the thigh. The deep fibular nerve **(answer d)** is also involved, but does not explain all the boy's findings. The tibial nerve (**answer b**) runs more medially through the popliteal fossa, and therefore is not involved.

463. The answer is e. (*Moore, p 726.*) Each of the muscles listed (**answers a, b, c, and d**) in the question is innervated by the deep branch of the radial nerve or its terminal portion, the posterior interosseus nerve. The deep radial nerve passes between the deep and superficial layers of the supinator muscle and lies on a bare area of the radius where it may be compressed by action of the supinator or damaged by a fracture of the radius.

464. The answer is b. (*Moore, p 684.*) The horizontal direction of the fibers of the clavicular head of the pectoralis major muscle draws the humerus medially and causes the distal fragment of the bone to sublux. The sternal head of this muscle also has the effect of pulling the arm medially, an effect that is normally offset by the strut-like action of the clavicle. The pectoralis minor muscle (**answer c**) is a much smaller muscle and has a minor role in subluxation compared to the pectoralis major. The deltoid (**answer a**) muscle would not cause inferior subluxation. The sternocleidomastoid (**answer d**) and the trapezius (**answer e**) muscles would not cause inferior subluxation.

465. The answer is d. (*Moore, p 684.*) Because large and important neurovascular structures pass between the clavicle and first rib, including the subclavian artery and vein, clavicular fractures may rarely produce life-threatening bleeding into the pleural cavity. The subscapular artery (**answer a**) and lateral thoracic artery (**answer c**) are both branches of the lateral one-third of the axillary artery, so are not likely injured. The thoracocervical trunk (**answer e**) is medial to the first rib, thus is also not likely to be threatened by clavicular fracture. The cephalic vein (**answer b**) is superficial and lateral, therefore it is not involved in clavicular fractures.

466. The answer is b. (*Moore, pp 685-686.*) Colles fracture is a compression/displacement of the distal end (within 2-3 cm) of the radius resulting a classic dinner fork deformity (thus not **answers a, c, and e**). Colles fracture also may involve the distal portion of the ulna (sometimes just the ulnar styloid process) if osteoporosis is present or if the forces are sufficient. It has been estimated that Colles fractures represent up to 80% of fractures of the radius. While falling on an outstretched hand can result in scaphoid fractures (**answer c**), they rarely occur at the same time as a distal radial fracture. Fractures of the trapezium (**answer d**) are relatively rare.

467. The answer is c. *(Moore, pp 817-818.)* The lunate bone tends to dislocate anteriorly into the transverse carpal arch, thereby entrapping the tendons of the extrinsic digital flexors and compressing the median nerve, producing symptoms of carpal tunnel syndrome (thenar weakness and paresthesia over the lateral 2.5 fingers). The capitate (**answer a**) is frequently fractured, but does not tend to dislocate into the carpal arch. The hamate (**answer b**) provides an anchor for the transverse carpal ligament and is, therefore, located lateral to the carpal tunnel. The scaphoid (navicular) bone (**answers d and e**) has a tendency to fracture but does dislocate into the carpal tunnel. This is a relatively uncommon cause of Carpal tunnel syndrome, but is called "carpal dislocation."

468. The answer is b. *(Moore, pp 551-556, 560.)* The way to remember the relationship of the femoral nerve, artery, and vein to the inguinal ligament is to remember NAVEL from lateral to medial, for femoral Nerve, outside the sheath (on top of the iliopsoas muscle), femoral Artery, femoral Vein, then an "Empty space" (filled with lymph nodes) and then, most medial the Lacunar ligament as the inguinal ligament attaches to the pubic tubercle at the lateral aspect of the pubic symphysis. The femoral artery (which is normally easily palpable because of its pulsation) is about half way along the inguinal ligament, which is attached to the pubic tubercle medially and the anterior superior iliac spine laterally. None of the other answers are correct (**answers a, c, d, and e**).

469. The answer is c. *(Moore, p 686.)* The scaphoid (EF) is the most frequently fractured bone of the hand. Other labeled structures are as follows: **A**, ulna; **G**, lunate; **H**, triquetrum; **I**, pisiform; **B**, ulna styloid process; **C**, radius; **D**, radial styloid process; **E**, scaphoid; **F**, tubercle of scaphoid; **J**, trapezium; **K**, trapezoid; **L**, capitate; **M**, hook of hamate; **N**, first metacarpal; **O**, first proximal phalange; **P**, first distal phalanges; **Q**, sesamoid bones; **R**, third proximal phalange; **S**, third middle phalange; and **T**, third distal phalange.

470. The answer is b. *(Moore, pp 817-818.)* Subluxation of the head of the radius from the annular ligament can be relocated by flexing the elbow at 90° and fully supernating the hand. This type of injury is called "nursemaid's elbow" or "pulled elbow" and is common in toddlers and young girls as their forearm gets suddenly pulled too hard, causing an incomplete dislocation of the circular head of the radius. The radius pulls out of the annular ligament, which attaches it to the proximal ulna, and allows it to articulate with the capitulum of the distal end of the humerus. Bruising of the coronoid fossa (**answer a**) only occurs during hyperflexion of the elbow. Subluxation of the head of the radius is not treated by hyperextending the elbow joint (**answer c**), which is painful. The radius does not articulate with the trochlea of the humerus (**answer d**). Dislocation of the ulna from the olecranon fossa (**answer e**) is quite painful and requires pain relief during relocation.

471. The answer is c. (*Moore, pp 684-685, 743.*) The radial nerve innervates extensors of the upper extremity. Damage to the radial nerve in the radial groove is frequently caused by supporting the arm in an outstretched position as may be encountered when an inebriated college student passes out on her friend's sofa. This is sometimes referred to as "Saturday night palsy." The median nerve (**answer a**) supplies the pronators (teres and quadratus) and the flexors of the fingers, thumb, and wrist. The ulnar nerve (**answer b**) supplies the flexor carpi ulnaris and a portion of flexor digitorum profundus. The axillary nerve (**answer d**) innervates the deltoid and teres minor and is thus involved in abduction of the arm. The musculocutaneous nerve (**answer e**) innervates flexors of the elbow joint (eg, biceps brachii).

472. The answer is b. (*Moore, pp 581-582.*) The boy has lost partial function of the gluteus medius muscle causing hip drop on the opposite side, which is called a "positive Trendelenburg sign." The gluteus medius (thus not **answer c**) is innervated by the superior gluteal nerve. The nurse who performed the injections likely injected too far medially within the buttock. Normally all injections should be performed in the upper lateral quadrant of the buttock, to avoid the sciatic nerve and superior and inferior gluteal nerves that exit the pelvis through the greater sciatic notch. The lateral cutaneous nerve of the thigh (**answer a**) provides general sensation to the anterior region of the thigh. The superior clunial (cluneal) nerves are the cutaneous innervation over the gluteus maximus and medius muscles. The inferior gluteal nerve (**answer d**) innervates the gluteus maximus muscle. The sciatic nerve (**answer e**) is not damaged because the pain does not extend down the back of the boy's leg and he has normal function of his hamstring muscles, which flex the leg at the knee.

473. The answer is b. (*Moore, p 679.*) The flexor pollicis brevis has t heads and there is a sesamoid bone associated with each of the tendons these heads. Sesamoid bones are isolated islands of bone that may occur in tendons passing over joints. The patella is the classic example. The adductor pollicis (**answer c**) also has two heads (transverse and oblique), but they are not associated with sesamoid bones. (**Answers a, d, and e** are not correct.)

474. The answer is d. (*Moore, pp 769-770.*) The ulnar nerve descends along the postaxial (ulnar) side of the forearm. It passes lateral to the pisiform bone and under the carpal volar ligament, but superficial to the transverse carpal ligament. In the hand it divides into superficial and deep branches. The median nerve (**answer a**) lies deep to the transverse carpal ligament where it is protected from superficial lacerations. Emerging from the carpal tunnel, it gives off the vulnerable recurrent branch (**answer b**) to the thenar eminence. The superficial branch (**answer c**) of the radial nerve (**answer e**) supplies the dorsolateral aspects of the wrist and hand.

475. The answer is a. (*Moore, pp 659-660.*) Fractures of the femoral neck, commonly called "hip fractures" are extremely common in older women as a consequence of osteoporosis. Since the woman was still able to bear some weight on her leg it is very unlikely that she had complete displacement of the femoral neck (**answer b**), rather a compression fracture with the fall. None of the symptoms are consistent with fracture in either the shaft (**answer c**) or distal portion (**answers d and e**) of the femur.

476. The answer is e. (*Moore, pp 684, 729-730.*) The clavicle is the most frequently broken bone in the body. Greenstick fractures of the clavicle are extremely common in children as a result of falling on outstretched arms. The fractures are called greenstick because one side of the bone breaks and separates when bent, but the other side does not separate, like a tree branch that bends but does not break completely. Colles fracture is also common from falling on outstretched arms, but there are no physical findings to support a Colles fracture ([**answer a**]; fracture of the distal radius, occasionally including the ulna) in this boy (nor scaphoid fracture [**answer b**]). The sternoclavicular joint (**answer d**) is extremely stable and is rarely dislocated. Fracture of the surgical head of the humerus (**answer c**) is not indicated by the physical findings.

77. The answer is d. (*Moore, pp 684-685.*) Breaks of the mid-shaft of the humerus are most likely due to damage to the radial nerve and deep artery of the arm (profunda brachii artery). The radial nerve **(answer c)** runs within the radial groove on the posterior surface of the humerus (mid-shaft) along with the deep artery of the arm. Because the radial nerve innervates all the extensors of the arm and forearm, the observation that the teenager suffers from wrist drop is expected. Normally the nerve to the posterior compartment of the arm, the extensors of the elbow joint, will be spared in such an injury. Since the left forearm and hand felt slightly cooler than the right this suggests that the deep artery of the arm is also compromised by the displaced fracture. The axillary nerve damage **(answers a and b)** would result in reduced shoulder movement, which is normal. The median nerve and brachial artery **(answer e)**, run along the medial aspect of the arm.

478. The answer is b. (*Moore, pp 684-685.*) Fractures of the femoral neck (cervical) will completely interrupt the blood supply to the femoral head in adults. If the capsular retinaculum also is torn, avascular necrosis of the head will occur because the only remaining blood supply to the head (through the ligamentum teres) is inadequate to sustain it. The nearer the fracture to the femoral head, the more likely the disruption of the retinacular blood supply. None of the other choices **(answers a, c, d, and e)** are correct.

479. The answer is e. (*Moore, pp 536-537.*) The lateral femoral cutaneous nerve passes beneath the inguinal ligament just medial to the anterior superior iliac spine. It innervates the lateral aspect of the thigh. The iliohypogastric nerve **(answer c)** innervates a portion of the gluteal, inguinal, and pubic regions. The ilioinguinal nerve **(answer d)** and the femoral branch of the genitofemoral nerve **(answer a)** supply the upper portions of the anterior thigh. The sensory distribution of the femoral nerve **(answer b)** innervates the anterior thigh and medial leg.

480. The answer is b. (*Moore, pp 554-555.*) Flexion of the thigh would be normal or unaffected by the reduced blood flow. The lesion involves the common iliac artery just proximal to its division into the internal and external iliac branches. Blood flow would be compromised to the external iliac artery and its downstream branches including the femoral, deep

femoral, popliteal, tibial, fibular, and plantar arteries. Blood flow w̧
also be diminished to branches of the internal iliac artery, including gluț
(**answer a**) and visceral arteries. One of the most powerful flexors of th̦
thigh is the psoas muscle, which originates from the lumbar vertebrae and
receives most of its blood from the aorta and common iliac artery and thus
would be unaffected by the lesion. All functions more distal to the blockage would likely be affected (thus not **answers c, d, and e**).

481. The answer is b. (*Moore, pp 662-663.*) The excess ability to displace
a flexed leg anteriorly is the anterior drawer sign, used to test for disruption
of an ACL tear. If the ACL is torn, when the knee is flexed, the cranial part of
the leg may be pulled forward excessively. Medial displacement (**answer e**)
would not be affected. If the posterior cruciate ligament, structure 12 were
torn, then **answer a** would have been correct. Excess ability to displace the
ankle medially (**answer c**) or laterally (**answer d**) would arise if the lateral
and medial collateral knee ligaments were torn, respectively. The other
numbered structures are as follows: 1, femur; 2, tibia; 8, patella; 9, ACL;
10, popliteal artery and vein; 11, head of the gastrocnemius muscle; and
12, posterior cruciate ligament.

482. The answer is a. (*Moore, p 529.*) The calcaneus is the most frequently fractured of the tarsal bones. The weight of the body is transmitted
down the tibia and onto the talus, which acts as a wedge cracking the calcaneus inferiorly. Unfortunately, this fracture normally involves the cartilaginous articular surface, complicating the healing process, increasing the
likelihood of developing an arthritic subtalar joint. Those fractures often
must be held together with screws or plates for optimal healing. Since the
pain extends across the foot, only the calcaneus crosses the heel, none of
the other bones (**answers b, c, d, and e**) listed are possible sites of fracture.
The distal end of the tibia (**answer c**) would have carried the bulk of the
force, but the pain location is inconsistent with a distal tibial fracture.

483. The answer is d. (*Moore, p 526.*) Semitendinosus, semimembranosus, and biceps femoris are the hamstring muscles that originate from
the ischial tuberosity. Avulsion fractures of the ischial tuberosity are common in runners, hurdlers and jumpers, and especially adolescents whose
bones are still growing. As the water skier was traveling backwards, his left
ski caught the water and suddenly his left leg was carried forward, as in

den hip flexion. The hamstring muscles contracted to slow the leg ..own, but were torn from their origin on the ischial tuberosity. Avulsion fractures almost always heal faster by reattaching the fragment with a surgical screw. The semitendinosus muscle originates at the ischial tuberosity and inserts at the pes anserine; the semimembranosus muscle originates at the ischial tuberosity and inserts at the posterior medial tibia. The biceps femoris muscle has a long head that originates at the ischial tuberosity and a short head at the posterolateral femur that inserts into the head of the fibula. The gracilis muscle (**answers a and e**) has its origin along the inferior ramus of the pubis. The adductor magnus muscle (**answers a, b, and c**) also has its origin along the inferior ramus of the pubis.

484. The answer is b. (*Moore, pp 554-555.*) Perforating branches of the deep femoral artery are the principal blood supply to the posterior thigh. The other arteries supply anterior (**answer d**), medial (**answer c**), and gluteal (**answer a**) regions of the thigh. The obturator artery (**answer e**) supplies the medial thigh.

485. The answer is d. (*Moore, pp 605-606.*) Compression of the common fibular (peroneal) nerve would affect all muscles innervated by this nerve, including tibialis anterior, fibularis (peroneus) longus, and extensor digitorum longus. Loss of dorsiflexion and eversion is usually complete. The extensors of the knee joint ([**answer a**] quadriceps femoris) are supplied by the femoral nerve, whereas the flexors of the knee joint ([**answer c**] the hamstrings and gracilis) are supplied by the tibial nerve and obturator nerve, respectively. The gastrocnemius and soleus muscles are the principal plantar flexors of the foot (**answer b**) and are innervated by the tibial nerve. The popliteus is the prime medial rotator of the tibia (**answer e**) and is also innervated by the tibial nerve.

486. The answer is c. (*Moore, pp 582, 660-661.*) About 85% of hip dislocations occur in a posterior direction as the head of the femur slips out of the acetabulum. This stretches the ischiofemoral ligament, which makes up the posterior aspect of the joint capsule. Posterior displacement is also the typical direction of force resulting from the striking of one's knee on the dashboard in a head-on car accident. Anterior hip displacement is unusual since the very strong iliofemoral ligament stabilizes the joint anteriorly and also limits hip extension. The sciatic nerve passes just posterior to the hip joint and may be damaged when the hip is displaced posteriorly, thus compromising innervation to the hamstring and posterior compartment of the leg. The obturator nerve (**answer a**) exits the pelvis through the obturator foramen and into the medial compartment of the thigh, so it is not nearby. The pudendal nerve (**answer b**) innervates the external genitalia, so it would also be unaffected. The femoral nerve (**answer d**) exits the pelvis under the inguinal ligament and into the anterior compartment, thus it will be anterior to any damage in this case. The superior gluteal nerve (**answer e**) exits the greater sciatic notch, but is cranial to a posteriorly displaced head of the femur and is mobile enough that it is unlikely to be damaged. Therefore, this is the second best answer.

487. The answer is e. (*Moore, p 529.*) The middle portion of the fibula is often used for bone grafting of other long bones. The fibula is a non-weight bearing bone that mainly serves as a site of muscle attachment and adds stability to the ankle joint. The middle portion of the fibula has the best blood supply (a branch of the fibular artery) and so is used for bone grafts. The distal portion of the tibia (**answer a**) while a long bone, would not be used as it is weight bearing. Neither the iliac crest (**answer b**), mandible (**answer c**), nor scapula (**answer d**) are long bones and thus are not suited for this type of bone graft. The iliac crest is often used to repair damaged vertebra, but is not used for long bone repair. Ribs are rarely used for repair of long bones as they are not sturdy enough, lacking sufficient compact (cortical) bone.

488. The answer is b. (*Moore, p 530.*) The fibularis (peroneus) brevis, a pronator and everter of the foot, inserts into the tubercle at the base of the fifth metatarsal. Inversion of the foot is a common means of avulsing this tendon from the tuberosity of the fifth metatarsal and is called *Jones fracture* for the doctor that caused his own fracture while dancing around a pole. It is normally treated by placing the patient in a short walking cast. The fibularis (peroneus) longus (**answer c**) passes under the tarsal arch to insert onto the plantar aspect of the first metatarsal. The tibialis posterior (**answer e**) inserts onto the navicular bone, whereas the tibialis anterior (**answer d**) inserts into the first cuneiform and first metatarsal. The abductor digiti minimi (**answer a**) inserts onto the proximal phalanx of the fifth toe.

489. The answer is b. (*Moore, pp 522-523.*) The navicular bone (**B**) articulates with both the talus and the three cuneiforms, which are distal. Other labeled structures are as follows: **A**, talus; **C**, calcaneus; **D**, cuboid; and **E**, fifth metatarsal.

490. The answer is c. (*Moore, pp 480-481.*) Kyphosis is an excessive anterior curvature of the spine, usually in the upper thoracic and lower cervical regions. Often this abnormal curvature is due to osteoporosis, especially in women, but also may be due to weakening of musculature and decrease height of the intervertebral discs. Lordosis **(answer a)** is an abnormal secondary curvature of the lumbar region of the spine and often occurs with pregnancy. Scoliosis **(answer b)** is abnormal lateral curvature of the spine that often appears during adolescence. Neither rheumatoid arthritis **(answer e)** nor osteoarthritis **(answer d)** is associated with height loss in the elderly.

491. The answer is d. (*Moore, pp 605-606.*) The common fibular (peroneal) nerve is the lateral terminal branch of the sciatic nerve. After arising near the apex of the popliteal fossa, it descends on the popliteus muscle and winds superficially around the fibular neck. It is extremely vulnerable in this position and is the most often injured nerve in the lower extremity. The common fibular nerve innervates all muscles in the anterior and lateral compartments of the leg. In addition, it provides sensory innervation to the dorsum of the foot and the anterolateral surface of the legs via the superficial and sural **(answer c)**/lateral sural cutaneous nerves, respectively. The tibial nerve innervates plantar flexors of the posterior compartment. The sciatic nerve **(answer a)** divides into the tibial **(answer e)** and common peroneal nerves superior to the popliteal fossa. Damage to it might result in deficits in both plantar flexion and dorsiflexion. The femoral nerve **(answer b)** innervates the quadriceps muscles of the anterior thigh. Damage to it would impair flexion of the thigh at the hip.

492. The answer is b. (*Moore, pp 620-621.*) The saphenous nerve accompanies the great saphenous vein along the medial aspect of the leg and foot as far as the great toe. The medial femoral cutaneous nerve **(answer a)** innervates the dorsal aspect of the leg. The superficial fibular nerve **(answer c)** innervates the central portion of the dorsum of the foot. The sural cutaneous nerve **(answer d)** innervates the lateral aspect of the foot. The medial and lateral plantar branches of the tibial nerve **(answer e)** supply the sole of the foot.

493. The answer is b. (*Moore, pp 622-623, 625.*) The dorsal pedal artery, a continuation of the anterior tibial artery, passes onto the dorsum of the

foot between the tendons of the extensor hallucis longus and exter
digitorum longus muscles. The dorsal pedal pulse may be palpated at th.
point before the artery passes beneath the extensor hallucis brevis muscle
The posterior tibial artery passes behind the medial malleolus, where the
posterior tibial pulse is normally palpable. None of the other answers
(**answers a, c, d, and e**) are correct.

494. The answer is e. (*Moore, pp 480-482.*) Idiopathic scoliosis presents
most frequently during the growth spurt for teenagers, 10 to 14 years for girls
and 12 to 15 for boys. Scoliosis is a lateral abnormal curvature of the spine and
ribs. It is often screened for by having a patient bend to touch their toes as the
relative height of the scapula is examined. Note that scoliosis often causes rib
deformity. Scoliosis (**answer d**) rarely develops in 4 to 8 year olds. Kyphosis
(**answer a**) is an excess anterior curvature of the spine in the upper thoracic
and cervical region and normally occurs in the elderly. Lordosis (**answers b
and c**) is an excess concavity of the spine in the lumbar region with the spinal
cord moving anteriorly. Lordosis most frequently presents in pregnant women.

495. The answer is d. (*Moore, pp 477-479.*) The fifth lumbar vertebra has
shifted anteriorly on top of the sacrum. This condition could also be
described as subluxation of the L5 vertebra on the sacrum. Spondylolisthesis
is often due to a fracture of the pars interarticularis, that portion of the vertebra arch, which forms the superior and inferior facet joints. This appears to
be the case in this image. The inferior facet joint on L5 has broken from the
lamina of the L5 and thus allowed the body and L5 to slide anteriorly and
inferiorly on top of the sacrum. Kyphosis (**answer a**) is an abnormal anterior
curvature, in the thoracic region of the elderly. Scoliosis (**answer b**) is an
abnormal lateral curvature and rotation of the vertebral column, most frequently initiates during adolescence, and involves both lumbar and thoracic
regions. Lordosis (**answer c**), an anterior convex curvature of the vertebral
column (so-called secondary curvature), most frequently occurs in adults
and within the lumbar region. Lordosis does not involve fracture of the vertebrae, as has occurred here. The sacrum (**answer e**) is not fractured.

496. The answer is d. (*Moore, p 442.*) The pedicle (**D** in the image in
Question 495) attaches to the vertebral body (**E**) and extends posteriorly.
Both the lamina and the transverse process (**C**) extend from that point. **A** is
the inferior articular facet of L2. **B** is the superior articular facet of L3.

7. The answer is b. (*Moore, pp 662-663.*) The medial meniscus is attached to the medial (tibial) collateral ligament, which holds it relatively immobile, making it more susceptible to damage. It is relatively immovable and, therefore, unable to evade damage such as occurred in this case. The medial meniscus is clearly not attached to the popliteus muscle **(answer a)** the ACL **(answer c)**, nor the femur **(answer e)**. The knee usually is hit laterally, causing more torsion on the medial meniscus **(answer d)**, making this the second best answer.

498. The answer is b. (*Moore, p 480.*) Articular branches of the dorsal rami carry pain fiber from facet joints. The woman's pain is likely coming from arthritic changes in her facet or zygapophysial joints that are innervated by articular branches of the dorsal rami. These joints limit the movement of the vertebral bodies with one another, such as when twisting her back. Since the woman does not have radicular pain, intervertebral disks **(answer d)** are an unlikely source of the pain. Anterior rami are spinal nerves that serve most of the body **(answer a and c [ventral])** and thus are unlikely to be involved. The pain is not within the neck region so the nuchal ligament **(answer e)** would not be involved.

499. The answer is b. (*Moore, pp 474-475.*) The deep incisure in the inferior border of the pedicle ensures that the spinal nerve associated with that vertebra will exit through the intervertebral foramen superior to the intervertebral disk so that it will not be affected by a herniation at that level. However, a posterolateral herniation (the usual direction) will impinge on the next lower nerve as it courses toward its associated intervertebral foramen. In this case, pain was distributed along the medial side of the leg and foot as far as the great toe, the distribution of the saphenous branch of the femoral nerve (L5). Herniation of the fourth lumbar intervertebral disk between vertebral bodies L4 to L5 would affect nerve L5. None of the other answers **(answers a, c, d, and e)** are correct.

500. The answer is b. (*Moore, pp 505-506.*) A horizontal line drawn across the posterior superior iliac crests crosses the fourth lumbar spinous process. Lumbar punctures (spinal taps) are performed at the L3 to L4 or L4 to L5 interspinous space since the spinal cord terminates by L2 in greater than 99% of the adult population. The ligaments that need to be penetrated in the midline include the supraspinous ligament, the interspinous ligament, and the ligamentum flavum (if slightly off the line). The needle must pierce both the dura mater and arachnoid mater order to collect cerebral spinal fluid (CSF), which should be clear. The sacr hiatus, which is marked by the sacral cornu and covered by the sacrococ-cygeal ligament, is used to gain access to the extradural space. None of the other answers (**answers a, c, d, and e**) are correct.

Bibliography

Abbas AK, Lichtman AH. *Basic Immunology: Functions and Disorders of the Immune System*. 3rd ed. Philadelphia, PA: Saunders/Elsevier; 2008.

Alberts B, Johnson A, Lewis J, Raff M, Roberts K, and Walter P. *Molecular Biology of the Cell*. 5th ed. New York, NY: Garland; 2008.

Avery JK, ed. *Oral Development and Histology*. 3rd ed. New York, NY: Thieme; 2002.

Casals T, Bassas L, Egozcue S et al, Heterogeneity for mutations the CFTR gene and clinical correlations in patients with congenital absence of the vas deferens. *Hum Reprod* 2000;15:1476-1483.

Costanzo LS. *Physiology*. 3rd ed. Philadelphia, PA: Saunders/Elsevier; 2006.

Fauci AS, Braunwald E, Kasper DL, et al, eds. *Harrison's Principles of Internal Medicine*. 17th ed. New York, NY: McGraw-Hill; 2008.

Favus MJ, ed. *Disorders of Bone and Mineral Metabolism*. 6th ed. Washington, DC: American Society for Bone and Mineral Research; 2006.

Fawcett DW. *The Cell*. 2nd ed. Philadelphia, PA: W. B. Saunders; 1981.

Ganong WF. *Review of Medical Physiology*. 22nd ed. New York, NY: Lange Medical Books/McGraw-Hill; 2005.

Gilbert SF. *Developmental Biology*. 8th ed. Sunderland, MA: Sinauer; 2006.

Greenspan FS, Gardner DG. *Basic and Clinical Endocrinology*. 8th ed. New York, NY: Lange Medical Books/McGraw-Hill; 2007.

Hansen JT, Lambert DR. *Netter's Clinical Anatomy*. Philadelphia, PA: Elsevier/ Saunders; 2008.

Johnson LR, ed. *Physiology of the Gastrointestinal Tract*. 3rd ed. New York, NY: Raven; 1994.

Mescher AL *Junqueira's Basic Histology: Text and Atlas*. 12th ed. New York, NY: McGraw-Hill; 2010.

Kandel ER, Schwartz JH, Jessell TM. *Principles of Neural Science*. 4th ed. New York, NY: McGraw-Hill; 2000.

Kierszenbaum AL. *Histology and Cell Biology*. 2nd ed. St. Louis, MO: Mosby; 2008.

Kindt TJ, Goldsby RA, Osborne BA. *Immunology*. 6th ed. New York, NY: W. H. Freeman and Company; 2007.

Kumar V, Abbas AK, Fausto N. *Pathologic Basis of Disease*. 8th ed. Philadelphia, PA: Elsevier/Saunders; 2010.

Lebenthal E. *Human Gastrointestinal Development*. New York, NY: Raven; 1989.

Lobov IB, Brooks PC, Lang RA. Angiopoietin-2 displays VEGF-dependent modulation of capillary structure and endothelial cell survival in vivo. *Proc Natl Acad Science USA.* 2002;99:11205-11210.

Mayne R, Burgeson RE, eds. *Structure and Function of Collagen Types.* New York, NY: Academic; 1987.

Mole SE. The genetic spectrum of human neuronal ceroid-lipofuscinoses. In: Symposium, "The neuronal ceroid-lipofuscinoses (NCL)—a group of lysosomal disease come of age." *Brain Pathol.* 2004;14:70-76.

Moore KL, Dalley AF, Agur AMR: *Clinically Oriented Anatomy.* 6th ed. Philadelphia, PA: Lippincott Williams & Wilkins; 2010.

Moore KL and Persaud TVN. *The Developing Human: Clinically Oriented Embryology.* 8th ed. Philadelphia, PA: W. B. Saunders; 2008.

Parmely MJ. *USMLE Roadmap Immunology.* New York, NY: Lange Medical Books/McGraw-Hill; 2006.

Reszka AA, Rodan GA. Mechanism of action of bisphosphonates. *Curr Osteoporos Rep.* 2003;1:45-52.

Riordan-Eva P, Whitcher JP. *Vaughan & Asbury's General Ophthalmology.* 17th ed. New York, NY: Lange Medical Books/McGraw-Hill; 2008.

Ross MH, Pawlina W. *Histology: A Text and Atlas.* 5th ed. Baltimore, MD: Lippincott Williams & Wilkins; 2006.

Rubin E. *Rubin's Pathology: Clinicopathologic Foundations of Medicine.* 4th ed. Baltimore, MD: Williams & Wilkins; 2005.

Sadler TW. *Langman's Medical Embryology.* 11th ed. Baltimore, MD: Williams & Wilkins; 2010.

Schoenwolf GC, Bleyl DB, Brauer PR, Francis-West PH. *Larsen's Human Embryology.* 4th ed. New York, NY: Churchill Livingstone; 2009.

Strauss JF, Mastroianni L, Barbieri R. *Yen and Jaffe's Reproductive Endocrinology.* 5th ed. Philadelphia, PA: Saunders/Elsevier; 2004.

Waxman SG. *Clinical Neuroanatomy.* 26th ed. New York, NY: McGraw-Hill; 2010.

Young B, Lowe JS, Stevens A, Heath JW. *Wheater's Functional Histology.* 5th ed. New York, NY: Churchill Livingstone; 2006.

Index